Bruce W. Konigsmark, M.D.

Late Associate Professor of Pathology and
Director of the Division of Neuropathology
Temple University Health Sciences Center
Philadelphia, Pennsylvania

Robert J. Gorlin, D.D.S., M.S.

Professor and Chairman, Division of Oral Pathology
University of Minnesota School of Dentistry;
Professor of Otolaryngology, Professor of Pediatrics,
Professor of Pathology, Professor of Dermatology,
Professor of Obstetrics and Gynecology
University of Minnesota School of Medicine
Minneapolis, Minnesota

1976

W. B. SAUNDERS COMPANY

Philadelphia, London, Toronto

GENETIC
AND
METABOLIC
DEAFNESS

W. B. Saunders Company: West Washington Square
Philadelphia, PA 19105

1 St. Anne's Road
Eastbourne, East Sussex BN21 3UN England

833 Oxford Street
Toronto, Ontario M8Z 5T9, Canada

Genetic and Metabolic Deafness   ISBN   0-7216-5489-4

Last digit is the print number: 9   8   7   6   5   4   3   2   1

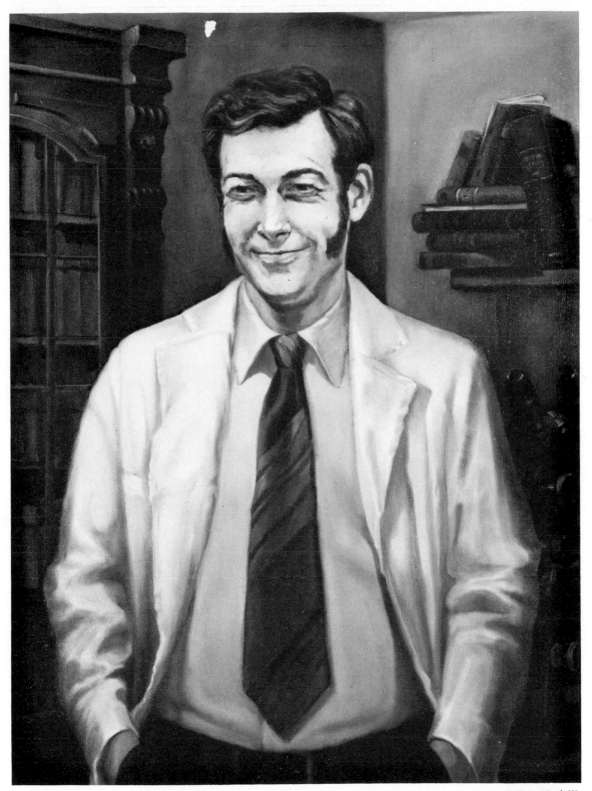

BRUCE W. KONIGSMARK (1928–1973)

FOREWORD

by MICHAEL M. PAPARELLA, M.D.

There are three reasons why I consider myself privileged to have been asked to contribute a brief introduction to this book: first, because the book is timely; second, because the authors are uniquely qualified to combine their talents in this effort; and third, because the many forms of hereditary hearing loss, as seen in the chapter headings, have been categorized and extensive references to the literature have been provided.

This book is timely because we are, I believe, on the threshold of a much greater understanding of all forms of hearing loss. This book represents the best study, compilation, and organization of hereditary deafness forms described in the literature to date, or for that matter, in the history of otology. As such, it should serve as a landmark reference for all students of hearing loss now and for many years to come. The reader is advised, however, to approach this book with a discerning "wait and see" attitude regarding the many types of hereditary hearing loss described and the many references to the literature. It should not be assumed naively that all of the types of hearing loss syndromes described in the literature represent established entities. Nevertheless, the book admirably describes the current state of the art regarding hereditary hearing loss and should serve as an important impetus to further study and to a continued separation of established syndromes from those unable to stand the test of time.

It is axiomatic in medicine that unless the etiology and pathogenesis of a disease are understood, there is little likelihood that the disease will be prevented or treated effectively. This same principle holds true for hearing loss and especially for hereditary hearing loss. In Chapter 1, reference is made to the woeful lack of knowledge regarding the incidence of hearing loss in general and, the various causes of hearing loss, in particular. This lack is due to two factors: absence or inadequacy of studies to collect data on incidence of hearing loss, and incomplete understanding of specific hearing losses, especially sensorineural types, as seen in our patients. It has been variably estimated that 15 to 20 million Americans have a "significant" hearing loss. The question of what constitutes a "significant" hearing loss is arguable. Thus, one could say that the incidence could be higher, based on the recognition that all of us gradually lose a bit of high-frequency hearing, in varying degree, beyond young adulthood. Would it not be useful if we knew what percentage of "significant" hearing loss was sensorineural as compared to conductive and what percentage of sensorineural hearing loss, in particular, was hereditary? In our clinics we see many patients, especially adults, with sensorineural hearing losses that defy diagnosis according to our present understanding of extrinsic etiologies. We continue to use clumsily such catch-all descriptive terms as "idiopathic" or "presbycusis." We have a special interest in studying adults with isolated sensorineural hearing loss and, when available, the pathology of their temporal bones. We surmise that in the absence of other factors, many of these patients have hereditary hearing loss (Paparella and Shumrick, 1973; Paparella et al., 1975). In addition, it seems that patients with presbycusis, or so-called aging deafness (a group that constitutes a very large percentage of geriatric patients with hearing loss), should be considered as any other group for whom a specific diagnosis is sought (Cawthorne and Hinchcliffe, 1957). It appears reasonable that many patients with presbycusis have some form of hereditary loss that manifests itself in the twilight of life. This explanation would help to account for one 70-year-old patient having relatively good hearing and another, with no discernible cause, having very poor hearing. In time, it is conceivable, indeed desirable, that the term "presbycusis" will become obsolete and that more specific etiologies, such as heredity, environmental noise, and infection, will be employed. Severe hereditary hearing loss in children is better understood than genetic hearing loss in adults, and as implied briefly herein, it appears that hereditary hearing loss constitutes a much greater percentage of currently undiagnosable sensorineural hearing loss for all age groups. Thus, this book serves as a timely reference to assess our current knowledge of inherited deafness and will help to define the role of genetic factors in hearing loss in the future.

The authors are uniquely qualified to contribute this reference. I know of no researcher other than Dr. Bruce W. Konigsmark more dedicated to the study of hereditary forms of hearing loss. His contributions to the literature and to our understanding of this kind of hearing loss were manifold. His scholarly pursuits were extensively devoted to this subject. It is a special tragedy, therefore, that Dr. Konigsmark's death occurred at such an early age and at a point when his contributions to our knowledge were cresting. This book serves as a dedication to his efforts and as a challenge to a legion of student-scholars who, it is hoped, will pick up Dr. Konigsmark's banner and will continue to contribute further to this important subject. As a scholar of the many syndromes described in the literature Dr. Robert Gorlin, in my view, has no peer. He has been especially interested in head and neck syndromes, having written a useful reference book on the subject (Gorlin et al., 1976). He has studied and continues to study new and old syndromes occurring in patients as well as the many phenotypic characteristics of these disorders. A number of new deafness syndromes have been originally described by him.

The third reason I am honored to contribute this introduction is the organization of content in this book. Out of chaos (the many descriptions of possible hereditary hearing loss and syndromes) has come some order. The ultimate goal of scholarly efforts in the study of hereditary hearing loss—for that matter, any hearing loss—is to provide a means of diagnosing these problems in our patients. This improvement in diagnosis in turn leads to an improved opportunity for treatment or prevention, as the case warrants. A proper diagnosis should be made as early as possible to prevent unnecessary retardation of social, cultural, or educational development. Certainly, diagnosis includes early identification of the disorder and studies of the conductive or sensorineural characteristics of the hearing loss. When a patient with a hearing loss such as a sensorineural deafness presents himself, it is the diagnostician's responsibility to make every effort to search for an etiologic diagnosis. This is of obvious importance for proper management. The first question one must ask is, "Is this patient's deafness congenital or is it of delayed onset?" Congenital deafness implies aplasia or dysgenesis of the organ of Corti and/or related structures. For that reason, the deafness should not be progressive. Delayed deafness relates to degenerative changes of the sense organ and may be progressive. The second question is, "Is the deafness genetic (hereditary) or is it nongenetic?" This is important, since approximately one half of all profound deafness disorders in children are genetic in origin. The third question is, "What other anomalies occur with the deafness and can be seen in congenital deafness or in acquired or delayed hearing loss?"

There is a great need for continued investigation of the pathology of hereditary deafness. The classically described pathologies, especially as seen in congenital genetic sensorineural deafness, include Michel's deafness (total aplasia of the bony and membranous labyrinth), Mondini's aplasia (partial aplasia of the bony and membranous labyrinth), Scheibe's aplasia (cochleosaccular aplasia), and Alexander's or Bing-Siebenmann's aplasia (aplasia of the cochlear duct and especially of the organ of Corti in the basal turn). Many authors have contributed to our understanding of the pathology of hereditary hearing loss; only a few of these investigators can be mentioned here: Nager, Fraser, Guild, Lindsay, and Schuknecht.

The chapter headings as outlined in this book describe, in general, types of hereditary hearing loss occurring alone or with associated abnormalities. Within each chapter, the reader will find many individual types of hearing loss described in the literature. This information provides a thorough and comprehensive assessment of our current state of knowledge regarding hereditary hearing loss and will be helpful in diagnosing and managing patients with hearing loss now and in the future.

REFERENCES

Cawthorne, T. E., and Hinchcliffe, R., Familial perceptive deafness. *Pract. Otorhinolaryngol. (Basel), 19*:69–83, 1957.

Gorlin, R. J., Pindborg, J. J., and Cohen, M. M., Jr., *Syndromes of the Head and Neck,* 2nd Ed. New York, McGraw-Hill Book Co., 1976.

Paparella, M. M., Hanson, D. G., Rao, K. N., and Ulvestad, R., Genetic sensorineural deafness in adults. *Ann. Otol. Rhinol. Laryngol., 84*:459–472, 1975.

Paparella, M. M., and Shumrick, D. A., *Otolaryngology, Volume II: Ear.* Philadelphia, W. B. Saunders Company, 1973, p. 333.

PREFACE

Hearing loss due to genetic defects is frequently undiagnosed, and many of those patients with a family history of hearing loss are never examined for possible hereditary deafness. The aims of this volume are to focus more attention on hereditary deafness and to aid in the diagnosis of specific types of genetic hearing loss.

Hereditary hearing loss is becoming progressively important, if one assumes that there is a greater proportion of persons with auditory deficit, since medical and surgical therapy is becoming more effective. Furthermore, genetic hearing loss is probably being diagnosed earlier and more often because of elementary school screening tests.

As employed in this text the words "deafness," 'hearing loss," and "hearing deficit" are to be understood as synonymous. Although this may meet with objection by some, this text is meant to appeal to individuals with diverse backgrounds: otolaryngologists, audiologists, pediatricians, speech pathologists, and geneticists. We also have considered the terms "neural," "sensorineural," and "perceptive" to be interchangeable, although this usage may not please the purist.

We have attempted to be as complete in our coverage of genetic and metabolic deafness as time and energies permitted. Perhaps we have fragmented where division was illusory or have grouped entities not easily separable. While these are no mere peccadilloes, we beg the indulgence of the reader.

This project would not have been possible without the aid of Mrs. Terry Crouthamel, Mrs. Carol Gear, Mrs. Jeanne Brandt, and Ms. Alice Preston, who arranged patient scheduling for tests and completed lengthy literature searches. We appreciate the help of the following audiologists who gave their time and support: Dr. Salah Salman, Dr. and Mrs. Salah Soliman, Mrs. Judy Yieces, Mrs. Diane Thompson, Miss Sandra Perkins and Mrs. Anita Pikus.

We are especially indebted to Dr. Marion Talbot, Dr. Charles Berlin, and Miss Harriet Haskins for reviewing and interpreting audiologic test results and to Dr. Donna Haciska and Dr. Joseph Toglia for performing and interpreting the vestibular tests. We thank Mrs. Barbara Worthington for numerous critical editorial comments. The Information Center for Hearing, Speech, and Disorders of Human Communication aided in literature searches in several translations.

Dr. John E. Bordley, Dr. William Hardy, Dr. Victor McKusick, Dr. Irving Shapiro, Dr. Susanne Ullman, Dr. Arndt Duvall, Dr. Alfred Michael, and Dr. Karlind Moller generously reviewed the manuscript and offered critical comments. Alice Preston, Bridget Stellmacher, and Virginia Hansen deserve special recognition for endless retyping and editing of the manuscript.

The financial support of the Social Rehabilitation Service, the John A. Hartford Foundation, The National Institute of Neurological Diseases and Stroke, and the United States Public Health Service (DE-1770) was greatly appreciated.

Finally, we wish to express our profound gratitude to Dr. LaVonne Bergstrom for her critical review of the entire text.

ENCOMIUM

Bruce Konigsmark was educated at Stanford University School of Medicine. His postgraduate training was in neurophysiology, pathology, clinical neurology, and neuropathology at UCLA, Johns Hopkins, Massachusetts General Hospital, and Harvard Medical School. He joined the Johns Hopkins faculty in 1963 as Associate Professor of Laryngology and Otology. Between 1963 and 1972 he developed an otoneuropathology laboratory at Johns Hopkins and initiated studies of hereditary deafness. In 1972 he was called to Temple University to organize a Division of Neuropathology. His untimely death in 1973 from leukemia cut short a highly productive career.

In his approach to hereditary deafness, Konigsmark proposed to study the great many types of deafness and to localize the defect to specific areas of the temporal bone and brain. As groundwork for this he realized the need to delineate, on clinical and genetic grounds, the many forms known or suspected to exist. In this effort the clinic and the library were his laboratory. In each he accumulated extensive material. On the clinical side he described many "new" or almost "new" entities: hereditary olivopontocerebellar atrophy with retinal degeneration, familial hearing loss associated with atopic dermatitis, recessive early onset sensorineural deafness, recessive conductive hearing loss with malformed external ears, congenital deafness and multiple lentigines, dominant mid-frequency hearing loss, familial congenital moderate sensorineural hearing loss, hereditary nephritis with sensorineural deafness, familial low-frequency hearing loss, dominant spinopontine atrophy, dominant congenital deafness and progressive optic nerve atrophy, and others.

Bruce's long-range objective — to define the neuropathology of hereditary deafness — was frustrated by the malignancy to which he succumbed. The tragedy of his death is evident to workers in the field. The tragedy is compounded for us who knew him as a valued colleague, friend, and warm human being.

Victor A. McKusick, M.D.

CONTENTS

Chapter 1

GENETIC HEARING LOSS

Each year between 2000 and 4000 profoundly deaf infants are born in the United States (Bergstrom *et al.*, 1971). Approximately 35 to 50 per cent of the cases of profound childhood deafness may be classified as genetic, and probably over one third of these cases are syndromal, i.e., associated with other anomalies. Thus, hereditary deafness is not rare, occurring somewhere between 1 in 650 and 1 in 2000 school children in the United States (Sank and Kallman, 1963; Brown, 1967).

The development and function of the ear are dependent upon hundreds or even thousands of genes interacting with each other and with the intra- and extrauterine environment. The form of the pinna, for example, is dependent upon many genes (multifactorial inheritance), but it may be grossly altered by single-gene mutation. The same applies to the external auditory canal, the ossicles, the oval window, the eustachian tube, the bony and membranous labyrinth, the semicircular canals, the utricle and saccule, and the auditory nerve. It is likely that the perilymph-endolymph balance and cochlear antigens are also under genetic control.

Although hereditary deafness syndromes are rather well-defined as a result of the anomalies associated with the hearing deficit, unassociated hearing loss, which accounts for less than two-score of the entities in this text, undoubtedly represents marked genetic heterogeneity. We have little doubt that in future years many of these "entities" will have been fragmented into new disorders, distinguishable by subtleties, clinical features, new and more sophisticated audiometric and vestibular function tests, temporal bone tomography, and temporal bone histopathology and/or histochemistry; in the case of recessive disorders, they may be distinguished by the identification of a specific enzyme defect (Anderson and Wedenberg, 1968; Kloepfer *et al.*, 1970). The reader will note that for most of the entities described in this text, even audiometric study has been incomplete.

Although over the past few years there have been rapid advances in our knowledge of the causes of congenital, childhood, and adult hearing loss, much remains to be known. Because the etiologic factors vary with age, it is easiest to consider separately hearing loss which is (a) congenital or of early onset and (b) of later onset.

CONGENITAL AND EARLY-ONSET HEARING LOSS

Since this text is concerned with hereditary deafness, we will not consider such nonheritable factors in congenital and early-onset hearing loss as infectious disease (rubella, otitis media, meningitis), ototoxic drugs, anoxia or birth injury, erythroblastosis, or maldevelopment of unknown origin. Technically, however, susceptibility to streptomycin ototoxicity and even to rubella may have a genetic basis (Anderson *et al.*, 1970).

There have been numerous studies on the causes of congenital and early-onset

1

deafness (Zonderman, 1959; Livingstone, 1961; Barton *et al.*, 1962; Robinson *et al.*, 1963; Fowler and Basek, 1964; Fraser, 1964; Johnston, 1968; Vernon, 1968; Bergstrom *et al.*, 1971; Gamstorp, 1971). These data, not surprisingly, are widely disparate because of the varying completeness of examination, the differences in populations studied, the different years in which the surveys were conducted, and the varying definitions regarding acceptance of one or another etiologic factor. For example, congenital ear malformations are cited as accounting for 2 to 8 per cent of those persons with congenital or early-onset deafness. Although congenital ear anomalies are found in several hereditary syndromes of hearing loss, it is evident that malformations of the ear may occur with no known cause, e.g., oculoauriculovertebral syndrome, idiopathic microtia, and anotia. Therefore, the estimate of 2 per cent (Zonderman, 1959; Fraser, 1964) is probably more accurate.

Genetic factors have been implicated in 5 to 65 per cent of the cases studied (Bordley and Hardy, 1951; Arnvig, 1954; Hopkins, 1954; Van Egmond, 1954; Barton *et al.*, 1962; Danish *et al.*, 1963; Whetnall and Fry, 1964; Proctor and Proctor, 1967; Danish and Levitan, 1967; Pellegrini, 1967; Johnston, 1968; Brown, 1969; Bergstrom *et al.*, 1971). This wide range is based essentially on the degree of diligence with which the examiners have looked for a hereditary background. Where histories have been scanty, heritable loss has been given more weight than all other factors since the investigator grouped together as "genetic" most cases in which etiology was unknown. As shown in Gamstorp's (1971) study, with some diligence a familial history of congenital severe hearing loss could be obtained in about 25 to 30 per cent of patients. An additional 5 to 10 per cent were classified as having a hereditary deafness syndrome because of associated physical or laboratory findings. Thus, about 35 per cent of patients were considered to have hereditary deafness.

Several studies have indicated that an even greater proportion of those with severe congenital hearing loss had a hereditary basis. Lindenov (1945), studying the deaf-mute population of Denmark, concluded on the basis of family history of 480 subjects that 45 per cent of the cases were hereditary. Fraser (1964), in his study of 2355 severely deaf children in 18 residential schools throughout Great Britain and Ireland, found about 30 per cent to have definite evidence of a hereditary basis for the hearing loss. This 30 per cent comprised 6 per cent with autosomal dominantly transmitted deafness, 0.5 per cent with X-linked hearing loss, and 23 per cent with evidence of autosomal recessively transmitted deafness. Since the majority of recessively transmitted cases are sporadic, Fraser determined by segregation analysis that approximately 40 per cent of the children with sporadic deafness had autosomal recessive hearing loss. This group, together with those with known autosomal recessive hereditary deafness, made a total of 38 per cent — a grand total of approximately 45 per cent of the 2355 children having hereditary deafness.

Sank (1963) conducted a genetic analysis of 688 adults who had early-onset total deafness. Among this group, 85 had deaf sibs but normal-hearing parents, 45 had one or both deaf parents, 47 had other deaf relatives, and 501 cases were sporadic. Using Haldane's method for determining recessiveness, Sank concluded that approximately 50 per cent of the cases of early-onset total deafness were genetic — 40 per cent being transmitted by recessive genes and 10 per cent by dominant genes.

Brown (1969) and Chung *et al.* (1969), in their survey at the Clarke School for the Deaf, found that approximately 70 per cent of the persons observed had hereditary deafness.

For historical interest, the reader is referred to the observations on the hereditary nature of deafness by Paulus Zacchias (1584–1659) (Cranefield and Federn, 1970).

The causes of hearing loss vary from region to region, country to country, and community to community. Communities in which marriage to close relatives is prevalent have a higher frequency of hereditary deafness. Dar and Winter (1969), in their study in Israel where parental consanguinity is common in communities of North African Jewish stock, found that in approximately 70 per cent of cases of deafness there is a recessive mode of inheritance. Furthermore, it is interesting to note that the prevalence rate for deafness in the United States is about 0.4 per 1000 as compared to an inbred Amish group of 1.8 per 1000. In various surveys consanguinity has usually ranged from 7 to 12 per cent (Hopkins, 1954; van Egmond, 1954; Brown, 1969).

In summary, until better data become available, it is currently estimated that of those born deaf in the United States about 50 per cent have hereditary hearing loss, making this the most important cause of congenital deafness. In perhaps 25 to 30 per cent the cause is entirely unknown. Some of these cases may be genetic. Most surveys have estimated that among congenital or very-early-onset hereditary deafness, autosomal recessive genes are responsible for 60 to 70 per cent, autosomal dominant genes for 20 to 30 per cent, and X-linked genes for about 2 per cent of hearing loss (Sank, 1963; Rosin, 1963; Fraser, 1964, 1965; Lumio, 1966; Brown, 1969; Chung *et al.*, 1969).

LATE-ONSET HEARING LOSS

A major cause of late-onset hearing loss is genetic. Since reliable data are not available, we will not attempt to cite the prevalence of the various types of deafness and their importance in causing 10 to 15 per cent of the adult population in the United States to develop hearing loss; all we are able to state is that the leading causes of late-onset deafness are heredity, presbycusis, infection, and environmental noise pollution (Collen *et al.*, 1970). Again, we can consider only hereditary factors in this text.

It must remain a blot on the medical and audiological professions that the only significant data on etiology of late-onset hearing loss in the United States are taken from interviews carried out by household survey (National Center for Vital Health Statistics, 1967, 1968). In this survey, infection was the cause of hearing loss in about 20 per cent of the cases and injury in approximately 7 per cent. "Other and ill-defined conditions," which included old age, heredity, and noise trauma, accounted for approximately 35 per cent. In another 35 per cent of the cases the cause was stated to be "unknown." These figures showed that in 1962–63 there were about 8.5 million persons in the United States with some degree of hearing loss (45.7 per 1000), that infection and unknown causes were the most frequent in producing hearing loss, and that the prevalence rate per 1000 population increased 36-fold with increasing age—from about 10 per 1000 for those under 25 years to about 360 per 1000 for those 75 years or older. Clearly, to diagnose and treat the causes of hearing loss arising in later years, one must have much better data on the etiology of late-onset deafness.

PATTERNS OF INHERITANCE

At the risk of offending some readers, we are presenting a brief review of single gene inheritance.

Autosomal Dominant Inheritance

Typically, one parent expresses the trait, which he transmits to 50 per cent of his progeny (one must remember that this is merely a probability estimate). In a small family of two children, for example, none, one, or both offspring may be affected. Yet, for each pregnancy the chances are 50 per cent for the child to have the trait. Males and females are equally affected. The trait is, therefore, carried vertically from one generation to the succeeding one. Failure of the trait to be expressed at all is spoken of as "lack of penetrance." An isolated example of a condition known to be autosomal dominant may represent a new mutation or a misrepresentation of paternity. Autosomal dominant disorders often vary in severity among the affected persons; this phenomenon is spoken of as "variable expressivity."

Autosomal Recessive Inheritance

The parents of children with autosomal recessive traits characteristically are clinically normal. They are carriers (heterozygotes) who transmit the homozygous condition to 25 per cent of their children, according to probability estimates. If the gene is quite rare, parental consanguinity is frequently found. Although two deaf parents, having the same recessive gene, ought to have only deaf children, this is by no means the case. There are many types of as yet indistinguishable forms of recessive deafness, and this information should be taken into account by the individual giving genetic counselling.

X-linked Inheritance

X-linked traits are transmitted from a carrier mother (heterozygote) to 50 per cent of her sons (hemizygotes). An affected male transmits the carrier state to all of his daughters but to none of his sons, i.e., there is never father-to-son transmission. Females may manifest X-linked disorders in modified form, since they are heterozygous and one X-chromosome is randomly "turned off" (heteropyknosis). This is known as the Lyon hypothesis. Rarely, an affected female results from the union of an affected male and a female heterozygote.

GENERAL CONSIDERATIONS

Most cases of hereditary profound childhood deafness are sensorineural rather than conductive in nature. Again, most examples of hereditary hearing loss are recessive. Recessive deafness characteristically is associated with retention of hearing of low-frequency tones. Presumably, this is due to the fact that most cases of recessive deafness are associated with the Scheibe type of change (predominantly affecting the organ of Corti, stria vascularis, and tectorial membrane of the basal coil of the cochlea). Secondary atrophy of the afferent neural structures supplying that area may also be seen. Presumably, as in deaf mice, degeneration of the organ of Corti proceeds from the base to the apex, the apical portion being responsible for transmission of low tones.

In dominantly inherited deafness, the audiogram is generally flat. However, in Waardenburg syndrome the audiogram pattern and pathologic changes are the same as those seen in recessively inherited deafness (Ormerod, 1960; Fraser, 1964).

In X-linked recessive deafness, some retention of hearing at all frequencies is common.

There seems to be little validity to Langenbeck's law of symmetry, i.e., that there is similar bilateral hearing loss in inherited deafness, and dissimilar bilateral hearing loss in acquired deafness. Although reduction of vestibular function is more common in postnatally acquired deafness than in genetic deafness, vestibular dysfunction is common in several heritable syndromes, such as the Usher and Waardenburg syndromes.

Although hereditary nerve deafness is usually bilateral, unilateral deafness clearly can be inherited as an autosomal dominant trait even though the gene is not always penetrant.

That there is considerable genetic heterogeneity among autosomal recessive hearing loss has been amply demonstrated in offspring of individuals with recessive deafness. While theoretically all offspring should be affected, there are, in fact, numerous pedigrees in which all of the children have been normal (Kraatz, 1925; Dahlberg, 1931; Macklin et al., 1946; Fraser, 1964; DeHaas et al., 1970).

There have been several informative studies of deafness in offspring of the deaf (Fay, 1898; Stevenson and Cheeseman, 1956; Sank, 1963; Brown, 1967). The largest study was that of Fay (1898), who examined 1391 matings between deaf parents. In only 14 per cent were all the progeny deaf; 79 per cent produced offspring whose hearing was normal, and 7 per cent had some children whose hearing was normal and other children who were deaf. The last group probably resulted from one of the parents having a new dominant mutation. One cannot, of course, exclude the possibility that one parent may have been heterozygous for the recessive gene affecting deafness in the partner (pseudodominance), especially in inbred kindreds.

Chung et al. (1959), employing statistical techniques based on the frequency of parental consanguinity in relation to the incidence of deafness in the population and using the frequency of complementation in matings of recessively deaf parents estimated that there may be as many as 24 to 48 different types of recessive hearing loss. They estimated further that one in eight individuals is heterozygous for at least one of this plethora of recessive genes that can effect deafness! Re-examination of the same population in 1970 suggested that the number of recessive genes involved was about five (Chung and Brown, 1970).

REFERENCES

Anderson, H., Barr, B., and Wedenberg, E., Genetic disposition—a prerequisite for maternal rubella deafness. *Arch. Otolaryngol., 91*:141–174, 1970.
Anderson, H., and Wedenberg, E., Audiometric identification of normal hearing carriers of genes for deafness. *Acta. Otolaryngol. (Stockh.), 65*:535–554, 1968.

Arnvig, J., Causes of deafness among pupils of state schools for the deaf during 1952–1953. *Ugeskr. Laeger, 116*:449–454, 1954.

Barton, M. E., Court, S. D., and Walker, W., Causes of severe deafness in school children in Northumberland and Durham. *Br. Med. J., 1*:351–355, 1962.

Bergstrom, L., Hemenway, W. G., and Downs, M. P., A high risk registry to find congenital deafness. *Otolaryngol. Clin. North Am., 4*:369–399, 1971.

Bordley, J. E., and Hardy, W. G., The etiology of deafness in young children. *Acta Otolaryngol. (Stockh.), 40*:72–79, 1951.

Brown, K. S., The genetics of childhood deafness. In *Deafness in Childhood.* McConnell, F., and Ward, P. H. (eds.), Nashville, Tenn., Vanderbilt University Press, 1967, pp. 177–202.

Brown, K. S., Genetic and environmental factors in profound prelingual deafness. *Med. Clin. North Am., 53*:741–772, 1969.

Chung, C. S., and Brown, K. S., Family studies of early childhood deafness ascertained through the Clarke School for the Deaf. *Am. J. Hum. Genet., 22*:630–644, 1970.

Chung, C. S., Robinson, O. W., and Morton, N. E., A note on deaf mutism. *Ann. Hum. Genet., 23*:357–366, 1969.

Collen, M. F., Feldman, R., Siegelaub, A. B., and Crawford, D., Dollar cost per positive test for automated multiphonic screening. *N. Engl. J. Med., 283*:459–463, 1970.

Cranefield, P. F., and Federn, W., Paulus Zacchias on mental deficiency and on deafness. *Bull. N. Y. Acad. Med., 46*:3–21, 1970.

Dahlberg, G., Eine statistische Untersuchungen über die Vererbung der Taubstummheit. *Z. Menschl. Vererb. Konstit.-lehre, 15*:492–517, 1931.

Danish, J. M., and Levitan, M., Changing aspects of deafness in school-age children. *Arch. Otolaryngol., 86*:166–171, 1967.

Danish, J. M., Tillson, J. K., and Levitan, M., Multiple anomalies in congenitally deaf children. *Eugen. Quart., 10*:12–21, 1963.

Dar, H., and Winter, S. T., A genetic study of familial deafness. *Isr. J. Med. Sci., 5*:1219–1226, 1969.

DeHaas, E., van Lith, G., Rijnjers, J., Rumke, S., and Volmer, C., Usher's syndrome with special reference to heterozygous manifestations. *Doc. Ophthalmol., 24*:166–190, 1970.

Dolowitz, D. A., An appraisal of genetics in clinical otology. *Ann. Otol. Rhinol. Laryngol., 80*:264–268, 1971.

Fay, E. A., *Marriages of the Deaf in America,* Washington, D. C., Volta Bureau, 1898.

Fowler, E. P., Jr., and Basek, M., Causes of deafness in young children. *Arch. Otolaryngol., 59*:476–484, 1954.

Fraser, G. R., Profound childhood deafness. *J. Med. Genet., 1*:118–161, 1964.

Fraser, G. R., Sex-linked recessive congenital deafness and the excess of males in profound childhood deafness. *Ann. Hum. Genet., 29*:171–196, 1965.

Fraser, G. R., The role of genetic factors in the causation of human deafness. *Audiology (Basel) 10*:212–221, 1971.

Gamstorp, I., School children with perceptive deafness. *Dev. Med. Child. Neurol., 13*:490–496, 1971.

Hopkins, L. A., Heredity and deafness. *Eugen. Quart., 1*:193–199, 1954.

Johnston, P. W., Factors associated with deafness in young children. *Public Health Rep., 82*:1019–1024, 1968.

Kloepfer, H. W., Laguaite, J., and McLaurin, J. W., Genetic aspects of congenital hearing loss. *Am. Ann. Deaf., 115*:17–22, 1970.

Kraatz, J. J., Hereditary deaf-mutism. *J. Hered., 16*:265–270, 1925.

Lindenov, H., *The Etiology of Deaf-mutism, with Special Reference to Heredity.* Copenhagen, Munksgaard, 1945.

Livingstone, G., Hearing and speech disorders in childhood. *Dev. Med. Child. Neurol., 3*:46–51, 1961.

Lumio, J. S., Piirainen, H., and Paljakka, P., Marriages between the deaf and hereditary deafness in Finland. *Acta Otolaryngol. (Stockh.), 62*:265–276, 1966.

Macklin, M. T., Mann, H. B., and Whitney, R., Genetic analysis of data and pedigrees. *Laryngoscope, 56*:583–601, 1946.

National Center for Vital and Health Statistics, *Characteristics of Persons with Impaired Hearing.* United States, July 1962–June 1963, Ser. 10, No. 35, 1967, pp. 1–64.

National Center for Vital and Health Statistics, *Prevalence of Selective Impairments.* United States, July 1963–June 1965, Ser. 10, No. 48, 1968, pp. 8–10.

Ormerod, F. C., The pathology of congenital deafness. *J. Laryngol. Otol., 74*:919–950, 1960.

Pellegrini, A., The deaf child: diagnosis and causes of deafness. *Int. Audiology, 6*:127–129, 1967.

Proctor, C. A., and Proctor, B., Understanding hereditary nerve deafness. *Arch. Otolaryngol. 85*:23–40, 1967.

Robinson, G. C., Brummitt, J. R., and Miller, J. R., Hearing loss in infants and preschool children. *Pediatrics, 32*:115–124, 1963.

Rosin, S., Die statistische Erfassung exogener Fälle bei einfach rezessivem Erbang mit Anwendung auf die rezessive Taubstummheit. *Arch. Julius Klaus Stift. Vererbungsforsch., 38*:253–262, 1963.

Ruben, R. J., and Rozycki, D. L., Clinical aspects of genetic deafness. *Ann. Otol. Rhinol. Laryngol.,* *80*:255–263, 1971.

Sank, D., Genetic aspects of early total deafness. In *Family and Mental Health Problems in a Deaf Population.* Ranier, J. D., Altschuler, K., and Kallmann, F. (eds.), New York, New York Psychiatric Institute, 1963, pp. 28–81.

Sank, D., and Kallman, F. J., The role of heredity in early total deafness. *Volta Rev., 65*:461–470, 1963.

Stevenson, A. C., and Cheeseman, E. A., Hereditary deaf-mutism with particular reference to Northern Ireland. *Ann. Hum. Genet., 20*:177–231, 1956.

Van Egmond, A. J., Congenital deafness. *J. Laryngol. Otol., 68*:429–443, 1954.

Vernon, M., Current etiology factors in deafness. *Am. Ann. Deaf., 113*:106–115, 1968.

Whetnall, E., and Fry, D. B., *The Deaf Child.* London, William Heinemann, Ltd., 1964.

Zonderman, B., The preschool nerve-deaf child: Study of etiological factors. *Laryngoscope, 69*: 54–89, 1959.

Chapter 2

GENETIC HEARING LOSS WITH NO ASSOCIATED ABNORMALITIES

There are at least 16 types of hereditary hearing loss with no associated abnormalities. Many can be separated from each other by mode of transmission, age of onset, severity of hearing loss, and type of audiogram. Although there are several types of recessive congenital severe deafness, we are unable to separate these with present techniques.

DOMINANT CONGENITAL SEVERE SENSORINEURAL DEAFNESS

Congenital severe sensorineural hearing loss with dominant transmission was first described by Fay in 1898. Since then, numerous articles have appeared in which kindred with this type of hearing loss have been described. At present, it is not clear how many different genes may be involved in producing this type of deafness, since affected patients have no other abnormalities that may help to distinguish different genes.

CLINICAL FINDINGS

Auditory System. The hearing loss shows little variation from one person to another; all patients have a moderate to profound sensorineural hearing loss of from 60 to 100 dB. They have defective speech and language development unless given special speech training.

Vestibular System. Caloric vestibular testing generally shows normal responses. However, Müller (1936) presented a family with dominant hearing loss in which several members had vestibular disturbances. By caloric testing we found affected persons with vestibular hypofunction in two families. This area deserves more attention, since abnormal vestibular function may characterize a specific type of dominant congenital deafness.

LABORATORY FINDINGS

Roentgenograms. No radiographic studies on patients have been described. Temporal bone tomograms would be of con-

7

siderable interest, since these may show abnormalities in some families and may be helpful in distinguishing types of deafness in this category.

PATHOLOGY

Although temporal bone changes in a large number of patients with congenital deafness have been described, few of these cases have well documented dominantly transmitted congenital deafness. A probable example of this disorder was described by Altmann (1950). The patient was a 22-year-old deaf-mute woman who died of sarcoma. Both parents and most of her direct relatives over the past three generations were deaf-mutes. No other family history was available. Microscopic sections showed complete disappearance of the organ of Corti in the basal turn (Fig. 2–1A) with only a mound of undifferentiated cells representing the organ of Corti being evident in the apical and middle turns of the cochlea. The stria vascularis was atrophic in the lower half of the basal turn but was normal in the remaining turns. Ganglion cells were described in the basal turn. The saccule was collapsed and the macula was atrophic.

HEREDITY

A number of pedigrees showing dominant transmission of severe congenital deafness have been presented (Fay, 1898; Popow, 1935; Hopkins and Guilder, 1969; Fraser, 1964) (Fig. 2–1B). Since congenitally deaf persons usually marry other persons who are deaf, pedigrees are sometimes difficult to interpret.

There have been several studies to determine the incidence of hereditary congenital deafness. Sank (1963), in a survey of deaf residents in New York state, concluded that autosomal dominant genes accounted for about 10 per cent of all congenital deafness. Since there are about 38,000 students in schools for the deaf in the United States, about 3800 of these students are likely to have dominantly transmitted congenital hearing loss.

DIAGNOSIS

In diagnosing a child with congenital severe deafness, one should rule out meningitis, prenatal rubella, kernicterus, birth injury, administration of streptomycin or other ototoxic drugs, viral infections, and otitis media. A careful otologic examination and history should be taken to evaluate various possible causes of hearing loss. A family history is also important, since parents frequently attribute hearing loss to infection or trauma when the real cause may be heredity.

When it is determined that the congenital severe deafness may be hereditary, the pedigree must be carefully constructed to determine whether transmission is autosomal dominant, recessive, or X-linked. In dominantly transmitted deafness, taking a good family history is important; all members of the family with hearing loss must be identified along with the age of onset and the severity of the hearing loss. Even if both parents are deaf, the hearing loss may be recessively transmitted (Mengel *et al.*, 1967).

A thorough physical and neurological examination should be done to search for other possible anomalies associated with the deafness that may help to define the disease. To differentiate congenital from early-onset recessive deafness, a history concerning the degree of development of the patient's speech may help in differential diagnosis. In cases where speech did begin to develop and where some evidence of facility with speech is present, the diagnosis of early-onset recessive deafness can be considered.

In all cases, it is important to carry out vestibular testing to determine the intactness of the vestibular system. This may help to distinguish dominant from recessive congenital severe deafness.

TREATMENT

For rehabilitation it is important that diagnosis be made early and that the child then be enrolled in a school for the deaf. In some cases, a hearing aid may help.

PROGNOSIS

Patients with this disorder are otherwise completely normal.

SUMMARY

Characteristics include: 1) autosomal dominant transmission, 2) congenital severe nonprogressive sensorineural deafness, and 3) variable vestibular responses.

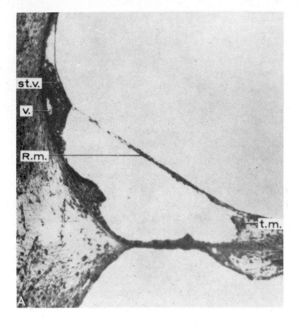

Figure 2-1 Dominant congenital severe sensorineural deafness. (A) Photomicrograph of section from temporal bone showing lower half of basal turn in organ of Corti. Reissner's membrane (R.m.) is adherent to stria vascularis (st. v.), which contains wide vascular space (v.). The organ of Corti has disappeared. The tectorial membrane (t.m.) is tucked into the internal sulcus. (From F. Altmann, *Arch. Otolaryngol., 51*:852, 1950.) *(B)* Pedigree of affected kindred. (Modified from E. Müller, *Arch. Ohren- Nasen- Kehlkopfheilkd., 142*:156, 1936.)

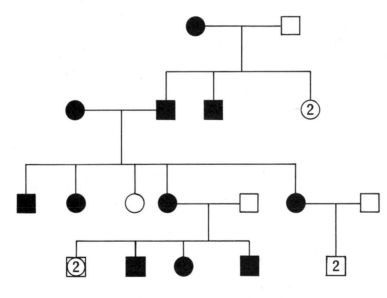

B

REFERENCES

Altmann, F., Histologic pictures of inherited nerve deafness in man and animals. *Arch. Otolaryngol., 51*:852–890, 1950.

Fay, E. A., *Marriages of the Deaf in America.* Washington, Volta Bureau, 1898.

Fraser, G. R., Profound childhood deafness. *J. Med. Genet., 1*:118–151, 1964.

Hopkins, L. S., and Guilder, R. P., *Clarke School Studies Concerning the Heredity of Deafness.* Northampton, Mass., Clarke School for the Deaf, 1969.

Mengel, M. C., Konigsmark, B. W., Berlin, C. I., and McKusick, V. A., Recessive early onset neural deafness. *Acta Otolaryngol. (Stockh.), 64*:313–326, 1967.

Müller, E., Vestibularisstörungen bei erblicher Taubheit. *Arch. Ohren-, Nasen-, Kehlkopfheilk., 142*:156–163, 1936.

Nance, W. E., and Sweeney, A., Genetic factors in deafness of early life. *Otolaryngol. Clin. North Am., 8*:19–48, 1975.

Popow, N. A., Hereditäre Atrophie der Hörnerven. *Z. Hals-, Nasen-, Ohrenheilk., 37*:407–413, 1935.

Sank, D., Genetic aspects of early total deafness. In *Family and Mental Health Problems in a Deaf Population.* Ranier, J. D., Altschuler, K., and Kallmann, F., (eds.), Springfield, Ill., Charles C Thomas, Publisher, 1963, pp. 28–81.

DOMINANT PROGRESSIVE EARLY-ONSET SENSORINEURAL HEARING LOSS

A form of hereditary deafness characterized by onset of a progressive sensorineural hearing loss in childhood or in early adult life has been described in several families. The most extensive pedigrees are those of Stephens and Dolowitz (1949), Johnsen (1952), Huizing *et al.* (1966), Teig (1968), Lenzi (1969), and Nance and Sweeney (1975). Other probable kindreds are those of Schneider (1937) and Wedenberg (1965).

CLINICAL FINDINGS

Auditory System. Auditory findings in affected persons in each of these reports were somewhat similar. Individuals in the first or second decade of life showed high-frequency sensorineural hearing loss with preservation of frequencies below 2000 Hz. The hearing loss progressed with gradual involvement of the middle frequencies until old age, when the hearing loss severely affected all frequencies (Fig. 2–2*A*). Huizing *et al.* (1966) divided the progression of hearing loss into five stages. In the first stage, the capacity to hear frequencies above 1000 Hz or 2000 Hz deteriorates. Thereafter, the hearing of mid and low frequencies becomes involved. By the fifth stage there is severe loss (70 to 80 dB) in all frequencies. Huizing and colleagues observed this stage only in persons over 45 years of age (Fig. 2–2*B*).

Teig (1968), studying a family with 25 affected persons, found a similar pattern of hearing loss. Follow-up studies of up to 15 years showed progressive deterioration of hearing. Recruitment tests performed on eight patients were positive. The positive recruitment tests suggested the existence of a degenerative lesion in the cochlea. The variable results of the tone-decay test indicated a possible retrocochlear lesion; this test, however, can be positive in cases with exclusive cochlear lesions. Recruitment was present in over 80 per cent of the cases studied by Lenzi (1969).

Vestibular System. Vestibular tests have been done on only a few affected persons. Ford (1960) found vestibular responses to be normal in two cases. We have identified and partially studied six families with dominantly transmitted progressive sensorineural hearing loss; some had vestibular abnormalities. Müller (1936) also found vestibular alterations. Nance and Sweeney (1975) reported dizziness and tinnitus. It is possible that several disease entities have been included in this category, distinguished by age of onset, severity of hearing loss, and involvement of the vestibular system.

LABORATORY FINDINGS

Roentgenograms. No radiographic findings have been described.

PATHOLOGY

The temporal bone changes in an 80-year-old woman with late onset of hearing loss were described by Gussen (1969). One of the patient's four children had progressive sensorineural hearing loss, which had begun at 17 years of age. The woman had two sons who exhibited onset of hearing loss at 4 and 6 years of age. The patient's hearing loss was noted when she was about 65 years old. An audiogram made when she was 76 years old showed a severe hearing loss of 60 to 100 dB affecting all frequencies.

Histologic sections of her temporal bone showed different stages of a process that appeared similar bilaterally. On the left side, there was marked hydrops of the saccule, whereas on the right side the saccule was collapsed, probably representing a later degenerative change. The left hydropic saccule herniated into the scala vestibuli causing partial collapse of the cochlear duct. The cochlear duct on the right side was distended. The sensory receptor areas of the saccule, utricle, and canal ampullae showed moderate to marked degeneration, which was more severe on the right side. The cochlear aqueduct aperture was obstructed by a fibrotic dura. There was marked loss of spiral ganglion cells bilaterally (Fig. 2–2*C*).

HEREDITY

In a Mormon family studied by Stephens and Dolowitz (1949) there were 62 affected members in six generations. There

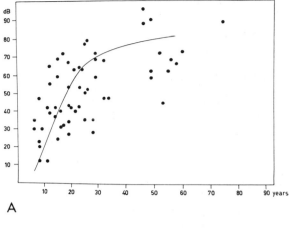

A

Figure 2-2 Dominant progressive early-onset sensorineural hearing loss. (A) Mean perceptive hearing loss as a function of age. Note rapid increase of hearing loss in first three decades.

(*B*) Characteristic audiometric stages of progression of the hearing impairment.

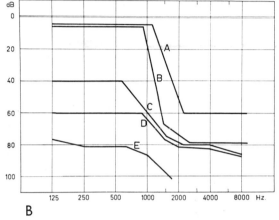

B

(*C*) Hydrops of saccule that almost fills vestibule. Arrows indicate Reissner's membrane showing marked extension of cochlear duct. The proximal part of the cochlear duct in the hook region (H) appears normal. There is marked loss of ganglion cells in the modiolus. (*A, B* from E. H. Huizing *et al., Acta Otolaryngol. (Stockh.), 61*:35, 1966; *C* from R. Gussen, *Arch. Otolaryngol., 90*:429, 1963.)

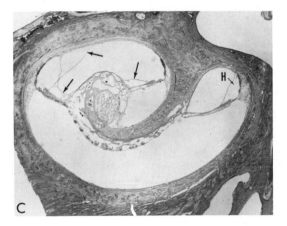

C

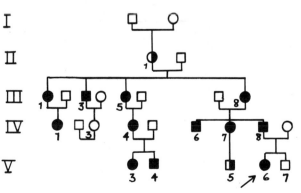

(*D*) Pedigree of affected kindred exhibiting autosomal dominant inheritance. (From W. E. Nance and A. Sweeney, *Otolaryngol. Clin. North Am., 8*:19, 1975.)

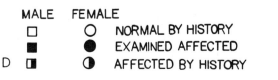

were 25 persons affected in five generations of the kindred described by Teig (1968). Huizing *et al.* (1966) described 67 individuals in five generations affected with progressive sensorineural hearing loss. Each family showed dominant transmission, with affected persons passing this abnormality to about half of their children (Fig. 2–2*D*).

DIAGNOSIS

Older patients with this type of hearing loss show findings quite similar to those patients who have dominant low-frequency or dominant mid-frequency hearing loss. Thus, it would be necessary to test younger affected persons in the families to determine which of these three types of hearing loss a patient may have.

TREATMENT

The deafness is best treated by use of a hearing aid as needed.

PROGNOSIS

The hearing loss is slowly progressive, resulting finally in severe deafness in the sixth or seventh decade of life.

SUMMARY

Characteristics include: 1) autosomal dominant transmission, and 2) childhood onset of a progressive symmetrical sensorineural hearing loss beginning with high frequencies and leading to severe hearing loss in old age.

REFERENCES

Dolowitz, D. A., and Stephens, F. E., Hereditary nerve deafness. *Ann. Otol. Rhinol. Laryngol.,* 70:851–859, 1961.

Ford, F. R., *Diseases of the Nervous System in Infancy, Childhood, and Adolescence.* 4th Ed., Springfield, Ill., Charles C Thomas, Publisher, 1960.

Gussen, R., Delayed hereditary deafness with cochlear aqueduct obstruction. *Arch. Otolaryngol.,* 90:429–436, 1969.

Huizing, E. H., van Bolhuis, A. H., and Odenthal, D. W., Studies on progressive hereditary perceptive deafness in a family of 355 members. *Acta Otolaryngol. (Stockh.),* 61:35–41, 161–167, 1966.

Johnsen, S., The heredity of perceptive deafness. *Acta Otolaryngol. (Stockh.),* 42:539–552, 1952. (Families 1, 2.)

Lenzi, P., Sulle sordità ereditarie (studio genètico e clinico di un ceppo familiare). *Arch. Ital. Otol.,* 80:453–485, 1969.

Müller, E., Vestibularisstörungen bei erblicher Taubheit. *Arch. Ohren-, Nasen-, Kehlkopfheilk.,* 142:156–163, 1936.

Nance, W. E., and Sweeney, A., Genetic factors in deafness of early life. *Otolaryngol. Clin. North Am.,* 8:19–48, 1975.

Schneider, K. W., Untersuchungen einer mit hereditärer degenerativer Innenohrschwerhörigkeit stark belasteten Sippe. *Z. Hals-, Nasen-, Ohrenheilk.,* 42:314–320, 1937.

Stephens, F. E., and Dolowitz, D. A., Hereditary nerve deafness. *Am. J. Hum. Genet.,* 1:37–51, 1949.

Teig, E., Hereditary progressive perceptive deafness in a family of 72 patients. *Acta Otolaryngol. (Stockh.),* 65:365–372, 1968.

Wedenberg, E., Hereditary deafness in the young deaf child: identification and management. *Acta Otolaryngol. (Stockh.), Suppl.* 206:26–27, 1965.

DOMINANT UNILATERAL SENSORINEURAL DEAFNESS

Although most types of hereditary deafness are bilateral with both ears equally affected, several types, including the Waardenburg syndrome and mandibulofacial dysostosis, may affect the ears unequally. Unilateral or bilateral severe sensorineural hearing loss with no other associated abnormalities was described by Smith (1939).

Everberg (1960a–c) documented cases of several families in which at least one person had unilateral hearing loss and other members had other hearing impairments. Only one of these families (Family XIII) appears to have the same type of hearing loss as that found in the kindred described by Smith.

CLINICAL FINDINGS

Auditory System. The tympanic membranes were normal in all five persons examined by Smith. Affected individuals were born deaf. In four, the right ear was involved and in four, the left; in one person the affected side was not determined and in another the hearing loss was bilateral. Audiometric results were not presented. Thus, it is possible that there may have been some hearing loss in the supposedly normal ear.

One of Everberg's probands was congenitally deaf only in the right ear, whereas the two sisters of the proband had bilateral congenital deafness and the mother had right-sided congenital deafness.

Vestibular System. Caloric vestibular tests were normal in the patients studied by Smith. In Everberg's series, vestibular function was absent on the deaf side in almost 30 per cent of the cases.

LABORATORY FINDINGS

Roentgenograms. Temporal bone roentgenograms on six affected persons showed no abnormalities.

PATHOLOGY

No histopathologic findings have been described.

HEREDITY

In the family studied by Smith there were 11 affected persons in four generations (Fig. 2–3). Involved were four of seven sibs, their mother, two maternal aunts, and their maternal grandfather. In a family described

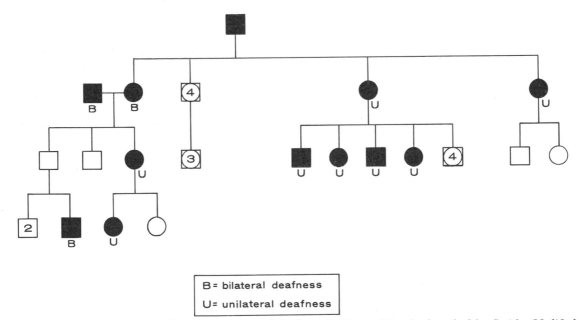

B = bilateral deafness
U = unilateral deafness

Figure 2–3 *Dominant unilateral sensorineural deafness.* Pedigree of family described by Smith. (Modified from A. B. Smith, *Lancet,* 2:1172, 1939.)

by Everberg there were five persons affected in three generations. The pedigree suggests that this form of deafness is transmitted by an autosomal dominant gene that shows variable expressivity, sometimes causing bilateral congenital deafness and sometimes only unilateral deafness.

DIAGNOSIS

Other factors that may cause unilateral deafness are various viral infections, meningitis, otitis media, head injury, or vascular disease. These types of unilateral deafness show a rather rapid onset and are not congenital.

TREATMENT

The deafness is best treated by use of a hearing aid, as indicated.

PROGNOSIS

There is no documented evidence that the hearing loss is progressive.

SUMMARY

Characteristics of this disorder include: 1) autosomal dominant transmission, 2) congenital moderate to severe unilateral or bilateral sensorineural hearing loss, and 3) normal vestibular function.

REFERENCES

Everberg, G., Unilateral anacusis. Clinical, radiological, and genetic investigations. *Acta Otolaryngol. (Stockh.), Suppl. 158*:366–374, 1960a.
Everberg, G., Etiology of unilateral total deafness. *Ann. Otol. Rhinol. Laryngol., 69*:711–721, 1960b.
Everberg, G., Further studies on hereditary unilateral deafness. *Acta Otolaryngol. (Stockh.), 51*:615–635, 1960c.
Smith, A. B., Unilateral hereditary deafness. *Lancet, 2*:1172–1173, 1939.

DOMINANT LOW-FREQUENCY SENSORINEURAL HEARING LOSS

Hearing loss first involving the low frequencies followed by the high frequencies in later years was described by Konigsmark, Mengel, and Berlin (1971) and by the Vanderbilt group (1968).

CLINICAL FINDINGS

Auditory System. Affected members in three kindreds described by Konigsmark *et al.* and in two kindreds studied by the Vanderbilt group showed somewhat similar audiologic findings but these may represent genetic heterogeneity. Otologic examinations showed no gross abnormalities of the ears, the external auditory canals, or the tympanic membranes.

The hearing loss is congenital or the onset is during infancy. Younger affected persons showed a pure-tone hearing loss most marked in low frequencies of 225 to 1000 Hz. In different individuals this loss ranged from about 20 dB to about 60 dB. Hearing in the higher frequencies, including 4000 and 8000 Hz, was normal in young affected persons. In the middle decades of life, hearing loss was found to be worse both in the low and high frequencies; hearing in the range of 2000 to 4000 Hz was relatively better preserved. Several members of a family tested by Konigsmark *et al.* had audiograms taken over a five- to six-year period that confirmed the slowly progressive hearing loss — affecting primarily frequencies around 8000 Hz. Older affected persons in each of the kindreds showed a hearing loss involving all frequencies ranging from 40 to 100 dB. Thus, it seems that the frequencies affected vary with age, beginning with low-frequency hearing loss in the first and second decades, followed by progressive high-frequency loss in the third and fourth decades, ultimately involving loss in all frequencies in the later decades of life. There were, however, moderate individual variations in severity of hearing loss, with some younger persons having a much more marked loss than older relatives.

Other audiometric testing showed the SISI test to be positive in six of nine cases and the tone decay test to be negative in nine of ten cases studied by Konigsmark *et al.* These results suggest a cochlear locus for the hearing loss. Speech discrimination tests were 90 per cent or less in 22 of 33 persons tested by the Vanderbilt group, and in eight of eleven cases tested in our kindred.

Vestibular System. Caloric vestibular tests were carried out in three individuals studied by Konigsmark *et al.* Two were normal and one was interpreted as mildly abnormal with a minimal rotatory component.

LABORATORY FINDINGS

Roentgenograms. Temporal bone tomograms done on three patients by the Vanderbilt group were normal.

Other Studies. Blood typing of three patients of the Vanderbilt group showed no evidence for genetic linkage between the low-frequency hearing loss locus and the ABO, Rh, or MNS loci.

PATHOLOGY

No histopathologic studies have been presented.

HEREDITY

Each of the kindreds with this syndrome exhibited autosomal dominant transmission (Fig. 2–4*B*).

DIAGNOSIS

Low-frequency hearing loss may be due to prenatal rubella. This diagnosis can be made by rubella titers, by history of maternal infection, or by associated visual and/or cardiac defects. Dominant mid-frequency sensorineural deafness shows some low-frequency hearing loss in earlier stages. It can be differentiated by the fact that the low frequencies of 250 and 500 Hz are not as severely involved as are frequencies of 1000, 2000, and 4000 Hz. In contrast, patients with dominant low-frequency sensorineural hearing loss have their most severe deficit in the 250 to 500 Hz range and show marked deterioration in the high frequencies (8000 Hz) in the third and fourth decades of life. In patients with mid-frequency sensorineural hearing loss this frequency is relatively well preserved. Dominant low-frequency sensorineural hearing loss may be heterogeneous. The deafness in the kindred described by the Vanderbilt group was not progressive and seemed to have its onset soon after birth. The family described by Konigsmark *et al.* developed hearing loss in the second or third decade and showed slow progression. Additional cases are necessary to document differences.

Iinuma *et al.* (1967) reported affected sibs and mentioned "familial occurrence," but because of insufficient information we cannot categorize these cases.

TREATMENT

Therapy consists of complete and periodic audiologic evaluation and use of a hearing aid as indicated.

PROGNOSIS

The evidence suggests that affected persons have rather severe hearing difficulties with increasing age. In the fifth or sixth decade a hearing aid is usually necessary. There is no evidence of other deficits in affected persons.

SUMMARY

Characteristics include: 1) autosomal dominant transmission, 2) moderate low-frequency sensorineural hearing loss with slow progression to moderately severe deafness involving all frequencies, and 3) normal vestibular responses.

REFERENCES

Iinuma, T., Shitara, T., Hoshino, T., and Kirikae, I., Sensorineural hearing loss for low tones. *Arch. Otolaryngol.*, 86:110–116, 1967.

Konigsmark, B. W., Mengel, M. C., and Berlin, C. I., Familial low frequency hearing loss. *Laryngoscope*, 81:759–771, 1971.

Vanderbilt University Hereditary Deafness Study Group, Dominantly inherited low-frequency hearing loss. *Arch. Otolaryngol.*, 88:242–250, 1968.

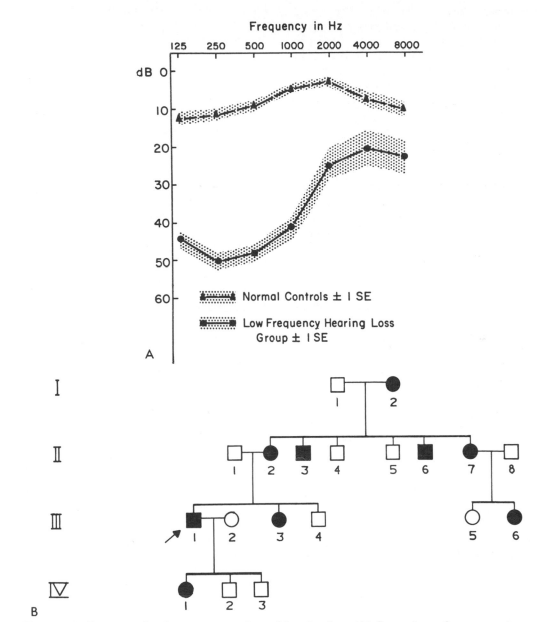

Figure 2–4 *Dominant low-frequency sensorineural hearing loss.* *(A)* Comparison of mean puretone audiograms in patients with hereditary low-frequency hearing loss and their normal relatives. (From Vanderbilt Group, *Arch. Otolaryngol., 88*:242, 1965.) *(B)* Pedigree of affected kindred showing autosomal dominant inheritance. (From B. W. Konigsmark *et al., Laryngoscope, 81*:759, 1971.)

DOMINANT MID-FREQUENCY SENSORINEURAL HEARING LOSS

Hearing loss involving the mid frequencies in childhood and progressing to involve all frequencies in adult life was described in single families by Mårtensson (1960), by Williams and Roblee (1962), and in additional families by Paparella *et al.* (1969) and Konigsmark, Salman, Haskins, and Mengel (1970).

CLINICAL FINDINGS

Auditory System. Williams and Roblee described a mother and three of her children who were affected with a similar type of mid-frequency hearing loss. Audiograms showed a 0 to 80 dB bilateral symmetrical sensorineural hearing loss, most severe at frequencies from 500 to 2000 Hz (Fig. 2–5A, B). A follow-up on these patients eight years later showed no progression of the hearing loss. In the family described by Mårtensson, 18 persons in six generations of a family were affected. Audiograms showed a saucer-shaped curve with hearing loss at 1000 to 2000 Hz most severe in younger persons. In older patients, all frequencies were affected. In four families studied by Konigsmark *et al.* younger affected persons also showed a sensorineural hearing loss of 10 to 60 dB, affecting primarily the frequencies from 1000 to 4000 Hz. Individuals in their fifth decade had more severe deafness involving all frequencies, with more marked loss in the high frequencies. Most affected persons indicated that hearing loss progressed slowly over the years. The degree of hearing loss varied considerably in different individuals of the same age, suggesting variable expression of the gene. The tone-decay test was negative in all affected persons in the families studied, whereas speech discrimination was generally normal. The SISI test was usually positive. These findings suggest that the lesion was not retrocochlear but rather involved the organ of Corti.

Vestibular System. Caloric vestibular tests done on 13 persons in four families studied by Konigsmark *et al.* showed normal vestibular responses. Vestibular tests were not described in the other families.

LABORATORY FINDINGS

No laboratory tests were described.

PATHOLOGY

Paparella, Sugiura, and Hoshino (1969) described the temporal bone pathology in a father and daughter with sensorineural hearing loss. The audiogram of the father showed a 55 to 100 dB sensorineural hearing loss with mild preservation at low frequencies and normal hearing at high frequencies (8000 Hz). From the data available, it appears that this father and daughter may have dominant mid-frequency hearing loss. The daughter's temporal bone showed complete loss of the organ of Corti in the basal turn with clumps of cells remaining in the middle and apical turns. The stria vascularis was atrophic. Spiral ganglion cells were deficient in the basal turn of the cochlea (Fig. 2–5C). It is difficult to correlate the marked involvement of the basal turn of the cochlea with the preservation of high-frequency hearing.

HEREDITY

The pedigrees of each of the persons of the kindred affected with mid-frequency hearing loss showed autosomal dominant transmission of the defect (Fig. 2–5D).

DIAGNOSIS

Mid-frequency sensorineural hearing loss may be caused by prenatal rubella, by ototoxins, or by noise trauma. A careful hearing history and family study will help to establish the familial characteristics of dominant mid-frequency sensorineural hearing loss. This form must also be differentiated from *dominant low-frequency sensorineural hearing loss.* In the latter disorder, the low frequencies of 250 and 500 Hz are the first affected, with preservation of the higher tones until about middle age, when the higher frequencies of 4000 and 8000 Hz begin to deteriorate at a rapid rate. In contrast, patients with dominant mid-frequency sensorineural hearing loss tend

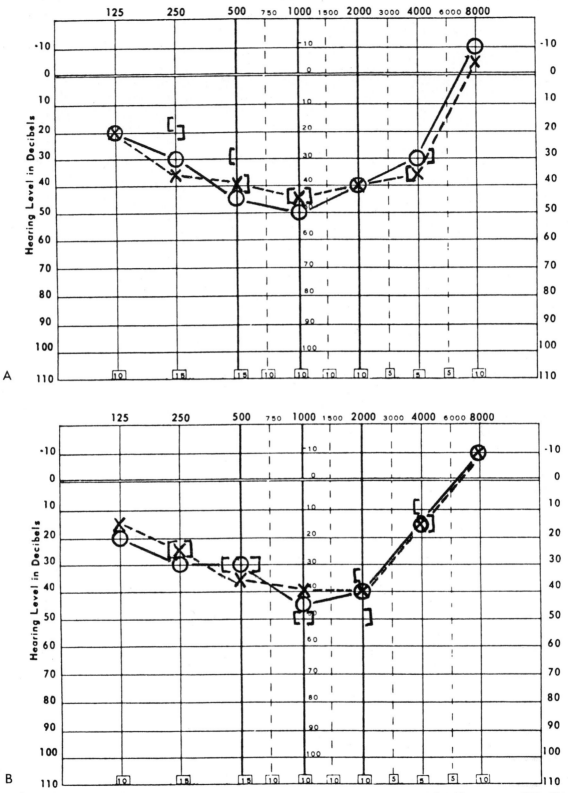

Figure 2–5 *Dominant mid-frequency sensorineural hearing loss. (A)* Audiogram of mother at age of 29; *(B)* Audiogram of son at age of 18. (From F. Williams and S. E. Roblee, *Arch. Otolaryngol.,* 75:69, 1962.)

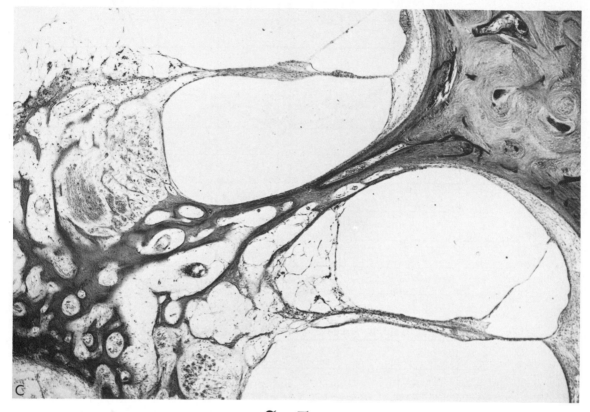

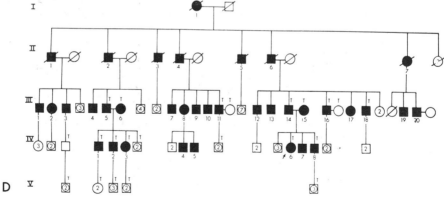

(C) Section of temporal bone showing marked loss of ganglion cells, atrophy of stria vascularis, and degeneration of organ of Corti. (From M. M. Paparella *et al.*, *Arch. Otolaryngol.*, 90:44, 1969.) (D) Pedigree of a family showing dominant transmission of mid-frequency sensorineural hearing loss. There are 35 affected persons in five generations. (From B. W. Konigsmark *et al.*, *Ann. Otol. Rhinol. Laryngol.*, 79:42, 1970.)

to preserve both low- and high-frequency hearing until the later years.

The mother and three daughters studied by Williams and Roblee, however, showed no increase in hearing loss over an eight-year period. It is possible that this family has a different form of deafness than that of the other kindreds or that some persons may show no progression of the deafness for longer periods of time.

TREATMENT

Treatment consists of the use of hearing aids as required.

PROGNOSIS

Affected persons in the families described by Konigsmark *et al.* showed some mild progression of hearing loss over periods of testing (6 to 15 years). The rate of progression may vary, remaining stable over a period up to possibly six years, as seen in one patient studied by Konigsmark *et al.* Older persons in the families studied by Mårtensson, Paparella *et al.*, and Konigsmark *et al.* showed a much more severe hearing loss than younger persons.

SUMMARY

The major characteristics include: 1) autosomal dominant transmission, 2) progressive sensorineural hearing loss involving mid frequencies in childhood and eventually all frequencies, and 3) normal caloric responses.

REFERENCES

Cawthorne, T. E., and Hinchcliffe, R., Familial perceptive deafness. *Pract. Otorhinolaryngol.,* *19*:68–83, 1957. (Same as Williams and Roblee.)
Konigsmark, B. W., Salman, S., Haskins, H., and Mengel, M. C., Dominant midfrequency hearing loss. *Ann. Otol. Rhinol. Laryngol., 79*:42–54, 1970.
Mårtensson, B., Dominant hereditary nerve deafness. *Acta Otolaryngol. (Stockh.), 52*:270–274, 1960.
Paparella, M. M., Sugiura, S., and Hoshino, T., Familial progressive sensorineural deafness. *Arch. Otolaryngol., 90*:44–51, 1969.
Williams, F., Lyons, J. P., Stein, S. P., and Roblee, L., Progressive hereditary nerve deafness. *Med. Ann. DC., 23*:681–683, 1954.
Williams, F., and Roblee, L. A., Hereditary nerve deafness. *Arch. Otolaryngol., 75*:69–77, 1962.

DOMINANT HIGH-FREQUENCY PROGRESSIVE SENSORINEURAL DEAFNESS

Although recognized as a possible distinct type of hearing loss by Crowe, Guild, and Polvogt (1934), abrupt dominant high-frequency progressive deafness was first demonstrated in four generations by Nance and McConnell (1974). Other examples are those of Glorig and Davis (1961) and Lenzi (1969).

CLINICAL FINDINGS

Auditory System. Among the individuals studied in four generations of one family by Nance and McConnell (1974), there was progression of hearing loss with age with involvement of lower frequencies. In the 6-year-old, there was abrupt loss above 2000 Hz; in the 28-year-old, above 1000 Hz; and in the 57-year-old, above 500 Hz. In childhood, this form of hearing loss may easily go undetected because of sufficient hearing in the speech range.

The SISI tests were positive at high frequencies, suggesting a localized cochlear lesion. Speech discrimination was poor.

Vestibular System. No studies have been reported.

LABORATORY FINDINGS

Roentgenograms. Tomographic studies were normal.

PATHOLOGY

Crowe *et al.* (1934) demonstrated a discrete area of atrophy in the basal turn of the organ of Corti together with atrophy of a portion of the eighth nerve supplying the basal turn.

HEREDITY

Autosomal dominant inheritance was documented by Nance and McConnell (1974).

DIAGNOSIS

It is not certain whether this represents a distinct entity. It may be the same as *dominant progressive early-onset sensorineural hearing loss.* Crowe showed that patients with dominant progressive early-onset sensorineural hearing loss show relatively normal histologic findings in the organ of Corti.

TREATMENT

Treatment consists of a hearing aid as indicated.

PROGNOSIS

The high-frequency loss becomes progressively marked with involvement of lower frequencies with age.

SUMMARY

Characteristics for this form are: 1) autosomal dominant inheritance, 2) abrupt high-tone sensorineural deafness, and 3) progression to lower frequency involvement with age.

REFERENCES

Crowe, S. J., Guild, S. R., and Polvogt, L. M., Observations on the pathology of high-tone deafness. *Bull. Johns Hopkins Hosp., 54*:315–380, 1934.

Glorig, A., and Davis, H., Age, noise, and hearing loss. *Trans. Am. Otol. Soc., 49*:262–280, 1961.

Lenzi, P., Sulle sordità ereditarie. *Arch. Ital. Otol. Rhinol. Laryngol., 80*:453–485, 1969.

Nance, W. E., and McConnell, F. E., Status and progress of research in hereditary deafness. *Adv. Hum. Genet., 4*:173–250, 1974.

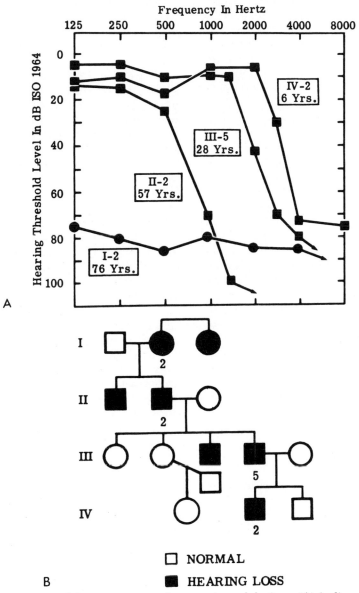

Figure 2-6 *Dominant high-frequency progressive sensorineural deafness. (A)* Audiogram showing abrupt loss of perception in various members of kindred. Note progression of loss with age. *(B)* Kindred showing autosomal dominant inheritance. *(A, B* from W. E. Nance and F . E. McConnell, *Adv. Hum. Genet., 4*:173, 1974.)

OTOSCLEROSIS

Otosclerosis is one of the major causes of hearing loss in the elderly. It has been the subject of over 1000 publications (Steinberg and Neumann, 1973). Guild (1944), studying 1100 pairs of temporal bones, found that 5 per cent had histologic evidence of otosclerosis. A somewhat higher incidence was found by Jørgensen and Kristensen (1967) in Denmark. Among 237 temporal bones, in general, 11 per cent showed otosclerosis; among patients above 60 years old, 18 per cent had otosclerosis.

CLINICAL FINDINGS

Auditory System. Although hearing loss from otosclerosis can be initiated in childhood, it usually begins in the second or third decades of life. In about 90 per cent of patients, symptoms are first noted between 15 and 45 years of age. The onset is insidious. Audiometric testing shows a conductive or a mixed sensorineural and conductive hearing loss, somewhat more marked in the higher frequencies. In some cases, the sensorineural component may be quite marked, with patients showing no response at higher frequencies to air or bone conduction (Myers *et al.*, 1963). Speech discrimination, tone decay, and SISI testing generally are normal.

Vestibular System. No vestibular abnormalities have been described in patients with otosclerosis.

LABORATORY FINDINGS

Polytomography of the temporal bone in otosclerosis has shown narrowing of the oval window and bridging bone covering the oval window (Brünner *et al.*, 1966).

PATHOLOGY

Careful examination of the stapes footplate shows "bridge formation" from the footplate to the oval window. This formation begins as a thickening of a portion of the footplate, progressing to involvement of the entire oval window (Gussen, 1969; Kelemen and Linthicum, 1969; Lindsay, 1973).

Histologically, otosclerosis consists of a focal spongy overgrowth of bone involving the bony labyrinth, usually beginning near the oval window. This spongy bone contains numerous small blood vessels and marrow and is sharply demarcated from surrounding normal bone. The otosclerotic change may spread from the oval window toward the round window and basal turn of the cochlea, and sometimes it may spread inward toward the posterior canal and cochlea. Nager and Fraser (1938) described six petrous bones in which the otosclerotic process involved the scala tympani, which was filled with bone in advanced cases. Wolff and Bellucci (1974) noted that six basic patterns could occur in one specimen. Bretlau (1971) suggested from his electron-microscopic studies that otosclerosis is an enzymatic disease whose destructive phase is associated with lysosomal hydrolases.

HEREDITY

Hammerschlag (1905) and Albrecht (1923) presented pedigrees showing autosomal dominant transmission of otosclerosis. Chumlea (1942) presented a family with nine persons affected in four generations, and Kabat (1943) described another kindred in which 19 persons had progressive hearing loss. Audiometric tests on several of the patients in the family studied by Kabat showed bilateral mixed hearing loss suggestive of otosclerosis. Pfändler (1949) investigated a Swiss family in which there were 15 cases of otosclerosis in five generations and concluded that otosclerosis was transmitted as a dominant trait with varying degrees of penetrance.

Larsson (1960) reviewed all cases of otosclerosis studied at the University of Göteborg Hospital from 1949 to 1957. In about 90 per cent of the 202 patients with otosclerosis, he was able to verify a family history of otosclerosis. Larsson concluded that otosclerosis was transmitted by an autosomal dominant gene with 25 to 40 per cent penetrance.

Morrison (1967) and Morrison and Bundey (1970) studied 150 patients with otosclerosis. About 70 per cent had a family history of otosclerosis. They also concluded that the disease is transmitted in an autosomal dominant manner, manifesting itself in about 40 per cent of the individuals carrying the abnormal gene.

Studies of monozygotic twins frequently show similarity in age of onset of otosclerosis (Juers, 1960). Nager (1955) reviewed 16 cases of identical twins with

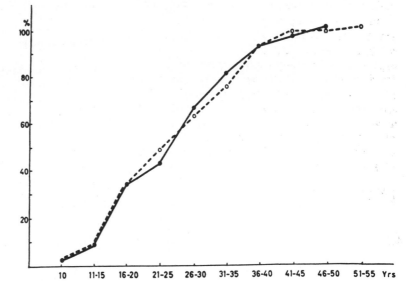

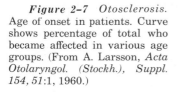

Figure 2-7 *Otosclerosis.* Age of onset in patients. Curve shows percentage of total who became affected in various age groups. (From A. Larsson, *Acta Otolaryngol. (Stockh.), Suppl. 154, 51*:1, 1960.)

clinical otosclerosis. In six pairs, loss of hearing occurred at the same age in both partners. In nine of the other ten pairs, the age of onset of the hearing loss varied between 3 and 16 years. Fowler (1966) found concordance in nearly all of 40 sets of identical twins.

There is no linkage between otosclerosis and the ABO, MN, and Rhesus blood groups, the secretor states, or haptoglobin genotypes (Morrison, 1967).

EPIDEMIOLOGY

Although about three per 1000 Caucasians have clinical signs of otosclerosis,

histologic otosclerosis is present in seven per 1000 according to Morrison (1967). Guild (1944), however, found histologic otosclerosis in 8 per cent of Caucasians and in 1 per cent of Afro-Americans.

Even though there seems to be a female predilection for this condition, the higher frequency of incidence probably reflects, in large part, the male-female ratio living at the late age of onset, since rarely are the data corrected for age.

DIAGNOSIS

A conductive progressive hearing loss may be caused by external auditory canal

Table 2-1   Penetrance of Gene in Otosclerosis*

RELATIONSHIP TO PROPOSITI	NUMBER AFFECTED	NUMBER NORMAL	TOTAL	EXPECTED RATIO	EXPECTED AFFECTED	DEGREE OF MANIFESTATION (per cent)
Parents	64	228	292	$\frac{1}{2}$	146	43·8
Grandparents	44	361	405	$\frac{1}{4}$	101·25	43·4
Aunts, uncles, nephews, nieces	100	864	964	$\frac{1}{4}$	241	41·5
Children	7	19	26	$\frac{1}{2}$	13	53·8
Siblings excluding propositi and sporadic families	75	250	325	$\frac{1}{2}$	162·5	46·1
Cousins	18	355	373	$\frac{1}{8}$	46·6	38·6
Totals	308				710·35	43·3

*From A. W. Morrison and S. E. Bundey, *J. Laryngol. Otol., 84*:921, 1970.

obstruction or by middle ear infection; these conditions can be diagnosed on otologic examination. Ankylosis of the stapediolabyrinthine joint, occurring in *osteogenesis imperfecta,* can be diagnosed on the basis of fragile bones, opalescent teeth, and blue scleras characteristic of this disease. Ankylosis or abnormalities of the middle ear bones are found in scores of disorders discussed in this text. McCabe (1966) has described an "otosclerotic inner ear syndrome" with associated vestibular findings.

TREATMENT

A hearing aid will help most patients with otosclerosis. In some cases, surgical therapy with stapedectomy may be carried out.

PROGNOSIS

The hearing loss is slowly progressive and is usually only moderate in degree. Pregnancy may accelerate the hearing loss.

SUMMARY

Characteristics of otosclerosis include: 1) autosomal dominant transmission with about 40 per cent penetrance, 2) gradual onset of hearing loss in the early decades of life, 3) slow progressive, conductive, or mixed symmetrical hearing loss of varying severity, and 4) normal vestibular response.

REFERENCES

Albrecht, W., Über die Vererbung der konstitutionell sporadischen Taubstummheit der hereditären Labyrinthschwerhörigkeit und der Otosclerose. *Arch. Ohr-, Nasen-, Kehlkopfheilk., 110*:15–48, 1923.

Bretlau, P., Otosclerosis. Electron microscopic studies of biopsies from the labyrinthine capsule. *Arch. Otolaryngol., 93*:551–562, 1971.

Brünner, S., Rovsing, H., and Jensen, J., Tomographic changes in otosclerosis. *Acta Radiol.* [Diagn.] *(Stockh.), 4*:632–638, 1966.

Chumlea, B. J., A pedigree of otosclerosis. *J. Hered., 33*:98–99, 1942.

Fowler, E. P., Otosclerosis in identical twins. A study of 40 pairs. *Arch. Otolaryngol., 83*:324–328, 1966.

Guild, S. R., Histologic otosclerosis. *Ann. Otol. Rhinol. Laryngol., 53*:246–267, 1944.

Gussen, R., The stapediovestibular joint: normal structure and pathogenesis of otosclerosis. *Acta Otolaryngol. (Stockh.), Suppl. 248*:1–38, 1969.

Hammerschlag, V., Zur Frage der Vererbbarkeit der Otosklerose. *Wien. Klin. Rdsch., 19*:5–7, 1905.

Jørgensen, M. B., and Kristensen, H. K., Frequency of histologic otosclerosis. *Ann. Otol. Rhinol. Laryngol., 76*:83–88, 1967.

Juers, A. L., Otosclerosis in identical twins. A review and report of two additional pairs. *Ann. Otol. Rhinol. Laryngol., 59*:205–214, 1950.

Kabat, C., A family history of deafness. *J. Hered., 34*:377–378, 1943.

Kapur, Y. P., and Patt, A. J., Otosclerosis in South India. *Acta Otolaryngol. (Stockh.), 61*:353–360, 1966.

Kelemen, G., and Linthicum, F. H., Labyrinthine otosclerosis. *Acta Otolaryngol. (Stockh.), Suppl. 253*:1–68, 1969.

Larsson, A., Otosclerosis, a genetic and clinical study. *Acta Otolaryngol. (Stockh.), Suppl. 154*:1–86, 1960.

Lindsay, J. R., Histopathology of otosclerosis. *Arch. Otolaryngol., 97*:24–29, 1973.

McCabe, B. F., Otosclerosis and vertigo. *Trans. Pac. Coast Otoophthalmol. Soc.,* 37–40, 1966.

Morrison, A. W., Genetic factors in otosclerosis. *Ann. R. Coll. Surg. Engl., 41*:202–237, 1967.

Morrison, A. W., and Bundey, S. E., The inheritance of otosclerosis. *J. Laryngol. Otol., 84*:921–932, 1970.

Myers, D., Wolfson, R., Tibbels, E., and Winchester, R., Apparent total deafness due to advanced otosclerosis. *Arch. Otolaryngol., 78*:52–58, 1963.

Nager, F. R., and Fraser, J. S., On bone formation in scala tympani of otosclerotics. *J. Laryngol. Otol., 53*:173–180, 1938.

Nager, G. T., Ein Paar weiblicher eineiiger Zwillinge mit klinisch sowie anatomisch konkordanter Otosklerose und ähnlichem Hörgewinn durch Fenestration. *Acta Otolaryngol. (Stockh.), 45*:42–58, 1955.

Pfändler, V., L'hérédité de l'otosclerose. *Schweiz. Med. Wschr., 79*:692–700, 1949.

Steinberg, D., and Neumann, O. G., Zur Genese der Otosclerose: eine Literatur Übersicht. *HNO, 21*:257–263, 1973.

Wolff, D., and Bellucci, R. J., Otosclerosis. Multiple manifestations of its basic pathology. *Arch. Otolaryngol., 79*:571–593, 1964.

RECESSIVE CONGENITAL SEVERE SENSORINEURAL DEAFNESS

Several studies have shown that a high percentage of congenital sporadic deafness is recessive in origin. Fraser (1965), adding his survey of 2300 children to the work of others, concluded that 38 per cent of profound childhood deafness is of autosomal recessive origin. Sank (1963), in a population survey and twin study of deaf residents of New York State, concluded that about 40 per cent of early total deafness is of autosomal recessive origin, whereas about 10 per cent is of dominant origin.

There is good evidence that several different recessive genes exist, each capable of producing this type of deafness.

CLINICAL FINDINGS

Auditory System. All persons studied who have this form of deafness have shown profound bilateral sensorineural hearing loss, although some affected persons have a minimal amount of residual hearing. Pure-tone audiograms show an 80 to 100 dB loss in all frequencies, with absent bone conduction. It is impossible to do other specialized audiometric tests, since too little residual hearing remains to carry out these tests. Examination of the external auditory canals and the tympanic membranes shows no abnormalities.

Vestibular System. Vestibular findings have been noted only among a few affected persons. In a study of two kindreds in Pennsylvania, Mengel *et al.* (1969) found vestibular function to be normal in 12 affected persons subjected to caloric vestibular tests. In another family personally studied, there was moderate to complete paresis of vestibular function. It is possible that this test may help to separate various types of recessive congenital deafness from others. Vestibular function was essentially normal in the kindred studied by McLeod *et al.* (1973).

Unfortunately, vestibular function is seldom evaluated in the congenitally deaf. Data concerning the frequency of vestibular disease, therefore, should be viewed with skepticism.

LABORATORY FINDINGS

Roentgenograms. No roentgenographic findings have been described.

PATHOLOGY

Pathologic changes involving the inner ear have been divided into five types and have been named for the author first describing these: Scheibe demonstrated a malformation limited to the epithelial structures of the pars inferior; Bing and Siebenmann described a normal bony labyrinth and immature development of the membranous parts of the inferior and superior labyrinth; Mondini-Alexander described a more severe abnormality with development of a single curved tube or shortened and flattened abnormal bony cochlea, sometimes associated with a dilated saccule and endolymphatic sac; Michel described temporal bones with a complete lack of development of the inner ear.

Although Altmann (1950, 1964) discussed the histopathologic changes in hereditary deafness in animals, he did not clarify the diagnosis in his four human cases. In three of the cases, there was no family history of deafness; in the fourth case, both parents and many other relatives were deaf.

Nager (1925) described the temporal bone findings in a 45-year-old congenitally deaf woman. Two of four of her sibs and two of four cousins were born deaf. Histologic examination of the patient's temporal bone revealed the Mondini type of change, with narrowing of the cochlear canal and endolymphatic sac and atrophy of the hair cells. There was atrophy of ganglion cells and nerve fibers, particularly in the basal turn of the cochlea.

Gray and Nelson (1926) reported the temporal bone findings in a 56-year-old deaf-mute. Although the patient's parents had normal hearing, one of his four brothers was born deaf. Examination of the temporal bones showed normal tympanic membranes and middle ears. The major pathologic changes included absence of the hair cells of the organ of Corti, collapse of Reissner's membrane, and a decrease in the number of spiral ganglion cells. The stria vascularis was atrophic in the apical turn but normal in the remaining two turns of the cochlea. Examination of the eighth nerve showed no abnormalities. The cochlear nuclei were also normal.

The temporal bone findings from one of the three congenitally deaf sibs from a sibship of nine, born of normal hearing parents, were described by Gulì and Bonetti (1956). The patient died at 64 years of age. Histologic examination of the temporal bones showed marked atrophy of the organ of Corti and stria vascularis in all turns of the cochlea. The cochlear ducts were small, with collapse of Reissner's membrane. There was moderate loss of spiral ganglion cells and nerve fibers.

HEREDITY

A large number of pedigrees have been presented showing recessive transmission of congenital severe sensorineural deafness (Albrecht, 1923; Undritz, 1928; Hopkins and Guilder, 1949; Stevenson and Cheeseman, 1955; Mengel et al., 1969). It is quite clear that several different genes may produce the same phenotype of congenital deafness. Mengel et al. (1969) studied the congenitally deaf persons in the Amish and Mennonite communities of Pennsylvania. Pedigree analysis showed that all 14 living deaf persons in the Amish isolate in Lancaster County could trace their ancestry through both parents to Christian Fischer, born in 1757. Pedigrees of affected persons in the Mennonite community could be traced to Jacob Kreytor, who died in 1742 or to Hans Weber, who died in 1730. In one case, an individual from the Mennonite group married a deaf person from the Amish kindred. Their three children had normal hearing. Since each pedigree exhibited autosomal recessive inheritance, the genes causing these two kinds of deafness must be at different genetic loci. Thus, they would be heterozygous for both types of deafness but phenotypically normal. Several other authors have presented pedigrees in which each of two deaf parents had autosomal recessive deafness. Children born of these unions had normal hearing (Mühlmann, 1930; Hammerschlag, 1934; Lehmann, 1950; and Stevenson and Cheeseman, 1956). Anderson and Wedenberg (1968) suggested that carriers could be detected by subtle audiometric changes, i.e., small but distinct dips in the middle-frequency range of the hearing threshold as well as abnormally high thresholds for the acoustically elicited stapedius reflex.

Several authors have addressed themselves to the question of the number of autosomal recessive genes involved in congenital deafness. Stevenson and Cheeseman (1956) found that in 12 matings of recessively deaf parents there were only five families in which all the children were deaf. The authors concluded that there are about six separate loci for recessive deaf-mutism. Fraser (1970), reviewing 3500 persons with profound hearing loss of early onset, estimated that the total number of such genes represented in his series was rather low (possibly four or five), but that one of these genes was relatively common. A similar estimate of six genes was made by Chung and Brown (1970).

EPIDEMIOLOGY

Lindenov (1945) found a range of 43 to 87 deaf-mutes per 100 thousand population in different countries. Autosomal recessive genes were responsible for a high percentage of this deaf-mutism. Sank (1963) in a population survey and twin study of deaf residents in New York State, concluded that about 40 per cent of all cases with early total deafness is of autosomal recessive origin. Fraser (1970) studied 2355 children in schools for the deaf and concluded that from 23 per cent to 30 per cent were deaf because of autosomal recessive inheritance.

DIAGNOSIS

In studying a child with congenital severe deafness, one should exclude the various causes of this type of hearing loss: meningitis, prenatal rubella, kernicterus, birth injury, administration of streptomycin or other ototoxic drugs, and viral infections such as measles and otitis media. A careful otologic examination and hearing history should be taken to evaluate these various possible causes of the hearing loss. A family history is also important, since frequently parents attribute hearing loss to infection or trauma although the true cause may be hereditary.

When it is determined that the congenital severe deafness is probably hereditary, a careful pedigree is necessary to determine whether transmission is autosomal recessive or dominant, or X-linked. A thorough physical and neurological examination should be done to search for other possible anomalies associated with the deafness that may help to define the disorder. To differen-

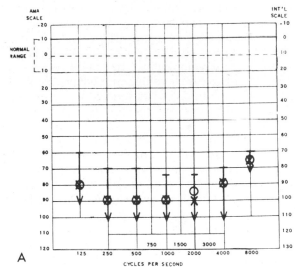

Figure 2–8   Recessive congenital severe sensorineural deafness. (*A*) Audiogram showing range of hearing loss in all affected persons tested. For proband, 0 = right ear, × = left ear.

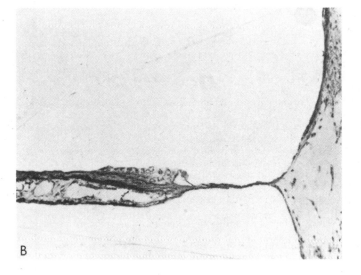

(*C*) Temporal bone section taken from patient with recessive congenital severe deafness. Section from basal turn of the cochlea showing atrophy of the stria vascularis and degeneration of the hair cells of the organ of Corti. (From E. Gulì and U. Bonetti, *Folia Hered. Pathol. (Milano),* 5:102, 1956.)

(*C*) Pedigree of Mennonite kindred with 12 congenitally deaf persons in eight generations. Arrow indicates proband. (*A, C* from M. C. Mengel *et al., EENT Monthly,* 48:301, 1969.)

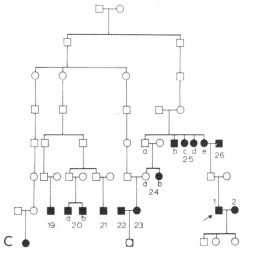

tiate congenital from *early-onset recessive sensorineural deafness*, it is helpful to take a careful history of the patient's development of speech, and to pay attention to the degree of development. In cases where speech began to develop and where some evidence of facility with speech is present, early-onset recessive sensorineural deafness is likely.

In all cases, it is important to do vestibular testing to determine the intactness of the vestibular apparatus, since this may help to define one or more of the types of recessive congenital severe sensorineural deafness.

TREATMENT

In the past, some congenitally deaf children have been sent to mental institutions. With the present day attention paid to diagnosis, this error should no longer occur. Affected persons usually have normal intelligence and can be trained in almost any type of work.

PROGNOSIS

Persons with congenital severe deafness who have no other abnormalities have a normal life span.

SUMMARY

Characteristics include: 1) autosomal recessive transmission, 2) congenital severe sensorineural hearing loss, and 3) normal vestibular function.

REFERENCES

Albrecht, W., Über die Vererbung der konstitutionell sporadischen Taubstummheit, der hereditären Labyrinthschwerhörigkeit und der Otosclerose. *Arch. Ohr-, Nasen-, Kehlkopfheilk., 110*:15–48, 1923.

Altmann, F., Histologic picture of inherited nerve deafness in man and animals. *Arch. Otolaryngol., 51*:852–890, 1950.

Altmann, F., The inner ear in genetically determined deafness. *Acta Otolaryngol. (Stockh.), Suppl.187*:1–39, 1964.

Anderson, H., and Wedenberg, E., Audiometric identification of normal hearing carriers of genes for deafness. *Acta Otolaryngol. (Stockh.), 65*:535–554, 1968.

Chung, C. S., and Brown, K. S., Family studies of early childhood deafness ascertained through the Clarke School for the Deaf. *Am. J. Hum. Genet., 22*:630–644, 1970.

Fraser, G. R., Sex-linked recessive congenital deafness and the excess of males in profound childhood deafness. *Ann. Hum. Genet., 29*:171–196, 1965.

Fraser, G. R., The causes of profound deafness in childhood. In *Sensorineural Hearing Loss.* Ciba Foundation Symposium, 1970, pp. 5–40.

Gray, A. A., and Nelson, S. H., The pathological conditions found in a case of deaf-mutism. *J. Laryngol., 41*:7–18, 1926.

Gulì, E., and Bonetti, U., Contributo allo studio dell' anatomia patòlogica del sordomutismo recessivo. *Folia Hered. Pathol. (Milano), 5*:102–150, 1956.

Hammerschlag, V., *Einführung in die Kenntnis einfacher Mendelistischer Vorgänge,* Vienna, Perles, 1934.

Hopkins, L. A., and Guilder, R. P., *Clarke School Studies Concerning the Hereditary Deafness.* Northampton, Mass., Edwards Brothers Inc., 1949.

Lehmann, W., Ein weiterer Beitrag zur Frage der Heterogenie der recessiven Taubstummheit. *Z. Menschl. Vererb. Konstit.-lehre, 29*:825–830, 1950.

Lindenov, H., *The Etiology of Deaf-mutism with Special References to Heredity.* Copenhagen, Munksgaard International Booksellers and Publishers, Ltd., 1945.

McLeod, A. C., Sweeney, A., McConnell, F., Kemker, F. J., Nance, W. E., and Webb, W. W., Autosomal recessive sensorineural deafness: a comparison of two kindreds. *South. Med. J., 66*:141–152, 1973.

Mengel, M. C., Konigsmark, B. W., and McKusick, V. A., Two types of congenital recessive deafness. *EENT Monthly, 48*:301–305, 1969.

Mühlmann, W. E., Ein ungewöhnlicher Stammbaum über Taubstummheit, *Arch. Rass. Ges. Biol., 22*:181–183, 1930.

Nager, F. R., Missbildungen der Schnecke und Hörvermögen. *Z. Hals-, Nasen-, Ohrenheilk., 11*:149–176, 1925.

Sank, D., The genetic aspects of early total deafness. In *Family and Mental Health Problems in a Deaf Population.* Ranier, J. D., Altschuler, K., and Kallmann, F. (eds.), New York, New York State Psychiatric Institute, 1963.

Stevenson, A. C., and Cheeseman, E. A., Hereditary deaf-mutism, with particular reference to northern Ireland. *Ann. Hum. Genet., 20*:177–231, 1956.

Undritz, W., Über die Bedeutung der Erbfaktoren bei verschiedenen oto-rhino-laryngologischen Erkrankungen. *Arch. Ohr-, Nasen-, Kehlkopfheilk., 119*:270–290, 1928.

RECESSIVE CONGENITAL MODERATE SENSORINEURAL HEARING LOSS

This disorder, characterized by congenital moderate nonprogressive sensorineural hearing loss, was found in two sibs in each of three sibships by Konigsmark, Mengel, and Haskins (1970). Additional sibships were contributed by Konigsmark (1971) and possibly by McLeod *et al.* (1973).

CLINICAL FINDINGS

Auditory System. Otologic examination showed normal auricles, external auditory canals, and tympanic membranes. By history, the hearing loss was noted in childhood, and all affected persons stated that there had been no progression of the loss. Follow-up audiograms were available on all cases for periods up to 16 years and showed no progression (Fig. 2–9*A*). The hearing loss in all cases was of moderate severity with a three-frequency average loss (500, 1000, 2000 Hz) of 30 to 50 dB. The hearing curves

were flat with minimal increase of hearing loss at higher frequencies. There was no air–bone gap. SISI tests were positive and tone-decay tests were negative, suggesting cochlear involvement.

Vestibular System. Caloric vestibular tests performed in five of six affected persons were normal.

LABORATORY FINDINGS

No laboratory tests were carried out.

PATHOLOGY

No histopathologic study of the temporal bones was carried out.

HEREDITY

In each of the three families, the remaining sibs and parents had normal hearing,

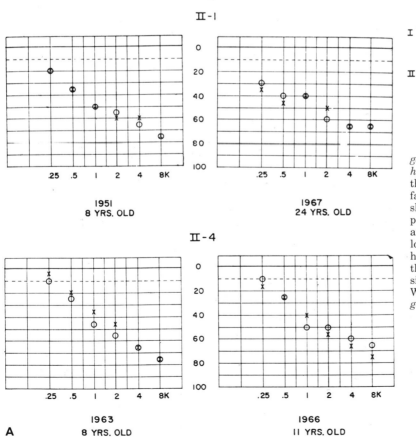

Figure 2–9 Recessive congenital moderate sensorineural hearing loss. (A) Audiograms of the two affected persons in one family. The upper audiograms show hearing loss over a 16-year period in one child; the lower audiograms show the hearing loss over a three-year period in her sib. (B) Pedigree showing the two affected persons among six sibs in one family. (From B. W. Konigsmark et al., J. Laryngol. Otol., 84:495, 1970.)

with the exception of one family in which the mother had otosclerosis (Fig. 2–9*B*). The involvement of two sibs with a quite similar sensorineural nonprogressive hearing loss in each of the sibships suggests that the deafness has autosomal recessive transmission.

DIAGNOSIS

Diseases, such as prenatal rubella, which cause congenital moderate sensorineural hearing loss should first be excluded. Recessive nonprogressive sensorineural hearing loss can be distinguished from *recessive early-onset sensorineural deafness* by a much more severe hearing loss in the latter disorder. When this nonprogressive hearing loss is sporadic, diagnosis is difficult. A careful family history that indicates either parental consanguinity or another affected person in the kindred could aid in the diagnosis.

SUMMARY

This form is characterized by: 1) autosomal recessive transmission, 2) congenital symmetrical nonprogressive moderate sensorineural hearing loss, which is more marked in higher frequencies, and 3) normal vestibular function.

REFERENCES

Konigsmark, B. W., Mengel, M. C., and Haskins, H., Familial congenital moderate neural hearing loss. *J. Laryngol., 84*:495–505, 1970.

Konigsmark, B. W., Congenital nonprogressive moderate neural hearing loss. *Birth Defects, 7*(4):140, 1971.

McLeod, A. C., Sweeney, A., McConnell, F. E., Kemker, J., Nance, W. E., and Webb, W. W., Autosomal recessive sensorineural deafness: a comparison of two kindreds. *South. Med. J., 66*:141–152, 1973.

RECESSIVE EARLY-ONSET SENSORINEURAL DEAFNESS

Early childhood onset of severe sensorineural hearing loss has been described in several kindreds (Barr and Wedenberg, 1964; Mengel *et al.*, 1967).

CLINICAL FINDINGS

Auditory System. Mengel, Konigsmark, Berlin, and McKusick (1967) studied ten affected persons in a Mennonite family. Each individual was found to have had at least some hearing at birth, responding to sounds and at times learning to articulate a few words. Progressive hearing loss developed rather rapidly between the ages of 1½ to 6 years, with severe hearing loss occurring in all affected persons by about 6 years of age. One child was able to attend a public school for several years before hearing loss forced her to transfer to a school for the deaf. Audiograms on the ten available affected family members showed a severe sensorineural hearing loss of 60 to 100 dB in all frequencies. Two individuals had a positive SISI score (90 to 100 per cent) bilaterally, suggesting cochlear origin of the hearing loss.

To document that there was some early hearing, Mengel *et al.* tested the speech of two affected persons. Their sonograms were compared with those made from a normal hearing person and from a congenitally deaf person (Fig. 2–10*B*). Sonograms from the congenitally deaf speaker, who had been trained in an oral school, showed absence of high frequencies and marked temporal elongation of speech, as compared with the normal control. Sonograms from the two persons with early-onset sensorineural deafness showed an intermediate type of speech pattern, much closer to normal than that of the congenitally deaf person. Skilled judges were also asked to evaluate the voice tape recordings to determine whether they thought that the subjects were essentially deaf since birth or previously had had some hearing. They judged that both patients must have had good low-tone hearing at least until their fifth to seventh year of life.

In the family presented by Barr and Wedenberg, four of seven sibs had hearing impairments. On admission to a school for the deaf, it was stated that they had a small degree of hearing and some speech. Their parents and other members of the family had normal hearing.

Vestibular System. Caloric vestibular tests done on affected persons in the Mennonite family showed a normal vestibular response.

LABORATORY FINDINGS

Roentgenograms. A tomogram done on the proband in the Mennonite family showed no temporal bone abnormality.

PATHOLOGY

No histopathologic findings were described.

HEREDITY

Sixteen members of the family reported by Mengel *et al.* were affected in three generations (Fig. 2–10*C*), males and females being equally involved. Although irregular dominant inheritance is possible, the proband's parents as well as the previous generations of the family were known to have essentially normal hearing. The pedigree is most compatible with autosomal recessive transmission. This mode of inheritance is also most probable for the four affected sibs in the family described by Barr and Wedenberg.

DIAGNOSIS

A detailed early history to determine whether the patient had any evidence of hearing loss in infancy and early childhood is essential for separating this disorder from the congenital forms of severe hearing loss. In later years, a sonogram or speech analysis may help in differential diagnosis by indicating that patients learned some speech during early infancy.

This disorder must also be differentiated from *X-linked sensorineural* forms of *deafness*. In the latter disorders, males are affected via transmission through their mothers.

TREATMENT

Although the hearing loss becomes quite severe at a very early age, during early childhood while hearing still remains the use of hearing aids would be quite beneficial for the child.

PROGNOSIS

The hearing loss is rapid in onset and profound, with essentially no hearing after 5 to 6 years of age.

SUMMARY

Characteristics of this form include: 1) autosomal recessive transmission, 2) early-onset severe sensorineural hearing loss with essentially no hearing after 5 to 6 years of age, and 3) normal vestibular function.

REFERENCES

Barr, B., and Wedenberg, E., Prognosis of perceptive hearing loss in children with respect to genesis and use of hearing aid. *Acta Otolaryngol. (Stockh.), 59*:462–474, 1964.

Mengel, M. C., Konigsmark, B. W., Berlin, C. I., and McKusick, V. A., Recessive early-onset neural deafness. *Acta Otolaryngol. (Stockh.), 64*:313–326, 1967.

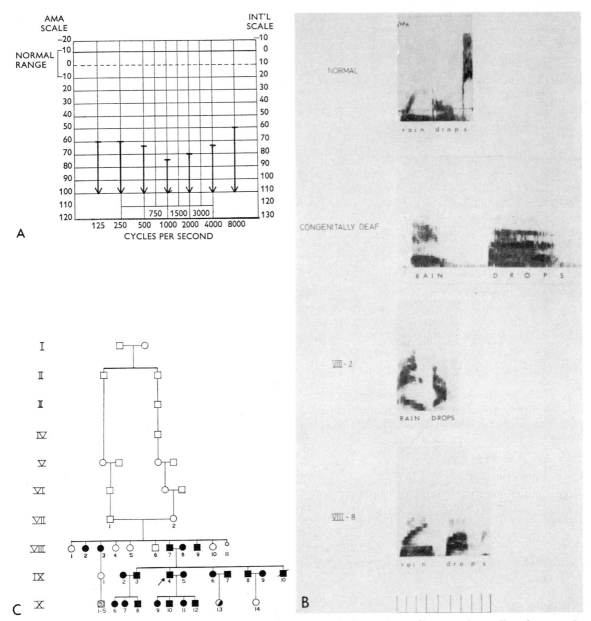

Figure 2–10 *Recessive early-onset sensorineural deafness. (A)* Composite audiogram of ten affected persons in a Mennonite kindred showing bilateral severe sensorineural hearing loss. *(B)* Sonograms on the same time base showing almost normal word duration in two affected persons (lower two sonograms) compared to prolonged duration of words in a congenitally deaf person. *(C)* Pedigree showing ten generations of a Mennonite family with 16 affected individuals in three generations. *(A, B,* and *C* from M. C. Mengel *et al., Acta Otolaryngol. (Stockh.), 64*:313, 1967.)

X-LINKED CONGENITAL SENSORINEURAL DEAFNESS

X-linked congenital hearing loss has been described in several families (Dow and Poynter, 1930; Mitsuda *et al.*, 1952; Sataloff *et al.*, 1955; Parker, 1955; Deraemaker, 1958; Richards, 1963; Fraser, 1965; McRae *et al.*, 1969). In each of these families, congenitally deaf males were found in several generations. These males were born of normal hearing mothers who often had deaf brothers.

CLINICAL FINDINGS

Auditory System. Audiograms on affected persons showed a 70 to 100 dB sensorineural hearing loss involving all frequencies (Fig. 2–11*A*). Because of the severity of the hearing loss, other audiometric tests could not be done. No abnormalities of pinnae, external auditory canals, or ear drums have been described.

Vestibular System. Vestibular tests have not been described.

Nervous System. In general, the intelligence of affected persons has been normal. However, two patients described in the family by Parker had marked to moderate mental retardation. The remaining affected persons had normal intelligence. The proband in the family described by McRae *et al.* had dull normal intelligence. Tests were not done on the remaining six affected men, but the clinical impression was that they were of normal intellect. Two of three affected persons in the family described by Deraemaker had severe mental deficiency, whereas the third had only mild mental retardation.

LABORATORY FINDINGS

Roentgenograms. No roentgenographic studies have been reported.

PATHOLOGY

No histopathologic study of the temporal bone has been noted.

HEREDITY

Each of the kindreds shows X-linked recessive transmission of the hearing loss. In the family described by Dow and Poynter there were nine deaf males in four generations. Sataloff *et al.* studied four generations of a family in which six males were deaf-mutes. All had normal mothers. In Deraemaker's kindred there were three deaf-mute male children in three generations. Parker presented a family with 14 affected members in three generations. Fraser reported several families showing X-linked transmission of congenital deafness. In the kindred described by Richards there were six deaf-mute males in three generations.

Whether all these cases represent the same disorder or whether there are several types of X-linked recessive congenital deafness cannot be stated at present.

Blood group tests were carried out on the family described by McRae *et al.* The Xg blood group results suggested that the gene locus is not closely linked to Xg.

INCIDENCE

Fraser (1965), studying about 2750 cases of profound childhood deafness, concluded that about 6.2 per cent of male patients had X-linked recessive deafness.

DIAGNOSIS

Other forms of X-linked deafness must be excluded. Causes of congenital deafness such as prenatal rubella, ototoxicity, hyperbilirubinemia, or congenital defects must be excluded. A careful family history must be obtained, since the disorder may be transmitted through several generations of unaffected females; if families have been small, there may have been no hemizygous affected males.

TREATMENT

The hearing loss is quite severe, precluding the use of hearing aids in treatment.

PROGNOSIS

Affected persons have no physical abnormalities other than the hearing loss; occasionally they show mental deficiency.

SUMMARY

Characteristics of this form of hearing loss include: 1) X-linked mode of transmission, 2) mental deficiency in some cases, 3) congenital severe sensorineural hearing loss, and 4) normal vestibular function.

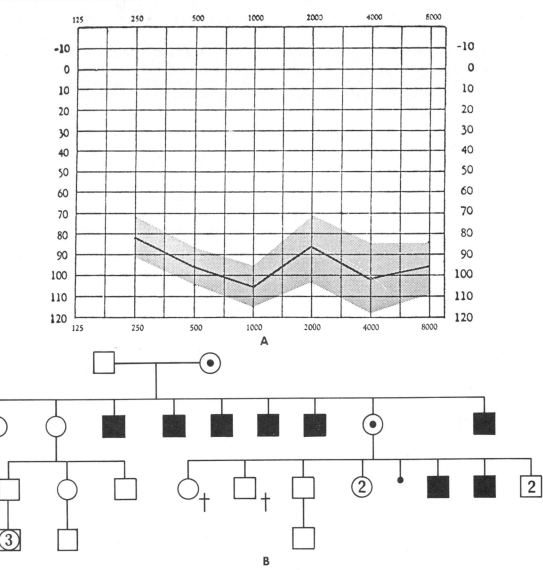

Figure 2–11 X-linked congenital sensorineural deafness. (A) Composite audiogram of affected males in kindred showing severe congenital sensorineural hearing loss. All had rudimentary speech development. (From N. Parker, *Am. J. Hum. Genet.*, 7:201, 1955.) (B) Pedigree of family showing eight affected males in two generations. (From K. N. McRae *et al., Am. J. Hum. Genet.,* 21:415, 1969.)

REFERENCES

Deraemaeker, R., Sex-linked congenital deafness. *Acta Genet. (Basel)*, 8:228–231, 1958.
Dow, G. S., and Poynter, C. I., The Dar family. *Eugen. News,* 15:128–130, 1930.
Fraser, G. R., Sex-linked recessive congenital deafness and the excess of males in profound childhood deafness. *Ann. Hum. Genet.*, 29:171–196, 1965.
McRae, K. N., Uchida, I. A., and Lewis, M., Sex-linked congenital deafness. *Am. J. Hum. Genet.,* 21:415–422, 1969.
Mitsuda, H., Inoue, S., and Kazama, Y., Eine Familie mit rezessiv-geschlechtsgebundener Taub-stummheit. *Jap. J. Genet.,* 27:142–147, 1952.
Parker, N., Congenital deafness due to a sex-linked hereditary deafness. *Amer. J. Hum. Genet.,* 7:201–203, 1955.
Richards, B. W., Sex-linked deaf-mutism. *Ann. Hum. Genet.,* 26:195–199, 1963.
Sataloff, J., Pastore, P. N., and Bloom, E., Sex-linked hereditary deafness. *Amer. J. Hum. Genet.,* 7:201–203, 1955.

X-LINKED EARLY-ONSET SENSORINEURAL DEAFNESS

X-linked early-onset sensorineural hearing loss was described by Mohr and Mageroy in 1960. All affected persons in this family had some hearing in early childhood, having developed speech in the early years. However, hearing loss limited further speech development in later childhood.

CLINICAL FINDINGS

Auditory System. The 11-year-old proband learned to speak, although somewhat loudly. At about 3 years of age, there was a decline in speech intelligibility until it was quite difficult to understand him at 12 years of age. Audiometric tests were not described. His 12-year-old cousin had similar difficulties learning to speak until 3 or 4 years of age when regression of speech and hearing were noted. Other affected persons in this pedigree also began speaking, but their capacity to speak deteriorated during childhood. One boy who was tested audiometrically when he was 13 years old showed a hearing loss of 80 dB or more in all frequencies.

Vestibular System. Vestibular tests were not described.

Other Findings. The proband had divergent strabismus and mild myopia. Intelligence was probably normal.

LABORATORY FINDINGS

Roentgenograms. Examination of the temporal bone and cranium showed normal structure.

Other Examinations. Electroencephalographic studies showed no abnormalities. Urine analysis and cerebrospinal fluid were normal.

PATHOLOGY

No histopathologic studies have been described.

HEREDITY

The pedigree shows only males affected in four generations of this kindred (Fig. 2–12). Transmission appears to be X-linked.

This disorder may be the same as *X-linked congenital sensorineural deafness*. However, two differences suggest that this is a different entity. Speech in all persons affected with X-linked congenital deafness has been undeveloped. In contrast, persons affected with X-linked early-onset sensorineural deafness showed evidence of progression of hearing loss at a very early age, after beginning speech was learned and before school age was reached. Thus, it seems reasonable to distinguish this type of hearing loss from the congenital severe and probably nonprogressive hearing loss described in other families.

DIAGNOSIS

The causes of childhood deafness such as meningitis, viral infection, and syphilis should be ruled out. A careful history to determine whether there is any evidence of progression of hearing loss in childhood is important in separating *X-linked congenital sensorineural deafness*, which is nonprogressive, from X-linked early-onset neural deafness, which shows progression in childhood.

TREATMENT

Treatment should be instituted by giving hearing aids to the very young child who might have available hearing. This must be instituted before the deafness is too marked for treatment.

PROGNOSIS

Individuals have progressive hearing loss.

SUMMARY

Characteristics of this type of hearing loss include: 1) X-linked transmission, and 2) moderate sensorineural loss in early childhood with essentially complete loss of hearing by school age.

REFERENCE

Mohr, J., and Mageroy, K., Sex-linked deafness of a possibly new type. *Acta Genet. (Basel)*, *10*:54–62, 1960.

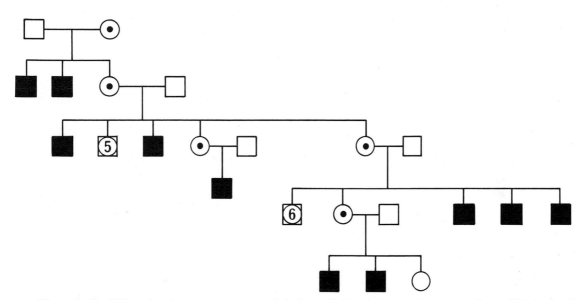

Figure 2–12 *X-linked early-onset sensorineural deafness.* Pedigree showing four generations of kindred with 10 persons affected by progressive hearing loss. (Adapted from J. Mohr and K. Mageroy, *Acta Genet. (Basel), 10*:54, 1960.)

X-LINKED MODERATE SENSORINEURAL HEARING LOSS

Livan (1961) described a kindred with slowly progressive moderately severe sensorineural hearing loss. Pelletier and Tanguay (1975) reported a somewhat similarly affected family.

CLINICAL FINDINGS

Auditory System. In four of five boys in the sibship reported by Livan (1961), hearing loss was first noted at 10 years of age and was slowly progressive. Audiograms done at 17 to 34 years of age showed a marked high-frequency hearing loss with normal hearing in low frequencies.

In the kindred of Pelletier and Tanguay (1975) there were eight affected males in four generations. Onset occurred around adolescence and did not progress beyond moderate impairment. SISI and tone-decay tests indicated cochlear pathology. Test results for retrocochlear pathology were negative.

Vestibular System. Caloric vestibular tests were normal.

LABORATORY FINDINGS

None were noted.

PATHOLOGY

No pathologic studies were described.

HEREDITY

The disorder, seen in four generations, was limited to males and was transmitted by female carriers, thus exhibiting an X-linked pattern.

DIAGNOSIS

There are several forms of X-linked deafness differing in onset (congenital, early-onset, etc.), type (sensorineural, mixed), and occurring with and without associated anomalies, which are discussed in this text.

TREATMENT

Hearing aids may be employed.

PROGNOSIS

The deafness is progressive.

SUMMARY

Characteristics of this form of deafness include: 1) X-linked inheritance, 2) adolescent onset of a slowly progressive moderate sensorineural hearing loss, and 3) normal vestibular responses.

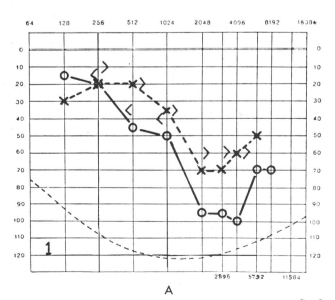

A

See legend on the opposite page

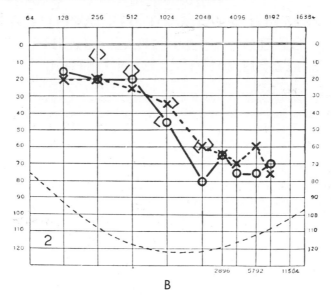

B

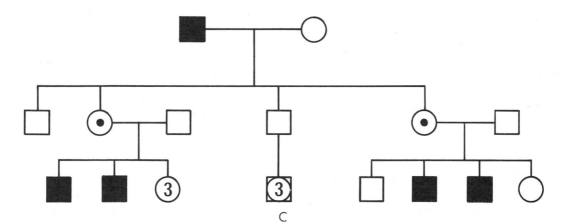

C

Figure 2–13 *X-linked moderate sensorineural hearing loss. (A, B)* Characteristic audiograms of two male sibs with X-linked moderate sensorineural hearing loss. (From A. Livan, *Arch. Ital. Otol.,* 72:331, 1961.) *(C)* Pedigree of family exhibiting X-linked moderate sensorineural hearing loss. (Redrawn from data contained in A. Livan, *Arch. Ital. Otol.,* 72:331, 1961.)

REFERENCES

Livan, M., Contributo alla conoscenza delle sordità ereditarie. *Arch. Ital. Otol.,* 72:331–339, 1961.
Pelletier, L. P., and Tanguay, R. B., X-linked recessive inheritance of sensorineural hearing loss expressed during adolescence. *Am. J. Hum. Genet.,* 27:609–613, 1975.

X-LINKED MIXED HEARING LOSS WITH CONGENITAL FIXATION OF THE STAPEDIAL FOOTPLATE AND PERILYMPHATIC GUSHER

This disorder is characterized by severe mixed hearing loss with vestibular abnormalities and X-linked inheritance (Nance *et al.*, 1971). A perilymphatic gusher usually occurs when stapedectomy is attempted. Other examples and families have been reported (Sooy, 1960; Shea, 1963; Ombrédanne, 1964; Wolferman, 1964; Fraser, 1965; Shine and Watson, 1968; Farrior and Endicott, 1971; Thorpe *et al.*, 1974; Nance and Sweeney, 1975).

CLINICAL FINDINGS

Auditory System. Audiometric testing was done on six affected males and five heterozygotic female carriers (Nance *et al.*, 1970). Affected males showed a 60 to 100 dB pure-tone hearing loss involving all frequencies (Fig. 2–14*A*). There was little change with age, with patients ranging in age from 3 to 51 years. Bone conduction showed a symmetrical 20 to 60 dB hearing loss. The mean speech reception threshold (SRT) in affected males was 83 dB. SISI, speech discrimination, and Békésy audiometric tests could not be done because of the severity of hearing loss.

Heterozygotic females had a variable mixed hearing loss, more marked in the lower frequencies (Fig. 2–14*A*). Pure-tone testing showed a 0 to 70 dB hearing loss, whereas bone conduction tests showed about half this degree of hearing deficit. SISI tests were positive in the low frequencies, suggesting cochlear involvement.

Exploratory tympanotomy of a 51-year-old affected male disclosed congenital fixation of the stapes with absence of the annular rim of the footplate. Clear fluid, presumably perilymph, welled into the middle ear when stapedectomy was attempted; when the procedure was terminated, there was no improvement (Nance *et al.*, 1971).

Impedance audiometry showed a variable degree of fixation of the stapedial footplate (Nance and Sweeney, 1975).

Vestibular System. Vestibular abnormalities were found in four of the five males tested. The abnormalities included absent or abnormal caloric responses or abnormality in Romberg testing (Nance *et al.*, 1971).

Nervous System. No other neurologic abnormalities were found. Psychologic testing, done on nine family members (affected males, heterozygous females, and normal members) showed normal intelligence in all.

LABORATORY FINDINGS

Roentgenograms. No roentgenographic findings were described.

Other Studies. Two patients received extensive clinical studies. No abnormalities were found in urinary or serum electrolytes, or in thyroid, liver, or renal tests. Electroencephalograms, electrocardiograms, and intravenous pyelograms were normal.

PATHOLOGY

Perilymphatic gusher was originally thought to be due to abnormal patency of the cochlear aqueduct (Rice and Waggoner, 1967), but recent evidence suggests that there is an abnormal communication between the internal auditory canal and the inner ear vestibule (Glasscock, 1973).

HEREDITY

Nance *et al.* (1971) suggested that this form is rather prevalent and may account for 0.5 per cent of profound childhood deafness. This figure is based on case reports of congenital fixation of the stapes with associated perilymphatic gusher but without family history. In several cases, a partial family history was given. Maternal half-brothers with congenital fixation of the stapes and perilymphatic gusher were described (Olson and Lehman, 1968).

Affected persons in the families described by Olson and Lehman (1968), Nance *et al.* (1971), and Thorpe *et al.* (1974) showed X-linked transmission of this disorder (Fig. 2–14*B*).

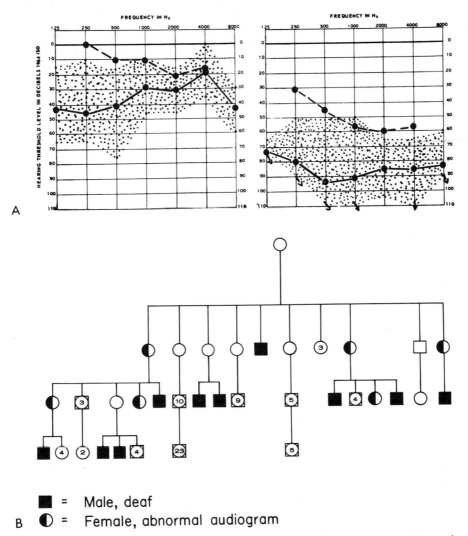

= Male, deaf

B ◑ = Female, abnormal audiogram

Figure 2-14 *X-linked mixed hearing loss with congenital fixation of the stapedial footplate and perilymphatic gusher.* (*A*) Audiograms showing comparison of average air and bone conduction thresholds in the ears of four carrier females (left) and six affected males (right). Stippled area indicates range of air conduction thresholds. (*B*) Modified pedigree showing X-linked inheritance. (*A,B* from W. E. Nance *et al., Birth Defects,* 7(4):64, 1971.)

DIAGNOSIS

There are several types of X-linked hearing loss: *X-linked pigmentary abnormalities and congenital sensorineural deafness, Norrie syndrome, Hunter syndrome,* etc. These can be differentiated from the X-linked mixed hearing loss with congenital fixation of the stapedial footplate and perilymphatic gusher because of their striking associated abnormalities. The other X-linked forms of deafness discussed in this chapter differ because of their age of onset, severity, normal vestibular function, and normal stapedial footplate.

TREATMENT

Affected persons can be helped with hearing aids. In the future, surgical procedures may be developed that will allow freeing of the stapes footplate; at present, this procedure is not practical. Attempts at surgical correction have currently been disappointing.

PROGNOSIS

There is little evidence that the hearing loss is progressive; study of patients over a longer period of time will be necessary for this to be determined. A vestibular defect was found in the four oldest of five patients tested. Although the deafness may be progressive, further tests are necessary to confirm this.

SUMMARY

The major characteristics of this disorder include: 1) X-linked transmission, 2) congenital fixation of the stapedial footplate, 3) perilymphatic gusher, 4) moderate to severe mixed hearing loss, and 5) vestibular hypofunction.

REFERENCES

Farrior, J. B., and Endicott, J. N., Congenital mixed deafness: cerebrospinal fluid otorrhea. Ablation of the aqueduct of the cochlea. *Laryngoscope, 81*:684–699, 1971.

Fraser, G. R., Sex-linked recessive congenital deafness and the excess of males in profound childhood deafness. *Ann. Hum. Genet., 29*:171–196, 1965.

Glasscock, M. E., The stapes gusher. *Arch. Otolaryngol, 98*:82–91, 1973.

Mossum, S. R., Personal communication, cited by Edwards, W. F.: Congenital middle ear deafness with anomalies of the face. *J. Laryngol., 78*:152–170, 1964.

Nance, W. E., Setleff, R. C., McLeod, A., Sweeney, A., Cooper, C., and McConnell, F., X-linked mixed deafness with congenital fixation of the stapedial footplate and perilymphatic gusher. *Birth Defects, 7*(4):64–69, 1971.

Nance, W. E., and Sweeney, A., Genetic factors in deafness of early life. *Otolaryngol. Clin. North Am., 8*:19–48, 1975.

Nance, W. E., Sweeney, A., McLeod, A. C., and Cooper, M. C., Hereditary deafness: a presentation of some recognized types, modes of inheritance, and aids in counseling. *South Med. Bull., 58*:41–49, 1970.

Olson, N. R., and Lehman, R. H., Cerebrospinal fluid otorrhea and the congenitally fixed stapes. *Laryngoscope, 78*:352–359, 1968.

Ombrédanne, M., Chirurgie des "aplasies mineures." Ses résults dans les grandes surdités congénitales par malformations ossiculaires. *Ann. Otolaryngol. (Paris), 81*:201–221, 1964.

Rice, W. J., and Waggoner, L. G., Congenital cerebrospinal fluid otorrhea via a defect in the stapes footplate. *Laryngoscope, 77*:341–349, 1967.

Shea, J. J., Jr., Complications of the stapedectomy operation. *Ann. Otol. Rhinol. Laryngol., 72*:1109–1123, 1963.

Shine, I., and Watson, J. R., A new syndrome of sex-linked congenital conductive deafness. Unpublished report, 1968.

Sooy, F. A., The management of middle ear lesions simulating otosclerosis. *Ann. Otol. Rhinol. Laryngol., 69*:540–558, 1960 (Case 3).

Thorpe, P., Sellars, S., and Beighton, P., X-linked deafness in a South African kindred. *S. Afr. Med. J., 48*:587–590, 1974.

Wolferman, A., Cerebrospinal otorrhea: a complication of stapes surgery. *Laryngoscope, 74*:1368–1379, 1964.

HEREDITARY MENIERE SYNDROME

Although most cases of Meniere syndrome are sporadic, persons affected with episodic vertigo and sensorineural hearing loss have been described in several kindreds (Brown, 1949; Bernstein, 1965).

CLINICAL FINDINGS

Auditory System. The 46-year-old proband reported by Brown (1945) had tinnitus in one ear for two years. There were recurrent episodes of vertigo and vomiting over the next two years. She had bilateral sensorineural hearing loss, more marked on one side. Her 32-year-old sister had similar episodes of vertigo and was found to have sensorineural hearing loss. A 35-year-old brother also experienced some tinnitus and episodes of vertigo. There was no history of hearing loss in their parents or in the parents' sibs.

In Family No. 4 of Bernstein (1965) the 25-year-old daughter had had mild attacks of vertigo and fluctuating hearing loss in one ear for two years. An audiogram showed mild high-tone loss, and vestibular tests exhibited hypofunction on one side. The mother and maternal aunt had a similar history of episodic vertigo and hearing loss. In Family No. 5 the 56-year-old male proband had a single episode of vertigo with nausea and vomiting followed by progressive hearing loss in one ear over a 20-year period. Hearing in the other ear began deteriorating at the age of 50 years. The audiogram showed severe hearing loss on one side and moderate hearing loss on the other. There was bilateral vestibular paresis. The patient's mother had a history of hearing loss with tinnitus and episodes of unsteadiness. A father and son were affected in Family No. 6. Over an eight-year period, the 34-year-old son had about 12 episodes of severe vertigo, tinnitus, and falling. An audiogram showed moderate sensorineural hearing loss in the right ear and a right vestibular paresis. The left ear was normal. The 70-year-old father had three severe episodes of vertigo over a period of 10 years. Hearing became progressively worse.

Headache. Both Brown and Bernstein noted a high incidence of migraine headaches in patients or family members. Brown described two brothers with an eight-year history of progressive sensorineural hearing loss and attacks of vertigo. One brother and the mother had migraine. The hearing status of the mother was not reported. In Family No. 2 described by Bernstein, 59- and 60-year-old sibs had a 20- and 10-year history of episodic vertigo and mild hearing loss. The 59-year-old proband, his father, and two paternal uncles had migraine headaches. In Family No. 3, a 50-year-old female had recurrent episodes of vertigo. There was no hearing loss, but caloric tests showed a right vestibular paresis. Two sisters had recurrent severe unilateral headaches. The son of the proband's oldest sister had a two-year history of episodic vertigo and hearing loss (it was not clear if this sister had vertigo). An audiogram showed moderate left-sided sensorineural hearing loss. Vestibular tests were normal. In Family No. 7, two sisters had recurrent episodes of vertigo, tinnitus, and mild hearing loss. One had mild hearing loss, the other, moderate hearing loss; both had unilateral vestibular paresis. One sister had severe right-sided headaches. The father had had unilateral hearing loss without vertigo for many years as well as recurrent unilateral headaches.

Vestibular System. Results were variable, as noted above.

HEREDITY

Brown (1949) described two sibships having this disorder. Two sisters and a brother, products of a first-cousin mating, as well as two maternal cousins were affected. Identical 47-year-old male twins with tinnitus and progressive bilateral sensorineural hearing loss beginning at about 30 years of age were also described by Brown. No further family history was noted.

Dominant transmission was suggested by several kindreds described by Bernstein (1965). His Family No. 4 consisted of affected female identical twins and the daughter of one twin.

DIAGNOSIS

True Meniere disease must be ruled out.

TREATMENT

Unfortunately, none of the descriptions have included clear definitions of the signs. Thus, it is difficult to confirm that these are truly migraine headaches. Relief by ergotamine has not been mentioned. It is quite possible that these headaches are not true migrainous but are only severe unilateral headaches, possibly related in some ways to the vestibular disease.

PROGNOSIS

The hearing loss has been progressive in most cases.

SUMMARY

From these studies it appears likely that there is a type of hereditary deafness associated with vestibular abnormalities resulting, in some cases, in vertiginous attacks. One type of hearing loss appears to be recessively transmitted, whereas another is dominantly transmitted and may be associated with unilateral severe headaches.

REFERENCES

Bernstein, J. M., Occurrence of episodic vertigo and hearing loss in families. *Ann. Otol. Rhinol. Laryngol.*, *74*:1011–1021, 1965.
Brown, M. R., The factor of heredity in labyrinthine deafness and paroxysmal vertigo. *Ann. Otol. Rhinol. Laryngol.*, *58*:665–670, 1949.

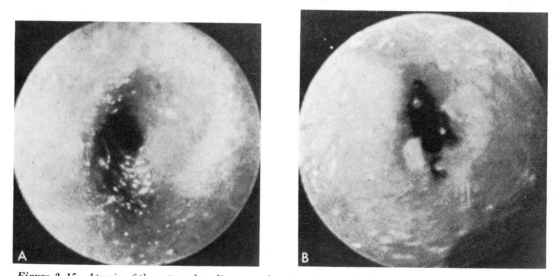

Figure 2–15   *Atresia of the external auditory canal and conduction deafness. (A, B)* Bilateral 2 to 3 mm. wide bony stenosis of external auditory canals. (From E. Hefter and H. Ganz, *HNO, 17*:76, 1969.)

ATRESIA OF THE EXTERNAL AUDITORY CANAL AND CONDUCTION DEAFNESS

Hefter and Ganz (1969) briefly described the combination of meatal atresia and conduction deafness in a mother and in three of her four children.

CLINICAL FINDINGS

Auditory Findings. There was such marked bony stenosis of the external auditory meatus that the eardrum was not visible.

Conduction deafness ranged in the various members from 10 to 60 dB. Some sibs exhibited mixed deafness.

LABORATORY FINDINGS

Roentgenograms. Roentgenographic examination of the mastoid processes showed them to be poorly pneumatized in most of the affected.

PATHOLOGY

Surgical examination showed the incus and malleus to be eroded and the stapes and tympanic membrane to be missing. The medial wall of the middle ear was covered with metaplastic epithelium and the floor of the middle ear was fused into a conglomerate mass. In another member of the family, the entire middle ear cavity was missing.

HEREDITY

The disorder appears to be inherited as a dominant trait.

DIAGNOSIS

The disorder appears to be unique.

TREATMENT

Surgical correction is possible in the less severely affected. A hearing aid may help.

PROGNOSIS

The more severe the bony meatal atresia, the poorer the surgical results.

SUMMARY

Characteristics include: 1) autosomal dominant inheritance, 2) meatal atresia, and 3) deafness, largely conductive.

REFERENCE

Hefter, E., and Ganz, H., Bericht über vererbte Gehörgangsmissbildungen. *HNO, 17:*76–78, 1969.

48

MISCELLANEOUS SYNDROMES

We have had occasion to examine a brother and sister, neither of whom had had a history of ear infections or injury. There were two normal sibs; the parents were nonconsanguineous.

Both manifested a moderate conduction deafness most severe in the 2000 to 8000 Hz range. The deafness was first noted when the patients were 10 to 12 years of age.

Tympanotomy revealed absence of the stapedial crura and a malformed incus. Both sibs had fixation of the footplate of the stapes. In one, there was no incudostapedial joint.

Inheritance of the deafness is presumably autosomal recessive.

Chapter 3

GENETIC HEARING LOSS WITH EXTERNAL EAR ABNORMALITIES

The external ear changes make these ten hereditary deafness syndromes easier to diagnose than those with no associated abnormalities. Seven of these syndromes are transmitted in an autosomal dominant and three in an autosomal recessive manner. In some, the hearing loss is congenital, in others, the loss is slowly progressive. The external ear abnormalities range from large prominent auricles to normal auricles (with preauricular pits or branchial fistulas) to anotia. Kleinfeldt and Dahl (1971) noted the frequent association of pinnal abnormalities with autosomal dominant sensorineural deafness, but they did not attempt to delineate further various entities within the group. The reader is referred to excellent general references for pinnal abnormalities (Lange, 1961).

REFERENCES

Kleinfeldt, D., and Dahl, D., Gehäuftes Auftreten von Veränderungen der Ohrmuscheln im Verbindung mit Gehörlosigkeit. *HNO, 19*:273–274, 1971.

Lange, G., Familienuntersuchungen über die Erblichkeit metrischer und morphologischer Merkmale des äusseren Ohres. *Z. Morphol. Anthropol., 57*:111–167, 1961.

OTOFACIOCERVICAL SYNDROME

A family having a syndrome with abnormalities of the external ear, face, and neck was described by Fára, Chlupáčková, and Hrivnáková (1967). Those affected were a father and four of his seven children.

CLINICAL FINDINGS

Physical Findings. The sunken nose root and narrow nose set in an elongated face were striking (Fig. 3–1A). The palate was highly arched and the mandible was somewhat small (Fig. 3–1C). The auricles were prominent and had large conchae. Preauricular fistulas were present just in front of the helix (Fig. 3–1A, B). In most cases, lateral cervical fistulas were also present.

The neck appeared long and the shoulders and clavicles sloped downward markedly. The scapulae were located more laterally than normal and showed mild winging (Fig. 3–1A). The neck musculature was weak, accounting for the lowered shoulders. All affected persons were short in stature.

Nervous System. There was a mild to moderate hyporeflexia, more marked in the arms. All those affected showed mild intellectual deficit.

Auditory System. Otologic examination revealed somewhat atrophic and irregularly thickened tympanic membranes. Audiometric tests done on four affected persons showed 60 to 70 dB bilateral conductive hearing losses, most marked in the low and high frequencies. A hearing loss of 40 to 50 dB was noted in the middle frequencies.

Vestibular System. Vestibular findings were not described.

LABORATORY FINDINGS

Roentgenograms. Roentgenograms were similar in all affected members. The skull showed narrowing in the middle-third of the face. The sella turcica was deep with a slanting clivus. There was a marked difference in the level of the orbital roof and the cribiform plate. The temporal pyramids were asymmetric with poor mastoid pneumatization (Fig. 3–1D). Roentgenograms of the carpal bones showed moderately retarded bone age in three children. The clavicles sloped obliquely downward (Fig. 3–1E).

Other Findings. Complete blood counts, urinalyses, and serum nonprotein nitrogen and cholesterol levels were normal. ^{131}I tests exhibited normal uptake. Dermatoglyphic abnormalities consisted of increased "atd" angles and an increased frequency of ulnar loops with central pockets.

Agenesis of one kidney was found in one of the four affected persons.

PATHOLOGY

No histopathologic findings were presented.

HEREDITY

The syndrome was observed in a father and in four of his seven children. The father stated that his mother showed similar facial and shoulder anomalies. However, she was not available for examination. The syndrome appears to be transmitted by an autosomal dominant gene having complete penetrance.

DIAGNOSIS

This syndrome, with its characteristic facies, sloping shoulders, auricular abnormalities, and hearing loss is unique. The other syndromes discussed in this section do not exhibit the facial or shoulder abnormalities found in this disorder.

TREATMENT

The conductive hearing loss can be minimized by a hearing aid. Tympanotomy with insertion of a prosthesis should be helpful. Surgical treatment includes excision of the fistulas and repair of the deformed ears.

PROGNOSIS

The hearing loss in each of the affected persons was noted in childhood. It is not clear whether the deafness was congenital or whether it progressed with age.

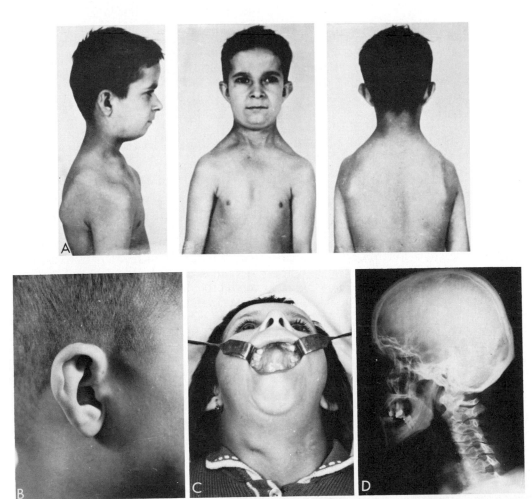

Figure 3-1 *Otofaciocervical syndrome.*
(A) Three views showing sloping shoulders and abnormal position of clavicles and scapulae. (B) Prominent ears, Darwinian tubercle, and fistula at insertion of helix. (C) Highly arched palate; right cervical fistula was present; left cervical fistula had been removed surgically. (D) Lateral view of father's skull showing vertical elongation of head, deep sella turcica, steep clivus, low sphenoid bone, and poor mastoid pneumatization. (E) Radiograph showing depressed position of the shoulders. The clavicles are at the level of the third rib, their outer ends running obliquely downward. The scapulae project at the level of the axillae. (From M. Fára *et al., Acta Chir. Plast. (Praha),* 9:255, 1967.)

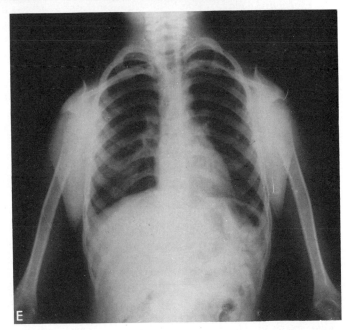

SUMMARY

The syndrome is characterized by: 1) autosomal dominant inheritance, 2) prominent auricles with deep conchae, 3) preauricular pits and lateral neck fistulas, 4) hypoplasia of the maxillozygomatic complex, 5) hypoplasia and weakness of cervical muscles, resulting in lowered shoulder girdle, 6) characteristic roentgenographic abnormalities, and 9) moderate to severe conductive hearing loss.

REFERENCE

Fára, M., Chlupáčková, V., and Hrivnáková, J., Dismorphia oto-facio-cervicalis familiaris. *Acta Chir. Plast.*, 9:255–268, 1967.

EAR MALFORMATIONS, CERVICAL FISTULAS OR NODULES, AND MIXED HEARING LOSS

A syndrome characterized by deformed auricles, preauricular appendages and/or pits, cervical fistulas or nodules, and hearing loss has been described in several kindreds (Hall and Zimmer, 1958; Martins, 1961; Wildervanck, 1962; McLaurin, Kloepfer, Laguaite, and Stallcup, 1966; Bourguet, Mazéas, and Lehuerou, 1966; Rowley, 1969; Shenoi, 1972; Henrot, Aladenine, and Inghel, 1972; Bailleul, Libersa, and Laude, 1972; Karmody and Feingold, 1974; Hunter, 1974; Melnick, Bixler, Silk, Yune, and Nance, 1975; Fitch, Lindsay, and Srolovitz, 1975.)

CLINICAL FINDINGS

External Ear. The ear deformities may be unilateral or bilateral—one ear usually being much more severely affected than the other. In mildly affected ears, the helix is usually thickened and the auricle is somewhat small. In the case of more severely affected ears, the entire auricle is thickened and quite small, alterations being more marked in the dorsal portion of the helix (Fig. 3–2A). Unilateral or bilateral preauricular pits have been present in about 75 per cent of affected persons (Fig. 3–2B). A few patients had a preauricular appendage (Fig. 3–2C) or atresia of the external auditory canal. One patient had low implantation of a malformed auricle (Wildervanck, 1962).

Auditory System. The hearing loss in these cases was variable, sometimes being more marked in the lower frequencies and ranging from 20 to 100 dB in severity. Usually, the hearing loss was somewhat more marked on the side with the more severely deformed auricle or external auditory canal. Five of seven patients studied by McLaurin *et al.* had unilateral or bilateral conductive hearing loss; one had bilateral sensorineural hearing loss; one had normal hearing. Only two patients in the family studied by Wildervanck had hearing loss—conductive, in both cases. Of seven patients tested by Bourguet *et al.* four had conductive hearing loss, two had sensorineural deafness, and one had mixed hearing loss. Conductive deafness was found in one individual and mixed hearing loss in five persons studied by Rowley. Speech discrimination varied from 34 per cent to 100 per cent in cases studied by McLaurin *et al.* Of ten patients in a kindred studied by Shenoi (1972) four had preauricular pits, three had deformed auricles, two had mixed deafness, and one had neural deafness. The deafness was first noted at puberty. Polytomography showed small cochleas (Karmody and Feingold, 1974). Melnick *et al.* (1975) reported stapes fixation and Mondini type of cochlear defect in their kindred. Fitch *et al.* found reduced numbers of cochlear neurons and degeneration of the stria vascularis.

Vestibular System. No vestibular findings were described.

Other Findings. Most patients have bilateral symmetrical cervical fistulas or nodules located anterior to the sternocleidomastoid muscle (Fig. 3–2D, E). Bourguet *et al.* (1966) noted facial paralysis in several of their affected patients, an observation also made by Hall and Zimmer (1958). Martins (1961), Melnick *et al.* (1975), and Fitch *et al.* (1975) found bilateral renal dysplasia and/or anomalies of the collecting system. Since this is a "silent component," it is conceivable that it has frequent associa-

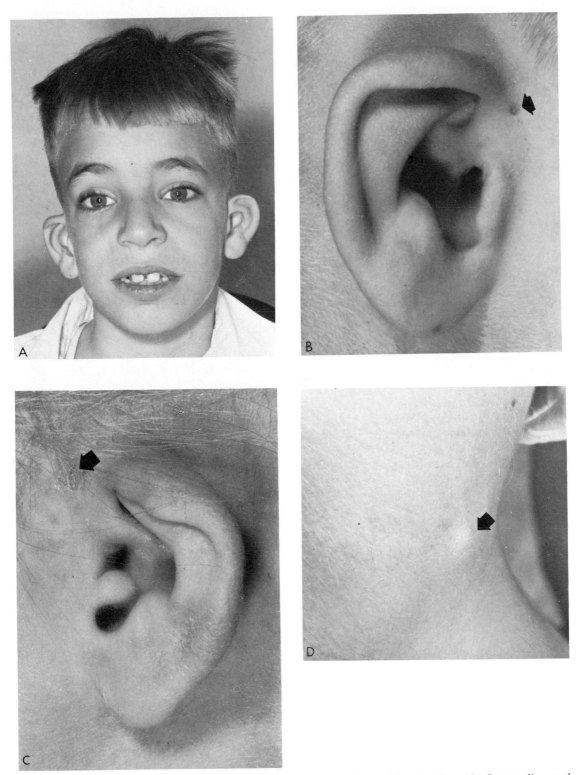

Figure 3–2 *Ear malformations, cervical fistulas or nodules, and mixed hearing loss. (A)* Outstanding malformed pinnae. *(B)* Preauricular pit, marked by arrow. *(C)* Auricular appendage, grossly malformed auricle and
preauricular pit. *(D)* Nodule anterior to sternocleidomastoid muscle.

Illustration continued on page 55

tion and should be looked for in other kindreds. An asthenic habitus and aplasia of the lacrimal ducts have also been reported (Melnick et al., 1975).

LABORATORY FINDINGS

No laboratory findings were noted.

PATHOLOGY

With one boy having a severe conduction hearing loss, explorations of the middle ear revealed similar changes bilaterally (McLaurin et al., 1966). The lenticular process of the incus was shortened, not reaching the head of the stapes. In a three-generation kindred studied by one of the authors (R.J.G.), one child had fixation of the footplate of the stapes and an enlarged, distorted, misplaced incus. Hall and Zimmer (1958) demonstrated rudimentary ossicles via tomography. Shenoi (1972) described a small malleus and incus, fusion of the incus and stapes, and absence of the oval window.

HEREDITY

All pedigrees have shown autosomal dominant transmission of this syndrome (Fig. 3–2F).

The origin of the auricular deformity is not clear. Since the auricle develops from mesenchymal hillocks near the margin of the first branchial groove, it would seem that the dominant gene responsible for this syndrome is involved with the organization of structures related to the first branchial groove and pouch.

DIAGNOSIS

This syndrome most closely resembles that of *preauricular pits, branchial fistulas, and sensorineural hearing loss,* differing only in that mixed or conductive loss is present in the syndrome considered here. They may, in fact, be identical, but whether they are cannot be answered at this time.

Malformed auricles have been described sporadically. These cases differ from the present syndrome in that there is no evidence of dominant transmission or hearing loss. Several families have been described with congenital dominantly transmitted cup-shaped deformity of the pinnae without associated hearing loss (Hanhart, 1949; Erich and Abu-Jamra, 1965; Kessler et al., 1971). Pretragal pits may also occur in an isolated case or in association with several syndromes discussed in this or in other chapters.

An isolated case of a girl with prominent ears, sensorineural deafness, slitlike ear canals, absent breasts, and chronic renal disease was described by Tawil and Najjar (1968). The deafness involved primarily the high frequencies.

TREATMENT

Plastic surgery may be considered for correction of auricular deformities, preauricular appendages, and cervical fistulas or nodules (Hall and Zimmer, 1958). Middle-ear exploration with possible insertion of a prosthesis should be considered where the conductive hearing loss is severe.

PROGNOSIS

The hearing loss in this syndrome is congenital with no evidence of progression.

SUMMARY

Characteristics of this syndrome include: 1) autosomal dominant transmission with variable expressivity, 2) unilateral or bilateral auricular deformities in 75 per cent of cases, 3) preauricular pits in about 75 per cent of cases, 4) unilateral or bilateral cervical fistulas in 50 per cent, 5) preauricular appendages in about 5 per cent, 6) atresia of the external auditory meatus in about 5 per cent, and 7) conductive or mixed hearing loss in about 50 per cent.

REFERENCES

Bailleul, J. P., Libersa, C., and Laude, M., Surdité et fistules auriculaires congénitales familiales. *Pédiatrie,* 27:739–747, 1972.

Bourguet, J., Mazéas, R., and Lehuerou, Y., De l'atteinte des deux premières fentes et des deux premiers arcs branchiaux. *Ann. Otolaryngol. (Paris),* 83:317–328, 1966.

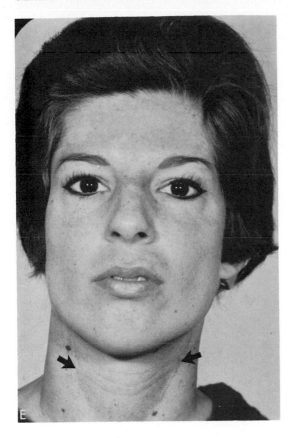

F

Figure 3-2 Continued (E) Patient in whom bilateral cervical fistulas had been surgically removed. (From P. T. Rowley, *Pediatrics, 44*:978, 1969.) *(F)* Pedigree of family exhibiting autosomal dominance and seen by one of the authors (R. J. G.). Members of kindred had variable expressivity of the syndrome.

Erich, J. B., and Abu-Jamra, F. N., Congenital cup-shaped deformity of the ears transmitted through four generations. *Mayo Clin. Proc., 40*:597–602, 1965.

Fitch, N., Lindsay, J., and Srolovitz, H., The temporal bone in the preauricular pit, cervical fistula syndrome. *Birth Defects,* in press.

Hall, J. G., and Zimmer, J., Congenital preauricular communicating fistulas: diagnosis, complications, and treatment. *Acta Otolaryngol. (Stockh.), 49*:213–220, 1958.

Hanhart, E., Nachweis, einer einfach-dominaten unkomplizierten sowie einer unregelmässigdominanten, mit Atresia auris, Palatoschisis, und anderen Deformationen verbundenen Anlage zu Ohrmuschelverkümmerung (Mikrotie). *Arch. J. Klaus Stift., 24*:374–398, 1949.

Henrot, H., Aladenine, J., and Inghel, J., Une surdité familiale de transmission. *Ann. Otolaryngol. (Paris), 89*:176–180, 1972.

Hunter, A. G. W., Inheritance of branchial sinuses and preauricular fistulae. *Teratology, 9*:225–228, 1974.

Karmody, C. S., and Feingold, M., Autosomal dominant first and second branchial arch syndrome: a new inherited syndrome? *Birth Defects, 10*(7):31–40, 1974.

Kessler, L., Wittwer, B., Rolfs, B., and Thomas, D., Klinish-genetisch Aspekte zum Missbildungsmuster der Mikrotien. *Z. Laryngol. Rhinol. Otol., 50*:234–242, 1971.

Martins, A. G., Lateral cervical and preauricular sinuses. *Br. Med. J., 1*:255–256, 1961.

McLaurin, J. W., Kloepfer, H. W., Laguaite, J. K., and Stallcup, T. A., Hereditary branchial anomalies and associated hearing impairment. *Laryngoscope, 76*:1277–1288, 1966.

Melnick, M., Bixler, D., Nance, W. E., Silk, K., and Yune, H., Familial branchio-oto-renal dysplasia. A new addition to the branchial arch syndromes. *Clin. Genet., 9*:25–34, 1976.

Peterson, D. M., and Schimke, R. N., Hereditary cup-shaped ears and the Pierre Robin syndrome. *J. Med. Genet., 5*:52–55, 1968.

Rowley, P. T., Familial hearing loss associated with branchial fistulas. *Pediatrics, 44*:978–985, 1969.

Shenoi, P. M., Wildervanck's syndrome. Hereditary malformations of the ear in three generations. *J. Laryngol. Otol., 86*:1121–1135, 1972.

Tawil, H. M., and Najjar, S. S., Congenital absence of the breasts. *J. Pediatr., 73*:751–753, 1968.

Wildervanck, L. S., Hereditary malformations of the ear in three generations. *Acta Otolaryngol., 54*:553–560, 1962.

Wirth, G., Aurikularanhänge auf dominanten Erbgrundlage. *Z. Laryngol. Rhinol. Otol., 41*:656–659, 1962.

PREAURICULAR PITS, BRANCHIAL FISTULAS, AND SENSORINEURAL HEARING LOSS

A syndrome that includes preauricular pits, sensorineural hearing loss, and branchial fistulas in 21 members of a family was studied by Fourman and Fourman in 1955. Of those affected, 17 had unilateral or bilateral branchial fistulas. A similar kindred was described by Brusis (1974).

CLINICAL FINDINGS

Ears. Affected persons had several types of ear anomalies, including small pits at the anterior margin of the helix on one or both sides in 17 persons (Fig. 3–3A), bilateral discharging branchial fistulas in one person, and a cartilaginous nodule at the lower end of the sternocleidomastoid muscle (Fourman and Fourman, 1955).

Auditory System. About 90 per cent of the affected persons had some hearing loss (Fourman and Fourman, 1955). Audiometric testing was performed in 17 affected family members, including 14 with preauricular pits and three without pits. Of the 14 persons with preauricular pits, 13 manifested mild to severe sensorineural hearing loss, and one was normal. Of the three persons without preauricular pits, two had hearing loss, one of whom had a branchial pit. The hearing of both low and high frequencies was involved, but hearing loss was more marked in the high frequencies. Hearing loss in those without preauricular pits was the same as in those with pits. Other audiometric tests were not described.

Although a few of those patients with hearing loss thought that it had been present from childhood, most stated that their hearing did not begin to deteriorate until they were about 20 years of age.

Vestibular System. Although Fourman and Fourman (1955) stated that there was no evidence of a vestibular disorder, the tests employed were not described. Brusis (1974), on the other hand, reported vestibular disturbances in his kindred.

LABORATORY FINDINGS

No laboratory findings were described.

PATHOLOGY

No histopathologic findings were presented.

HEREDITY

Affected persons were found in four generations of a family. In each generation transmission was from an affected parent to about half the children (Fig. 3–3B), the pedigree suggesting autosomal dominant transmission.

Although the preauricular pits probably represent persistence of the dorsal end of the first branchial groove, it is difficult to correlate the hearing loss to this first arch anomaly. The preauricular pits, branchial fistulas, and inner ear hearing loss probably are pleiotropic effects of a single dominant gene.

DIAGNOSIS

Preauricular pits are a rather common congenital anomaly, being seen in about 1 to 5 per cent of the white population (Ewing, 1946; Schachter, 1949; Gualandrini, 1969). The pits are bilateral in about one third of the cases. No associated hearing loss has been described in these cases. Přecechtěl (1927) reported a kindred with pretragal pits, cervical fistulas, and deafness, but he did not describe the type of hearing loss. Preauricular and branchial pits may also occur as isolated autosomal dominant anomalies (Pritchard, 1908; Schüller, 1929; Wheeler *et al.*, 1958; Böhme, 1960; Gundermann, 1965). The syndrome of *ear malformations, cervical fistulas or nodules, and mixed hearing loss* generally shows external ear abnormalities; some affected persons, however, have only preauricular pits. Furthermore, the hearing loss is conductive or mixed, in contrast to the sensorineural hearing loss observed in this syndrome. However, because of variable expressivity, it may represent the same entity. An isolated case of pretragal nodules, heterochromia iridis, branchial nodules, and sensorineural deafness was reported by Robinson and Wright (1968).

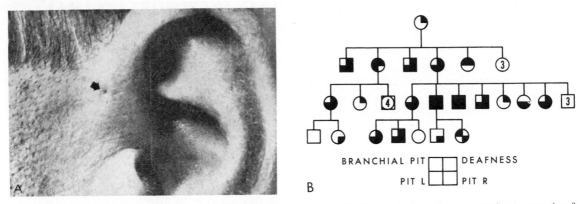

Figure 3–3 *Preauricular pits and sensorineural hearing loss. (A)* Preauricular pit just anterior to margin of helix. *(B)* Modified pedigree of family, described by Fourman and Fourman, with preauricular pits, branchial pits, and hearing loss. (*A* and *B* from P. Fourman and J. Fourman, *Br. Med. J., 2*:1354, 1955.)

TREATMENT

Since preauricular pits generally cause no difficulty, no treatment is necessary. When discharging branchial fistulas exist, surgical incision may be required (Murray, 1973). A hearing aid may be of use.

PROGNOSIS

Apparently the hearing loss is progressive, although this has not been documented.

SUMMARY

Characteristics of this syndrome include: 1) autosomal dominant transmission with variable expressivity, 2) unilateral or bilateral preauricular pits in about 85 per cent of affected persons, 3) unilateral or bilateral branchial fistulas in about 20 per cent of the patients, and 4) mild to severe progressive sensorineural hearing loss with onset in the first or second decade in about 90 per cent of affected persons.

REFERENCES

Böhme, G., Über einen Fall von bilateralen symmetrischen Ohr-Hals-Fisteln mit Heredität über vier Generationen. *HNO, 8*:359–360, 1960.

Brusis, T., Gleichzeitiges Vorkommen von degenerativer Innenohrschwerhörigkeit, Vestibularisstörung, beiderseitigen Ohr-und lateralen Halsfisteln bei mehreren Mitgliedern einer Familie. *Laryngol. Rhinol. Otol. (Stuttg.), 53*:131–139, 1974.

Ewing, M. R., Congenital sinuses of the external ear. *J. Laryngol. Otol., 61*:18–23, 1946.

Fourman, P., and Fourman, J., Hereditary deafness in a family with ear pits (fistulas auris congenita). *Br. Med. J., 2*:1354–1356, 1955.

Gualandrini, V., Ricerche genetiche sulla fistula auris congenita. *Acta Genet. Med. (Roma), 18*:51–68, 1969.

Gundermann, H., Die mediane und laterale Halsfisteln und-zysten in der Differentialdiagnostik der Halslymphknotenerkrankungen. *Z. Laryngol. Rhinol. Otol., 44*:174–180, 1965.

Murray, D. S., Marsupialization of preauricular sinuses. *Br. J. Plast. Surg., 26*:186–187, 1973.

Pritchard, E., Case of symmetrical bilateral helical fistulae, unilateral branchial fistula, and preauricular tubercle. *Proc. R. Soc. Med., 2*:227–228, 1908.

Přecechtěl, A., Pedigree of anomalies in the first and second branchial cleft. *Acta Otolaryngol. (Stockh.), 11*:23–30, 1927.

Robinson, G. C., and Wright, V. J., Sensorineural hearing loss and congenital heterochromia iridum. *Am. J. Dis. Child., 116*:106–109, 1968.

Schachter, M., Recherches sur les fossettes para-auriculaires, ou fistules auriculaires congénitales (fist. auris cong.). *Schweiz. Med. Wochenschr., 79*:343–345, 1949.

Schüller, J., Zur Vererbung der Fistula auris bzw. auriculae congenita. *Münch. Med. Wochenschr., 76*:160–162, 1929.

Wheeler, C. E., Shaw, R. F., and Cawley, E. P., Branchial anomalies in three generations of one family. *Arch. Dermatol., 77*:715–719, 1958.

THICKENED EAR LOBES AND INCUDOSTAPEDIAL ABNORMALITIES

A syndrome of hereditary conductive deafness characterized by thickened ear lobes and congenitally abnormal incudostapedial joints was described by Escher and Hirt (1968). A mother and two affected sons were reported by Wilmot (1970).

CLINICAL FINDINGS

External Ear. Thirteen of 14 affected persons had hypertrophic and thickened ear lobes (Fig. 3–4*A*). The rest of the auricle was normal in size and shape (Escher and Hirt, 1968). In the family described by Wilmot (1970), the changes in the pinnae were less marked.

Auditory System. Twelve of the affected persons reported by Escher and Hirt showed conductive hearing loss on audiometric testing. The severity of the hearing loss was not described, and other audiometric tests were not presented. The hearing loss was noted at an early age and was probably congenital. A 40 to 60 dB conductive loss was documented by Wilmot.

Vestibular System. No vestibular findings were described.

LABORATORY FINDINGS

No laboratory findings were reported.

PATHOLOGY

Bilateral tympanotomies were performed on one patient and unilateral tympanotomy on another by Escher and Hirt. The ossicular changes were very similar in each of the three ears observed. The malleus was normal; the long crus of the incus was curved into a long hook; the head of the stapes was absent (Fig. 3–4*B*). In each case, a fibrous band connected these two ossicles (Fig. 3–4*C*). The ossicular chain was restored, resulting in marked hearing improvement, but no documentation was presented to confirm this change. In Wilmot's family, tympanotomy in the mother showed a shortened long process of the incus. The stapes was mobile but headless and rotated with both crura imbedded in the promontory. Changes in the sons were similar to those observed in the mother. In one son the footplate was fixed.

HEREDITY

Both pedigrees showed dominant transmission of the syndrome.

It is interesting that although the major portion of the incus arises from the first visceral arch, the long crus arises from the second arch (Hanson *et al.*, 1962). During the sixth to seventh week of fetal life the joint between the incus and stapes dissolves, with a secondary reunion developing about the twenty-third week of gestation. It thus appears that the dominant gene causing this abnormality is related to the proper development of this joint during embryogenesis. Wilmot suggested that the anomaly developed prior to the sixth week of fetal development. Deafness has been reported in association with absence of the long process of the incus (White, 1964).

DIAGNOSIS

The external ear abnormality in this syndrome is only mild, in marked contrast to the moderate and severe auricular deformities seen in other syndromes described in this section. Some patients with this syndrome may have no external ear abnormality. The moderately severe conductive hearing loss differs from *otosclerosis* in that the syndrome is congenital and apparently nonprogressive. The definitive diagnosis requires examination of middle ear structures.

TREATMENT

Patients with the syndrome can benefit from tympanotomy with correction of the defect by a prosthesis or by restoration of the ossicular chain. The hearing loss is apparently congenital and nonprogressive.

PROGNOSIS

Prognosis is excellent. The cosmetic defect is minimal, and the deafness may be corrected.

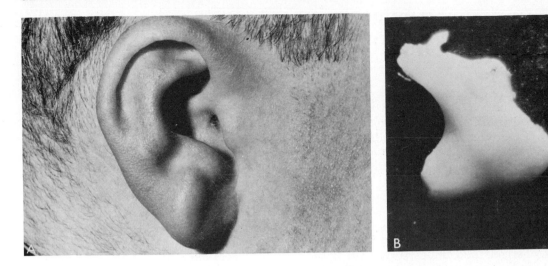

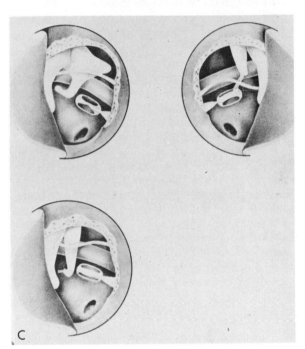

Figure 3–4 Thickened ear lobes and incudo-stapedial abnormalities. (A) Thickened ear lobe. (B) Incus with hook on distal end. (C) Diagram of three surgically treated ears showing missing connection between incus and stapes. (A, B, and C from F. Escher and H. Hirt, Acta Otolaryngol., 65:25, 1968.)

SUMMARY

The syndrome is characterized by: 1) autosomal dominant transmission with complete penetrance, 2) hypertrophic ear lobes in most cases, and 3) congenital conductive hearing loss due to malformation of the incudostapedial junction.

REFERENCES

Escher, F., and Hirt, H., Dominant hereditary conductive deafness through lack of incus-stapes junction. *Acta Otolaryngol. (Stockh.)*, 65:25–32, 1968.

Hanson, J. R., Anson, B. H., and Stickland, E. M., Branchial sources of the auditory ossicles in man. *Arch. Otolaryngol.*, 75:200, 1962.

Hough, J. V. D., Congenital malformations of the middle ear. *Proc. R. Soc. Med.*, 57:1145–1146, 1964.

White, J. W., Conductive deafness due to congenital absence of the long process of the incus. *Clin. Proc. Wash. D.C. Child. Hosp.*, 20:283–288, 1964.

Wilmot, T. J., Hereditary conductive deafness due to incus-stapes abnormalities and associated with pinna deformity. *J. Laryngol. Otol.*, 84:469–479, 1970.

LOP EARS, IMPERFORATE ANUS, TRIPHALANGEAL THUMBS, AND SENSORINEURAL DEAFNESS

Townes and Brocks (1972) described a family in which the father and five of his seven children displayed a syndrome of sensorineural deafness, satyr ears, imperforate anus, triphalangeal thumbs, and various other bony anomalies of the hands and feet.

CLINICAL FINDINGS

Physical Findings. All but one of the affected persons had imperforate anus with rectovaginal or rectoperitoneal fistula. In one child, the defect was limited to imperforate anus.

The skeletal anomalies were variable. All had pes planus. Three children had triphalangeal thumbs (Fig. 3–5E). In two of these children the thumb was bifid; in one child there were supernumerary thumbs. The father and three children had bilateral clinodactyly of the fifth toe.

Auditory System. All affected persons had folding of the superior helix (lop or satyr ears) (Fig. 3–5A, B, C). Auditory testing in the father and in three of the five affected children showed mild to moderate sensorineural deafness. The decibel loss was not specified. The other two children were not tested.

Vestibular System. No mention was made of vestibular testing.

LABORATORY FINDINGS

Roentgenograms. In addition to the skeletal changes noted above, pseudoepiphyses of the second metacarpals were observed in two children. Absent triquetrals were noted in two of the kindred. Short or fused metatarsals were found in the father and in two children (Fig. 3–5F).

PATHOLOGY

No histopathologic findings were presented.

HEREDITY

The syndrome has autosomal dominant inheritance with variable expressivity.

DIAGNOSIS

Imperforate anus as an isolated anomaly has been inherited as an X-linked recessive (Weinstein, 1965), autosomal recessive (van Gelder and Kloepfer, 1961; Cozzi and Wilkinson, 1968), or autosomal dominant trait (Kaijser and Malmstrom-Groth, 1957; Cozzi and Wilkinson, 1968). Imperforate anus may be part of a complex (VATER) association of vertebral defects, tracheoesophageal fistulas with esophageal atresia, and radial and renal defects (Quan and Smith, 1973).

Triphalangeal and/or bifid thumb may be inherited as a dominant isolated trait (Swanson and Brown, 1962) or in association with the Holt-Oram syndrome (Holmes, 1965) or the Blackfan-Diamond syndrome (Minagi and Steinbach, 1966). Aase and Smith (1961) described a combination of congenital anemia and triphalangeal thumbs as an autosomal recessive syndrome. Triphalangeal thumbs have also been reported in association with deafness (see Chap. 5).

TREATMENT

The lop ears and anorectal anomalies may be treated surgically.

PROGNOSIS

The hearing loss appears very early in life and is probably congenital. There is no evidence to suggest that it is progressive. The skeletal anomalies are in part correctible orthopedically.

SUMMARY

The syndrome is characterized by: 1) autosomal dominant inheritance with variable expressivity, 2) satyr ears, 3) imperforate anus with rectovaginal or rectoperitoneal fistula, 4) triphalangeal thumbs and various other bony anomalies, and 5) sensorineural deafness.

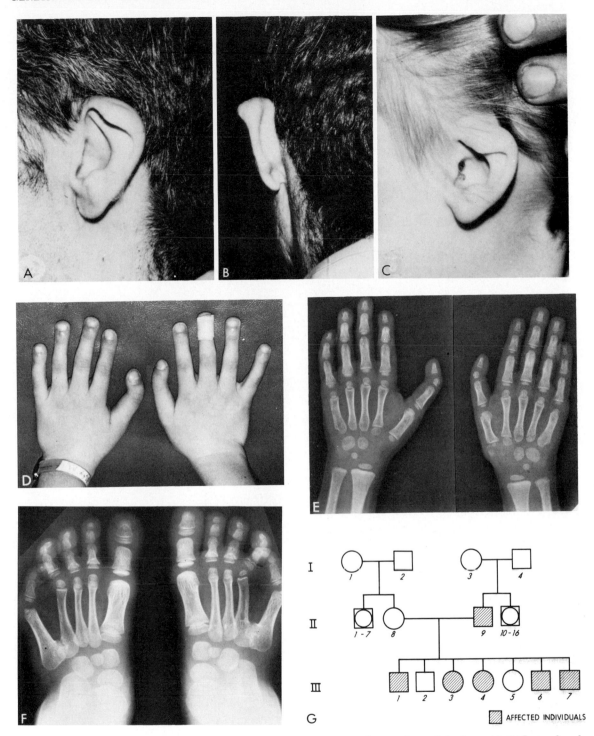

AFFECTED INDIVIDUALS

Figure 3–5   *Lop ears, imperforate anus, triphalangeal thumbs, and sensorineural deafness. (A, B)* Lateral and posterior view of father (II-9) showing satyr form of lop-ear deformity. *(C)* Lateral view of III-6 presenting similar abnormality. *(D)* Deviation of distal phalanges of thumbs. *(E)* Note triphalangeal thumbs. Supernumerary thumbs had been surgically excised. Note accessory carpal bone, and absence of triquetral bones. *(F)* Radiograph of feet of III-3. Note lateral displacement and fusion of proximal ends of fourth and fifth metatarsals. Also observe cone-shaped epiphyses at proximal end of first metatarsals and at proximal phalanges of second and third toes. *(G)* Pedigree showing autosomal dominant inheritance. *(A–G from P. L. Townes and E. R. Brocks, J. Pediatr., 81:321, 1972.)*

REFERENCES

Aase, J., and Smith, D. W., Congenital anemia and triphalangeal thumbs. *J. Pediatr.*, 74:471–474, 1961.

Cozzi, F., and Wilkinson, A. W., Familial incidence of congenital anorectal anomalies. *Surgery*, 64:669–671, 1968.

Holmes, L. B., Congenital heart disease and upper-extremity deformities. *N. Engl. J. Med.*, 272:437–444, 1965.

Kaijser, K., and Malmstrom-Groth, A., Ano-rectal abnormalities as a congenital familial incidence. *Acta Paediatr. Scand.*, 46:199–200, 1957.

Minagi, H., and Steinbach, H. L., Roentgen appearance of anomalies associated with hypoplastic anemias of childhood: Fanconi's anemia and congenital hypoplastic anemia. *Am. J. Roentgenol.*, 97:100–109, 1966.

Quan, L., and Smith, D. W., The VATER association. *J. Pediatr.*, 82:104–107, 1973.

Swanson, A. B., and Brown, K. S., Hereditary triphalangeal thumb. *J. Hered.*, 53:259–265, 1962.

Townes, P. L., and Brocks, E. R., Hereditary syndrome of imperforate anus with hand, foot, and ear anomalies. *J. Pediatr.*, 81:321–326, 1972.

Van Gelder, D. W., and Kloepfer, H. W., Familial anorectal anomalies. *Pediatrics*, 27:334–336, 1961.

Weinstein, E. D., Sex-linked imperforate anus. *Pediatrics*, 35:715–718, 1965.

CUP-SHAPED EARS, MIXED HEARING LOSS, AND THE LACRIMOAURICULODENTODIGITAL SYNDROME

Hollister, Klein, De Jager, Lachman, and Rimoin (1973) reported a Mexican family in which the father and five of his eight children showed a new disorder that they designated the lacrimoauriculodentodigital syndrome.

CLINICAL FINDINGS

Physical Findings. All but one of the affected persons had nasolacrimal duct obstruction with hypoplasia of the lacrimal puncta. This was manifested by chronic tearing and occasional discharge of pus, dacryocystitis, and conjunctivitis from early infancy (Fig. 3–6*A, B*).

Digital anomalies were variable: tapering of second and third fingers, tapering and/or duplication of terminal phalanges of thumbs, clinodactyly of fifth fingers, hypoplasia of thumbs, and syndactyly of second and third fingers (Fig. 3–6*C, D, E*).

The teeth were small with hypoplastic enamel, and the maxillary lateral incisors had conical crown form (Fig. 3–6*F*).

Auditory System. The auricles were cup-shaped in all affected persons (Fig. 3–6*A, B*). In some of the affected persons there was severe conductive or sensorineural loss; others manifested mild high or low sensorineural or conduction deafness. Stiffness of the conductive apparatus, ascertained by impedance audiometry, suggested otosclerosis or ossicular abnormalities.

Vestibular System. Vestibular function studies were not mentioned.

LABORATORY FINDINGS

Roentgenograms. Radiographs of the hands showed a wide variation in bony anomalies (Fig. 3–6*G*). Tomograms were unremarkable.

Other Findings. Unilateral renal hypoplasia or aplasia was noted in some of the sibs.

PATHOLOGY

Study of the temporal bones was not carried out.

HEREDITY

The syndrome was transmitted in an autosomal dominant manner (Fig. 3–6*H*).

DIAGNOSIS

Obstruction of the nasolacrimal duct occurs in 1 to 6 per cent of otherwise normal newborn infants. It is resolved by the third month of life by spontaneous rupture of the membrane of the nasal end of the duct (Viers, 1966). Absence of lacrimal puncta may be an isolated phenomenon or

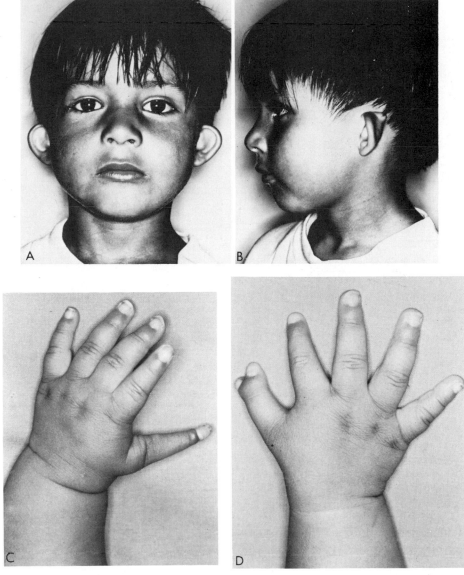

Figure 3-6   *Cup-shaped ears, mixed hearing loss, and the lacrimoauriculodentodigital syndrome. (A,B)* Prominent cup-shaped ears extend at right angles from the side of the head. The eyes have a watery, glistening appearance, and on the right there is an overflow of tears from the outer canthus. *(C, D)* Long, tapering thumbs with large nail, bifid thumb tip with extra ectopic nail and tapering of second and third digits bilaterally. *(E)* Right hand has long, tapering thumb with ectopic nail and syndactyly. Left hand has rudimentary thumb fused to index finger, prominent interdigital cleft between second and third fingers, and ulnar deviation of third digit.

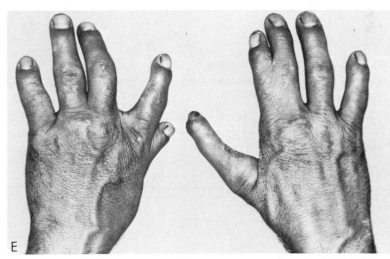

Illustration continued on the following page

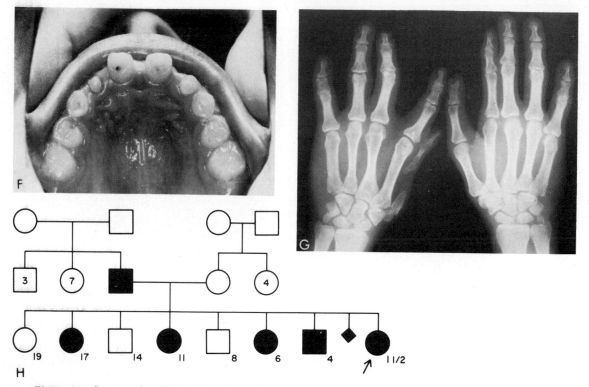

Figure 3–6 Continued *(F)* Maxillary lateral incisors have conical crown form. Premolar cusp patterns are abnormal and show excessive wear. *(G)* Radiograph of hands seen in *E*. Tip of right thumb has extra tuftlike ossification center. Left hand shows hypoplasia of greater multangular and phalanges of thumb. Metacarpal is represented by two widely separated ossification centers. *(H)* Pedigree of affected family. *(A–H* from D. Hollister *et al., J. Pediatr.,* 83:438, 1973.)

part of the ectrodactyloectodermal dysplasia–clefting syndrome (Gorlin, Pindborg, and Cohen, 1976). Agenesis of maxillary lateral incisors may be inherited as an autosomal dominant trait (Gorlin and Goldman, 1970). Cup-shaped auricles are found in several syndromes discussed in this chapter.

TREATMENT

The cup-shaped ears may be corrected for improved appearance. A hearing aid may be employed. The nasolacrimal duct atresia may be corrected surgically.

PROGNOSIS

Nasolacrimal duct atresia may result in dacryocystitis.

SUMMARY

The syndrome is characterized by: 1) autosomal dominant inheritance, 2) cup-shaped ears, 3) nasolacrimal duct obstruction and hypoplasia of lacrimal puncta, 4) various digital anomalies, 5) maxillary lateral incisors with conical crown form, 6) mild amelogenesis imperfecta, and 7) mixed hearing loss.

REFERENCES

Gorlin, R. J., and Goldman, H., *Thoma's Oral Pathology,* 6th Ed. St. Louis, The C. V. Mosby Company, 1970.

Gorlin, R. J., Pindborg, J. J., and Cohen, M. M., Jr., *Syndromes of the Head and Neck,* 2nd Ed. New York, McGraw-Hill Book Company, 1976.

Hollister, D. W., Klein, S. H., De Jager, N. J., Lachman, R. S., and Rimoin, D. L., The lacrimo-auriculo-dento-digital syndrome. *J. Pediatr.,* 83:438–444, 1973.

Viers, E. R., Disorders of the nasolacrimal apparatus in infants and children. *J. Pediatr. Ophthalmol.,* 3:32–34, 1966.

MALFORMED LOW-SET EARS AND CONDUCTION HEARING LOSS

A syndrome characterized by unilateral or bilateral malformed low-set ears and mild to severe conductive hearing loss was found in two sibships in a single kindred of Mennonites in Pennsylvania (Mengel, Konigsmark, Berlin, and McKusick, 1969).

CLINICAL FINDINGS

Physical Findings. The affected children were smaller than their unaffected sibs. Three of the six affected sibs had a highly arched palate, which was not present in their unaffected sibs.

External Ear. The auricles in all six affected children manifested mild to severe abnormality (Fig. 3–7A). The pinnae were small, and frequently the helix folded forward. In one case, the auricle was represented by a small amount of cartilaginous tissue surrounding the external auditory meatus. In four of the six children, one ear was located as much as 4 cm. below the other one (Fig. 3–7B). Usually, the malpositioned ear showed a greater auricular deformity than the more normally placed ear. In each case, the external auditory canal participated in the deformity, its opening being displaced with the ectopic auricle. There was no atresia of the canal.

Auditory System. Although hearing tests revealed marked variation in the degree of deafness, all six children had a 70 to 80 dB hearing loss in at least one ear. In some, the hearing loss was much more marked in one ear than in the other. Audiometric tests showed the deafness to be conductive. SISI tests, recruitment tests, and tone-decay tests were negative. The pure-tone audiometric results were confirmed by speech reception threshold values.

Vestibular System. Caloric vestibular tests were normal.

Mental Status. Intelligence tests on four of six children showed that three were severely retarded, whereas one was normal.

Cardiovascular System. A moderate systolic blowing murmur at the cardiac apex was found in five of six affected children. No unaffected sibs had a heart murmur. Electrocardiograms showed no abnormalities.

Reproductive System. Hypogonadism was found in three of four affected males; two of the boys had cryptorchidism.

LABORATORY FINDINGS

Roentgenograms. Skull roentgenograms obtained on two of the patients were not remarkable. Temporal bone polytomograms of the proband showed ossicular chain abnormalities.

PATHOLOGY

An ossicular chain deformity was found on exploratory tympanotomy in one patient. The malleus was slightly malformed and posteriorly positioned. Both the incus and stapes were absent. From the head of the malleus, a small fibrous band passed to the oval window area.

HEREDITY

The four patients in these two sibships were found to be descendants of a Swiss male who died in 1720 (Fig. 3–7D). It is most likely that the syndrome is transmitted by an autosomal recessive gene that was carried to the United States via one or more of the progenitor's four sons.

DIAGNOSIS

The auricular abnormality in this syndrome is similar to that described by Potter (1937), Romei (1959), and Kessler (1967) in several members of a family. Apparently, neither hearing loss nor low-set ears was associated with this auricular deformity. The syndrome of *ear malformations, preauricular cervical fistulas or nodules, and mixed hearing loss* shows somewhat similar auricular deformities. However, affected persons in the family described by Wildervanck (1962) did not have low-set ears, and the affected persons did not have mental retardation.

TREATMENT

The hearing loss may be aided by a hearing aid or by surgical therapy with

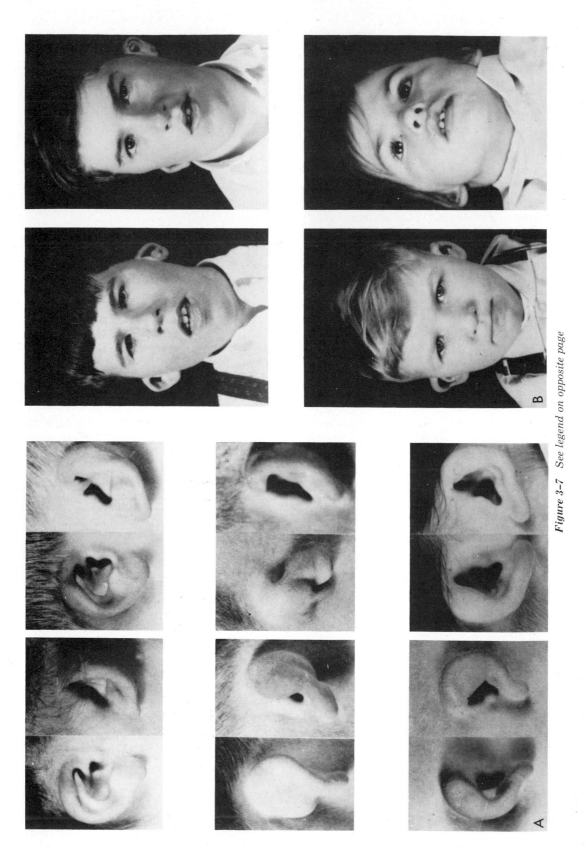

Figure 3-7   See legend on opposite page

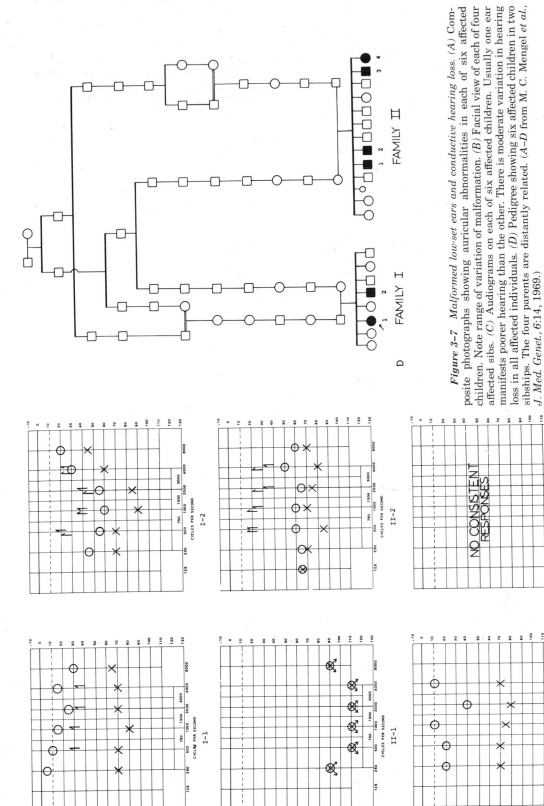

Figure 3–7 Malformed low-set ears and conductive hearing loss. (A) Composite photographs showing auricular abnormalities in each of six affected children. Note range of variation of malformation. (B) Facial view of each of four affected sibs. (C) Audiograms on each of six affected children. Usually one ear manifests poorer hearing than the other. There is moderate variation in hearing loss in all affected individuals. (D) Pedigree showing six affected children in two sibships. The four parents are distantly related. (A–D from M. C. Mengel et al., J. Med. Genet., 6:14, 1969.)

placement of a prosthesis in the middle ear. Replacement of the low-set ears may be considered; however, repositioning is impractical, since the canal is also malpositioned.

PROGNOSIS

The defects are congenital with no evidence of progression.

SUMMARY

Characteristics of this syndrome include: 1) autosomal recessive inheritance, 2) unilateral or bilateral low-set ears, 3) unilateral or bilateral malformed pinnae, 4) mental retardation in about 50 per cent of the cases, 5) cardiac murmur, 6) hypogonadism in males, and 7) mild to severe conductive hearing loss.

REFERENCES

Kessler, L., Beobachtung einer über 6 Generationen einfach-dominant vererbten Mikrotie 1. Grades. *HNO. 15*:113–116, 1967.
Mengel, M. C., Konigsmark, B. W., Berlin, C. I., and McKusick, V. A., Conductive hearing loss and malformed low-set ears as a possible recessive syndrome. *J. Med. Genet., 6*:14–21, 1969.
Potter, E. L., A hereditary ear malformation transmitted through five generations. *J. Hered., 28*:255, 1937.
Romei, L., Una famiglia con conformazione del padiglione auricolare del tipo de Potter (cup-shaped ear). *Acta Genet. Med. (Roma), 8*:483–486, 1959.
Wildervanck, L. S., Hereditary malformations of the ear in three generations. *Acta Otolaryngol. (Stockh.), 54*:553, 1962.

MICROTIA, MEATAL ATRESIA, AND CONDUCTION HEARING LOSS

Unilateral or bilateral microtia, external auditory canal atresia, and hearing loss were described in two sibships by Ellwood, Winter, and Dar (1968) and in sibs by Konigsmark, Nager, and Haskins (1972). An additional family was briefly reported by Dar and Winter (1973).

CLINICAL FINDINGS

External Ear. In one family described by Ellwood *et al.*, two of three sibs had similar anomalous external ears. The auricles were absent except for a slightly raised soft tissue mass beneath the skin at the usual sites. The external auditory meatus was represented by only a small dimple. The other facial features were entirely normal except for slight ocular hypertelorism in one patient. The two affected sibs in the second family exhibited defects only of their left ears, which were quite small, being represented by a small ridge of cartilage beneath the skin, as if the auricle were folded forward. In both sibs the right pinna was normal except for mild downward folding of the upper pole of the helix. One sib exhibited moderate atresia of the left external auditory meatus, whereas the other manifested atresia of the right auditory meatus.

Auditory System. Audiometric testing performed in one sib at 1 week of age showed a startle reaction to only those sounds exceeding 80 dB. At 4 months of age, the other sibs showed no reaction to strong sound stimuli. In the second sibship, both children had audiometric tests at about 18 months of age. The authors noted that one child had a 70 dB hearing loss by air conduction and a 30 to 50 dB loss by bone conduction. The second child was found to have normal hearing.

Konigsmark *et al.* (1972) described male sibs with severe microtia, rudimentary pinnae, and absence of external meatal openings. However, there was only moderate bilateral hearing loss. In one boy, audiometric testing showed a 40 to 60 dB conductive hearing loss with 100 per cent bilateral speech discrimination that did not diminish with age. The other male sib exhibited normal hearing in the right ear and severe sensorineural hearing loss in the left ear.

Vestibular System. Vestibular testing was not described.

LABORATORY FINDINGS

Roentgenograms. Roentgenograms showed no abnormalities other than pectus

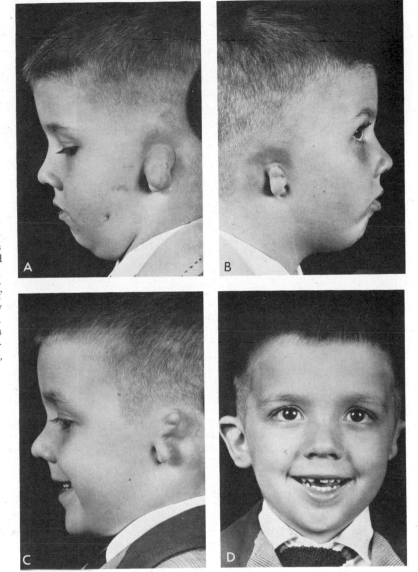

Figure 3–8 Microtia, meatal atresia, and conductive hearing loss. (A, B) Lateral views showing bilateral microtia and absent external meatal openings. (C, D) Normal right ear but microtic left with a rudiment of cartilage attached superiorly and a small lobule inferiorly. The external auditory canal was absent. (A–D from B. Konigsmark et al., Arch. Otolaryngol., 96:105, 1972.)

excavatum in one child and duplication of the thumb in another (Konigsmark et al., 1972).

PATHOLOGY

Two of the children described by Ellwood et al. (1968) died in infancy; autopsies were not performed.

HEREDITY

In both sibships, the parents were normal and there was no familial history of ear malformations or hearing loss. The parents of the second set of sibs were not known to be related although both the paternal and maternal grandparents were Ashkenazic Jews from Rumania. Thus, it is likely that the syndrome is transmitted in an autosomal recessive manner. Whether the syndrome described represents two different recessive diseases—one with severe bilateral involvement, the other with less severe unilateral involvement—is not known at the present time. In another family reported by Dar and Winter (1973), the parents of the affected sibs were consanguineous.

DIAGNOSIS

The syndrome of *ear malformations, preauricular pits, cervical fistulas or nodules, and mixed hearing loss* may be associated with meatal atresia and small malformed auricles. Case reports of sporadic congenital meatal atresia and microtia are not uncommon (Whetnall and Fry, 1964); some of these patients may have this syndrome. Hefter and Ganz (1969) described stenosis or narrowing of the external ear canal and conduction deafness in a mother and in three of her four children. However, no other anomalies were evident.

TREATMENT

The external ear abnormalities can be partially rectified by plastic surgery in which an auricle is constructed (Edgerton, 1969; Konigsmark *et al.*, 1972). A prosthesis may also be employed (Stallings *et al.*, 1971). The deafness can be helped by a hearing aid. Whether the hearing loss is the result of atresia of the external auditory meatus or

due to malformation of the ossicles is not known. Possibly, middle ear surgery may be of help.

PROGNOSIS

Although two children described by Ellwood *et al.* (1968) died in infancy, the cause of death appears to be unrelated to the ear defects. The deafness is congenital and nonprogressive.

SUMMARY

If we accept both sibships as having the same disorder, the major characteristics include: 1) autosomal recessive inheritance, 2) unilateral or bilateral anotia or microtia, 3) unilateral or bilateral external meatal atresia, and 4) moderate to severe congenital conductive deafness.

REFERENCES

Dar, H., and Winter, S. T., Letter to the editor. *J. Med. Genet.,* 10:305–306, 1973.
Edgerton, M. T., Ear construction in children with congenital atresia and stenosis. *Plast. Reconstr. Surg.,* 43:373–380, 1969.
Ellwood, L. C., Winter, S. T., and Dar., H., Familial microtia with meatal atresia in two sibships. *J. Med. Genet.,* 5:289–291, 1968.
Hefter, E., and Ganz, H., Bericht über vererbte Gehörgansmissbildungen. *HNO, 17:*76–78, 1969.
Konigsmark, B., Nager, G. T., and Haskins, H. L., Recessive microtia, meatal atresia, and hearing loss. *Arch. Otolaryngol.,* 96:105–109, 1972.
Stallings, J. O., Sessions, D. B., Howard, M. L., Beal, D. D., and Stewart, K. C., Congenital microtia. Reconstruction with a silicone rubber (Silastic) prosthesis. *Arch. Otolaryngol., 94:*176–179, 1971.
Whetnall, E., and Fry, D. B., *The Deaf Child.* Springfield, Ill., Charles C Thomas, Publisher, 1964, p. 96.
Wildervanck, L. S., Hereditary malformations of the ear in three generations. *Acta Otolaryngol. (Stockh.),* 54:553–560, 1962.

MICROTIA, HYPERTELORISM, FACIAL CLEFTING, AND CONDUCTION HEARING LOSS

Two sisters with a syndrome of hypertelorism, clefting of the lip and palate, and microtia were described by Bixler, Christian, and Gorlin (1969).

CLINICAL FINDINGS

Physical Findings. The 8- and 12-year-old sisters were below the third percentile for height and weight for their ages. Both were mildly microcephalic and mentally retarded. The head circumference of the younger girl was 45.5 cm., whereas that

of the older girl was 49 cm. — both being below the third percentile for their ages. The young girl had a mild bifid nose, and the older sib had a broad nasal tip. Both had broad nasal roots and ocular hypertelorism, but they both had normal vision. Unilateral right-sided complete cleft lip and palate were surgically repaired in both girls (Fig. 3–8*A–D*).

Auditory System. The external ears were markedly abnormal, with bilateral absence of the tragus and the anterior-superior helix. One ear was less severely in-

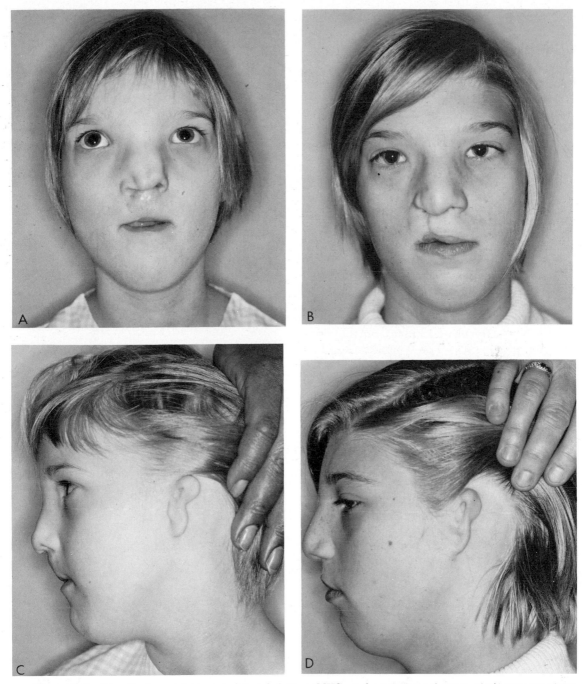

Figure 3–9 *Microtia, hypertelorism, and facial clefting (MHC syndrome).* Frontal views of (*A*) younger sister and (*B*) older sister. Prominent hypertelorism, broad nasal roots, and repaired cleft lips are evident. (*C,D*) Lateral facial views of sisters with the MHC syndrome showing microtia in younger (*C*) and older (*D*) sister. Both left ears show absent external meatuses. (*A-D* from D. Bixler *et al., Am. J. Dis. Child., 118:*495, 1969.)

volved in the younger sister. In both girls, one external auditory meatus was absent and the other was atretic (Fig. 3–9*A–D*). Temporal bone tomograms revealed bilateral atresia of the external auditory canals in the sisters. Hypoplasia of the left stapes and incus and of the right stapes and malleus was noted in one sister. The other girl was thought to have fusion of the ossicles on the left. The inner ears were normal. The sisters had bilateral conductive hearing loss, but the degree was not described.

Vestibular System. Vestibular tests were not reported.

Cardiovascular System. The sisters had congenital heart disease; an endocardial cushion defect was noted in the younger girl, and an atrial septal defect was found in the older girl. Three maternal uncles and an aunt as well as two first cousins also had congenital heart disease. Thus, the heart disease probably represents an independent genetic defect, which is not part of the syndrome.

Urinary System. Intravenous pyelograms revealed a pelvic kidney on the left and a normally placed kidney on the right in the older girl. The younger sib had crossed ectopia of the left kidney, positioned on the right side in the lumbar region.

Other Findings. Both girls had hypoplasia of the thenar eminences of both hands.

LABORATORY FINDINGS

Skull radiographs showed steep mandibular angle, short mandibular ramus, shortened upper facial height, depressed nasal floor, and decreased cranial flexure angle.

Roentgenograms of the long bones and vertebrae were essentially normal.

HEREDITY

This syndrome, involving two of four sibs with normal parents, strongly suggests autosomal recessive inheritance.

DIAGNOSIS

In the median cleft face syndrome (frontonasal dysplasia), patients have a wide spectrum of anomalies that includes marked hypertelorism, bifid nose, cranium bifidum occultum, and, occasionally, cleft lip and/or palate (Gorlin *et al.*, 1976).

Some similar features are found in *otopalatodigital (OPD) syndrome*: conduction deafness, cleft palate, and growth retardation. However, the facial and skeletal alterations found in the OPD syndrome are not found in the syndrome discussed in this section.

TREATMENT

The auricles as well as the cleft lip and palate should be corrected surgically.

PROGNOSIS

The deafness apparently is not progressive and may be treated surgically; a hearing aid may also be used.

SUMMARY

The characteristic features of the syndrome include: 1) autosomal recessive transmission, 2) microtia and meatal atresia, 3) ocular hypertelorism, 4) cleft lip and palate, 5) microcephaly and mental retardation, 6) ectopic kidneys, and 7) conductive hearing loss.

REFERENCES

Bixler, D., Christian, J. C., and Gorlin, R. J., Hypertelorism, microtia, and facial clefting. A newly described inherited syndrome. *Am. J. Dis. Child., 118*:495–498, 1969.

Gorlin, R. J., Pindborg, J. J., and Cohen, M. M., Jr., *Syndromes of the Head and Neck,* 2nd Ed. New York, McGraw-Hill Book Company, 1976.

LOP EARS, MICROGNATHIA, AND CONDUCTION DEAFNESS

We have had the opportunity to examine a mother and her son and daughter with prominent lop ears (corrected several years prior to our seeing them); long, thin nares; micrognathia; and nonprogressive mixed, mostly conductive hearing loss of 30 to 60 dB. There was no history of infections, tinnitus, or vertigo. There were two other normal sibs.

The external auditory canals were remarkably narrow. On tympanotomy both were found to have fixation of the footplate of the stapes. The posterior crura were about 65 per cent of their normal length and were not attached to the footplate. The stapedial muscle and tendon were rudimentary.

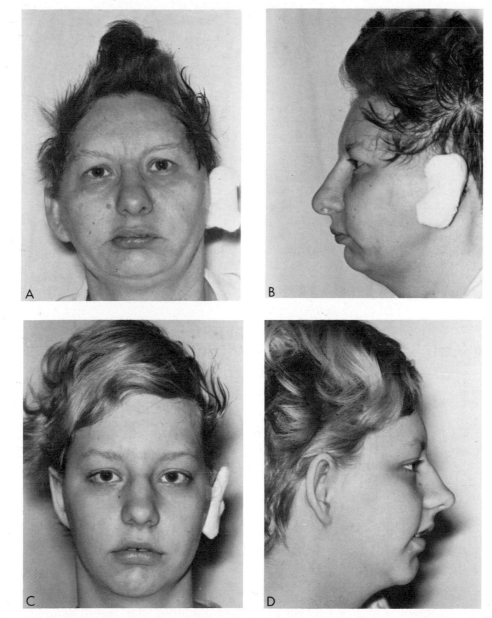

Figure 3-10 *Lop ears, micrognathia, and conduction deafness. (A–D)* Mother and daughter had bilateral lop and outstanding ears, which had been surgically corrected. A son had similar pinnal abnormalities. All had small mandibles and conductive hearing loss.

Chapter 4

GENETIC HEARING LOSS ASSOCIATED WITH EYE DISEASE

Usher syndrome is the most common disorder in this category. These patients are congenitally deaf and have a progressive visual loss caused by retinitis pigmentosa. The prevalence of this syndrome among profoundly deaf children may be as great as 10 per cent.

In addition to association with eye dis-

ease and hearing loss, some syndromes considered in this section involve the nervous system; some include diabetes mellitus. Although these syndromes might have been included in other sections, they shall be considered here because the eye signs are constant and reasonably obvious.

RETINITIS PIGMENTOSA AND CONGENITAL SENSORINEURAL DEAFNESS
(Usher Syndrome)

The Usher syndrome is characterized by congenital moderate to severe sensorineural hearing loss, vestibular hypofunction, and slowly progressive retinitis pigmentosa. Some patients show mental deficiency and later psychosis (Hallgren, 1959). It is possible that the Usher syndrome is a genetic heterogeneity and that the kindred described by Hallgren represents a separate entity (Hallgren syndrome).

The association of deafness and retinitis pigmentosa was described as early as 1858 by von Graefe and was recognized as having an unusually high incidence among the Jewish deaf. The significance of in-

creased consanguinity was pointed out by Liebreich (1861) and Hammerschlag (1907). The disorder was extensively documented by Usher (1914), who emphasized its genetic nature. Lindenov (1945) in Denmark and Hallgren (1959) in Sweden estimated its incidence in those countries at about 3 per 100,000 in the general population. A similar estimate was made by Kloepfer, Laguaite, and McLaurin (1966) of the incidence of the syndrome in the United States. Its prevalence among profoundly deaf children has been estimated by a number of investigators at 3 to 10 per cent (Vernon, 1959; Fraser, 1964).

74

CLINICAL FINDINGS

Separation of the Usher syndrome into subtypes will not be made. There is, in fact, evidence that expressivity can be quite variable (McLeod *et al.*, 1971).

Ocular System. Loss of vision generally is noticed by the age of 10 years; initial eye symptoms, however, may appear as early as preschool age in the form of night blindness. Vision deteriorates slowly, progressing to blindness in about 40 per cent of those with this syndrome in their fifth decade, in about 60 per cent of those in their sixth decade, and in about 75 per cent in their seventh decade (Hallgren, 1959). Ophthalmoscopic examination shows a typical slowly progressive retinitis pigmentosa, beginning with granular accumulations of pigment in the optic fundus and extending toward the periphery. The visual fields slowly constrict and are accompanied by decreasing visual acuity. The optic discs become pale and the arterioles become narrowed.

Other ocular findings include cataract, loss of color vision, and occasionally glaucoma. Capsular, cortical, and anterior or posterior cataracts were noted in about 10 per cent of patients by 20 years of age and in about 50 per cent of those over 40 years (Hallgren, 1959; Cherry, 1973).

Nervous System. Hallgren found mental retardation in about 25 per cent of 114 patients with this syndrome who were over 8 years of age. Vernon (1959) noted similar percentages in a much smaller series.

Psychosis was diagnosed in about 25 per cent of patients in Hallgren's group, as compared to 3 to 4 per cent in a rural Swedish population. Although schizophrenia was most common, several patients exhibited aggressiveness or periodic depression. Many reported auditory hallucinations. Bossu and Luypaet (1958) noted loss of olfactory sensitivity. Vernon's review of the literature indicated a similar prevalence of psychosis or other forms of disturbance in patients from New York. On the other hand, Nuutila (1970) did not find an increased frequency of mental retardation or psychosis.

Auditory System. About 90 per cent of 177 patients described by Hallgren (1959) had severe bilateral congenital deafness, whereas 10 per cent had moderate (30 to 70 dB) sensorineural hearing loss, more marked in the higher frequencies. Similar findings were noted by Landau and Feinmesser (1956), Kloepfer *et al.* (1966), and by McLeod *et al.* (1971). SISI scores were positive in the higher frequencies and Békésy tracings were type II, suggesting a cochlear origin for the deafness. Less severe hearing loss was noted by McGovern (1960) and by Goode *et al.* (1967).

Vestibular System. Vestibular responses to caloric testing generally are abnormal (Hallgren, 1959). All patients tested by Vernon (1959) and by McLeod (1971) showed defective vestibular function. In six patients tested by McLeod *et al.* (1971) caloric responses were normal in four, depressed in one, and absent in another. However, all six patients had some difficulty in balance. Whether vestibular or cerebellar abnormalities are the cause of the unsteadiness is not clear, but most investigators suggest labyrinthine abnormalities.

LABORATORY FINDINGS

Blood and urine analyses and skull roentgenographic studies have been normal. Electroencephalographic abnormalities have been an inconstant finding (Krill and Stamps, 1960).

PATHOLOGY

Temporal bone changes involve the cochlea and its nerve and vascular supply. There is marked atrophy of the organ of Corti and of the epithelium of the inner and outer sulci in the lower basal turn, the degeneration decreasing in the upper turns. In addition, there is severe atrophy of the spiral ganglion, its peripheral and central fibers, and the end branches of the labyrinthine vessels (Nager, 1927; Buch and Jorgensen, 1963). These changes are typical of the Scheibe type.

HEREDITY

Examples of affected sibs having normal parents and increased consanguinity together indicate autosomal recessive transmission (Kloepfer *et al.*, 1966; McLeod, 1971). An estimated 1 per 100 individuals is a carrier. Heterozygotes may exhibit gyrate atrophy (Holland *et al.*, 1972), elevated dark adaptation thresholds (de Haas *et al.*, 1970), or mild deafness (McLeod *et al.*, 1971).

DIAGNOSIS

In addition to diagnosis by ophthalmoscopy, the retinitis pigmentosa may be diagnosed by electroretinography, electrooculography, visual field tests, and dark adaptation recording.

Retinitis pigmentosa as an isolated finding can be inherited as an autosomal recessive, dominant, or X-linked condition (Vernon, 1959). In several syndromes, there is the combination of retinitis pigmentosa and hearing loss. In *Alström syndrome,* the patient is obese and may have diabetes mellitus. In *Refsum syndrome,* there is mental deterioration, progressive peripheral neuropathy, and elevated phytanic acid levels. In the Bardet-Biedl syndrome there is mental deficiency, obesity, hypogonadism, and polydactyly. Persons with the Laurence-Moon syndrome show mental retardation, hypogenitalism, and spastic paraplegia. Patients with *Cockayne syndrome* are distinguished by their small stature, severe mental deficiency, and birdlike facies.

Retinitis pigmentosa has been noted in *progressive external ophthalmoplegia, retinal pigmentary degeneration, cardiac conduction defects,* and *mixed hearing loss* (Kearns syndrome).

TREATMENT

In most cases, the deafness is so profound that the use of a hearing aid is not possible. There is no treatment for retinitis pigmentosa.

PROGNOSIS

Most patients are forced to retire from their occupations at 30 to 40 years of age, either because of advancing failure of vision or because of other disabilities associated with the condition.

SUMMARY

The syndrome is characterized by: 1) autosomal recessive inheritance, 2) progressive visual loss with retinitis pigmentosa, 3) mental retardation and/or psychosis (occasionally), 4) mild ataxia, congenital severe or moderate sensorineural hearing loss, and 5) absent vestibular response.

REFERENCES

Bossu, A., and Luypaet, R., Le syndrome d'Usher. *Ann. Ocul. (Paris), 191:*529–534, 1958.
Buch, N. H., and Jorgensen, M. B., Pathological studies of deaf-mutes. *Arch. Otolaryngol., 77:*246–253, 1963.
Cherry, P. M. H., Usher's syndrome. *Ann. Ophthalmol., 5:*743–752, 1973.
de Haas, E., Van Lith, G., Rijnders, J., Rümke, A., and Volmer, C., Usher's syndrome with special reference to heterozygous manifestations. *Doc. Ophthalmol.,28:*166–190, 1970.
Fraser, G. R., Profound childhood deafness. *J. Med. Genet., 1:*118–151, 1964.
Goode, R. L., Rafaty, F. M., and Simmons, F. B., Hearing loss in retinitis pigmentosa. *Pediatrics, 40:*875–880, 1967.
Hallgren, V., Retinitis pigmentosa combined with congenital deafness; with vestibulo-cerebellar ataxia and mental abnormality in a proportion of cases. A clinical and geneticostatistical study. *Acta Psychiatr. Scand., Suppl.138:*1–101, 1959.
Hammerschlag, V., Zur Kenntnis der hereditär-degenerativen Taubstummheit. V. Über pathologische Augenbefund bei Taubstummen und ihre differential-diagnostische Bedeutung. *Z. Ohrenheilk., 54:*18–36, 1907.
Holland, M. G., Cambie, E., and Kloepfer, W., An evaluation of genetic carriers of Usher's syndrome. *Am. J. Ophthalmol., 74:*940–947, 1972.
Kloepfer, H. W., Laguaite, J. K., and McLaurin, J. W., The hereditary syndrome of deafness in retinitis pigmentosa. *Laryngoscope, 76:*850–862, 1966.
Krill, A. E., and Stamps, F. W., The electroencephalogram in retinitis pigmentosa. *Am. J. Ophthalmol., 49:*762–773, 1960.
Landau, J., and Feinmesser, M., Audiometric and vestibular examinations in retinitis pigmentosa. *Br. J. Ophthalmol., 40:*40–44, 1956.
Liebreich, R., Abkunft und Ehen unter Blutsverwandten als Grund von Retinitis pigmentosa. *Dtsch. Klin., 13:*53–55, 1861.
Lindenov, H., *The Etiology of Deaf-Mutism with Special Reference to Heredity.* Copenhagen, Munksgaard, International Booksellers and Publishers, Ltd., 1945.
McGovern, F. H., The association of nerve deafness and retinitis pigmentosa. *Ann. Otol., 69:*1044–1053, 1960.
McLeod, A. C., McConnell, F., Sweeney, A., Cooper, M., and Nance, W., Clinical variation in Usher's syndrome. *Arch. Otolaryngol., 94:*321–334, 1971.

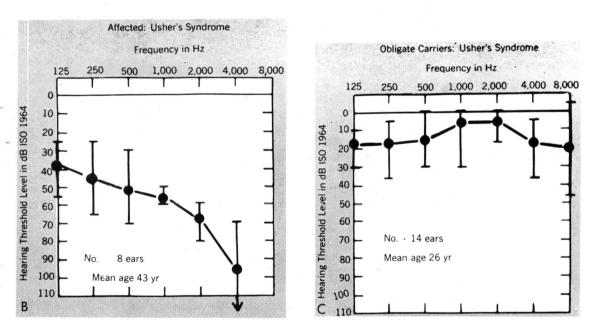

Figure 4-1 *Retinitis pigmentosa and congenital sensorineural deafness (Usher syndrome). (A)* Equatorial view of fundus showing typical bone spicule pigmentary changes clustered around vessels. *(B, C)* Mean audiograms in Usher syndrome. In affected individuals and in obligate heterozygotes. (From A. C. McLeod *et al., Arch. Otolaryngol., 94:*321, 1971.)

Nager, F. R., Zur Histologie der Taubstummheit bei Retinitis pigmentosa. *Beitr. Path.,* 77:288–303, 1927.

Nuutila, A., Dystrophia retinae pigmentosa-dysacusis syndrome (DRD). A study of the Usher—or Hallgren—syndrome. *J. Génét. Hum., 18:*57–88, 1970.

Usher, C. H., On the inheritance of retinitis pigmentosa, with notes of cases. *R. Lond. Ophthalmol. Hosp. Rep., 19:*130–236, 1914.

Vernon, M., Usher's syndrome—deafness and progressive blindness. Clinical cases, prevention, theory, and literature survey. *J. Chron. Dis., 22:*133–151, 1959.

von Graefe, A., Vereinzelte Beobachtungen und Bemerkungen. Exceptionelles Verhalten des Gesichtsfeldes bei Pigmentenartung der Netzhaut. *Albrecht von Graefes Arch. Klin. Ophthalmol., 4:*250–253, 1858.

RETINAL DEGENERATION, DIABETES MELLITUS, OBESITY, AND SENSORINEURAL HEARING LOSS

(Alström Syndrome)

A syndrome characterized by transient early obesity, loss of central vision due to atypical retinal degeneration, adult diabetes mellitus, and progressive sensorineural hearing loss was found in a Swedish kindred by Alström, Hallgren, Nilsson, and Åsander (1959). Other cases were described by Klein and Ammann (1969), Weinstein, Kliman, and Scully (1969), Lista, Podesta and Mazzei (1972), Goldstein and Fialkow (1973), and Edwards, Sethe, and Scoma (1973). One of the patients described by Klein and Ammann was noted earlier by Graf (1964). Less likely examples are the male sibs described by Boenheim (1929).

CLINICAL FINDINGS

Physical Findings. Mild to moderate truncal obesity has been a problem in all affected children between 2 and 10 years, but this condition usually disappeared with age. No adult male has been taller than 65 inches (165 cm.) and no adult female taller than 63 inches (160 cm.) (Fig. 4–2*A*, *B*).

Ocular System. Initial nystagmus with progressive visual loss began during the first two years of life in all patients. Vision slowly deteriorated; by the second decade there was almost total loss due to diffuse retinal degeneration with central and peripheral involvement. Posterior cortical cataracts of mild to moderate degree generally appeared during the second decade. Secondary changes have included optic atrophy, pigmentary alterations, dislocated lenses, and glaucoma (Goldstein and Fialkow, 1973).

Nervous System. Neurologic examination showed no abnormality except for eye and ear involvement. Intelligence was normal in all cases.

Integumentary System. Premature baldness in males and scanty hair or spotty alopecia in females have been noted in nearly all cases. Acanthosis nigricans has been present in the axillae of all patients examined.

Genitourinary System. Chronic renal disease is probably the most variable aspect of the syndrome. It may be mild, exhibiting only impaired glomerular and tubular function manifested by aminoaciduria and an inability to concentrate water, or it may be severe, resulting in death. The renal problems first become evident in the third decade (Goldstein and Fialkow, 1973).

Males have small testes but normal pubic hair and beard. Females have abnormal menstrual histories (oligomenorrhea, dysmenorrhea, hypermenorrhea, metromenorrhagia), and sparse axillary and pubic hair. They have not exhibited hypogonadism.

Auditory System. Sensorineural hearing loss has been first noted at about 7 years of age and has progressed, becoming moderately severe in the second and third decades. The Békésy, tone-decay, and SISI tests suggest cochlear involvement (Goldstein and Fialkow, 1973).

Vestibular System. No vestibular findings have been mentioned.

LABORATORY FINDINGS

Roentgenographic studies have demonstrated scoliosis and hyperostosis frontalis interna (Klein and Ammann, 1969; Goldstein and Fialkow, 1973).

Carbohydrate intolerance first becomes manifest in the third decade and has been present in 8 of 10 cases. Three patients exhibited fasting hyperglycemia; four showed carbohydrate intolerance on glucose loading, despite normal fasting blood sugars; and one was stated to have diabetes, but the condition was not documented (Weinstein *et al.*, 1969).

Renal impairment has been manifested by albuminuria, elevated blood urea nitrogen, aminoaciduria, hyperuricemia, and nephrogenic diabetes insipidus in several cases.

Hypertriglyceridemia with elevation of the pre-betalipoprotein fraction has been demonstrated in three of four patients investigated.

Urinary 17-ketosteroid levels have been decreased and urinary gonadotropin levels have been increased in males. Plasma testosterone levels have been low (Wein-

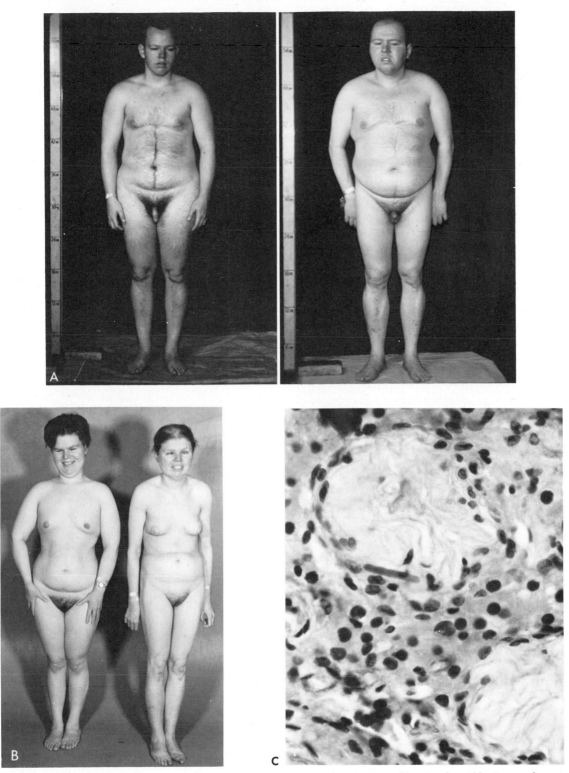

Figure 4-2 *Retinal degeneration, diabetes mellitus, obesity, and sensorineural hearing loss (Alström syndrome).*
(A) Nineteen-year-old and 33-year-old sibs exhibiting short stature, complete blindness, and partial hearing loss.
(From R. L. Weinstein *et al., N. Engl. J. Med., 281*:969, 1969.) *(B)* Thirty-six-year-old and 33-year-old female sibs
with Alström syndrome. Blindness was noted at about 1 year of age, deafness at 6 years; partial alopecia began at
20 years of age. Both had difficulties with their menses. Patient at left is wearing a wig. (From J. L. Goldstein and
P. J. Fialkow, *Medicine, 52*:53, 1973.) *(C)* Photomicrograph of testicular specimen showing pale hyalinized tubules.
Also note crystalloid of Reinke. (From R. L. Weinstein *et al., N. Engl. J. Med., 281*:969, 1969.)

stein *et al.,* 1969; Klein and Ammann, 1969).

PATHOLOGY

Testicular biopsy has shown small hyalinized tubules with occasional Leydig and Sertoli cells and thickening of the lamina propria (Fig. 4–2C). Biopsy of the ovaries of a 16-year-old girl dying of unstated causes showed no abnormalities.

Histologic sections of the kidneys showed chronic nephropathy manifested by thickening of glomerular and tubular membranes. Many glomeruli were hyalinized (Goldstein and Fialkow, 1973).

HEREDITY

Although pathogenesis is not presently understood, resistance to the action of several polypeptide hormones (insulin, vasopressin, and gonadotropins) is thought to account for the diabetes mellitus, nephrogenic diabetes insipidus, and primary hypogonadism. Goldstein and Fialkow (1973) suggested that generalized membrane thickening and hyalinization of connective tissue may be important consequences of the basic abnormality.

In all cases, the parents of affected children have been normal. The occurrence of the syndrome in sibs of both sexes and the increased rate of consanguinity strongly indicate autosomal recessive inheritance.

DIAGNOSIS

Patients with the Laurence-Moon syndrome have retinitis pigmentosa, mental retardation, hypogenitalism, and spastic paraplegia. Those with the Bardet-Biedl syndrome show obesity and retinitis pigmentosa in association with polydactyly, hypogonadism, and mental retardation. Individuals with the Alström syndrome do not have mental retardation or polydactyly. Deafness and diabetes mellitus are rare in either the Laurence-Moon or the Bardet-Biedl syndrome (Burn, 1950; Garstecki *et al.,* 1972). Furthermore, the age of onset of total blindness is before the second decade in the Alström syndrome in contrast to

being the fourth decade in the Laurence-Moon and Bardet-Biedl syndromes. The sisters reported by Weiss (1932) had obesity, hypogonadism, mental retardation, and sensorineural deafness, but no retinitis pigmentosa. At present, they cannot be classified.

Primary hypogonadism, which occurs in the Reifenstein syndrome, myotonic dystrophy, and germinal cell aplasia, must be excluded. The separation on clinical and microscopic grounds has been clearly discussed by Weinstein *et al.* (1969).

We cannot easily classify the two brothers with infantile diabetes, optic atrophy, hypogonadism, and sensorineural deafness reported by Codaccioni *et al.* (1969). These may represent a separate syndrome, since there is no evidence of retinitis pigmentosa.

TREATMENT

A hearing aid may be used for the progressive hearing loss. Although a major portion of the visual deficit is due to atypical retinitis pigmentosa, that portion caused by polar cataracts may be improved by removal of the lens. The obesity may be controlled by diet, the diabetes mellitus, by appropriate medical therapy.

PROGNOSIS

Little hope can be offered to these patients, since vision and hearing deteriorate progressively. Intelligence, however, remains normal. The life span may be shortened by the renal dysfunction.

SUMMARY

Characteristics of this syndrome include: 1) autosomal recessive inheritance, 2) onset in infancy of retinitis pigmentosa with loss of central vision, 3) onset in childhood of diabetes mellitus, 4) transient obesity, 5) onset in the second decade of posterior cortical cataract, 6) onset in the third decade of nephropathy, 7) acanthosis nigricans, and 8) onset in late childhood of progressive sensorineural hearing loss.

REFERENCES

Alström, C. H., Hallgren, B., Nilsson, L. B., and Åsander, H., Retinal degeneration combined with obesity, diabetes mellitus, and neurogenous deafness. *Acta Psychiatr. Neurol. Scand., 34(Suppl. 129)*:1–35, 1959.

Boenheim, F., Zur Kenntnis der Laurence-Biedlschen Krankheit. *Endokrinologie, 4*:263–273, 1929. (Cases 3, 4.)

Burn, R. A., Deafness and the Laurence-Moon-Biedl syndrome. *Br. J. Ophthalmol., 34*:65–88, 1950.

Codaccioni, J. L., Mattei, A., Jubelin, J., Carlon, N., and Luciani, J. M., Hypotrophie testiculaire primitive chez deux frères atteints de diabète infantile, atrophie optique familial et surdité neurogène pour l'un. *Ann. Endocrinol., 30*:669–676, 1969.

Edwards, J. A., Sethe, P. K., and Scoma, A., An Alström-like syndrome in three black sibs. In *American Society of Human Genetics Abstracts, 25th Meeting,* Atlanta, Georgia, October 24–27, 1973.

Garstecki, D., Borton, T., Stark, E., and Kennedy, B., Speech, language, and hearing problems in the Laurence-Moon-Biedl syndrome. *J. Speech Hear. Disord., 37*:407–413, 1972.

Goldstein, J. L., and Fialkow, P. J., The Alström syndrome. *Medicine, 52*:53–71, 1973.

Graf, K., Schwerhörigkeit als Symptom familiärer heredodegenerativer Erkrankungen (Abiotrophien). *Pract. Otorhinolaryngol. (Basel), 26*:46–54, 1964.

Klein, D., and Ammann, F., The syndrome of Laurence-Moon-Bardet-Biedl and allied diseases in Switzerland: clinical, genetic, and epidemiological studies. *J. Neurol. Sci., 9*:479–513, 1969.

Lista, G. A., Podesta, H. A., and Mazzei, C. M., El sindrome de Alström. *Prensa Med. Argent., 59*:253–254, 1972.

Weinstein, R. L., Kliman, B., and Scully, R. E., Familial syndrome of primary testicular insufficiency with normal virilization, blindness, deafness, and metabolic abnormalities. *N. Engl. J. Med., 281*:969–977, 1969.

Weiss, E., Cerebral adiposity with nerve deafness, mental deficiency, and genital dystrophy: a variant of the Laurence-Biedl syndrome. *Am. J. Med. Sci., 183*:268–272, 1932.

RETINITIS PIGMENTOSA, NYSTAGMUS, HEMIPLEGIC MIGRAINE, AND SENSORINEURAL DEAFNESS

Young, Leon-Barth, and Green (1970) reported a syndrome in four members of a family who were affected by hemiplegic migraine and nystagmus. Two of these individuals also had sensorineural deafness and retinitis pigmentosa.

PHYSICAL FINDINGS

Ocular System. Prior to the migrainous attack, the altered vision consisted of a sensation of whirling lights, blurred vision, and dark spots in all fields of vision. Upon clearing, this was followed by headache on the side contralateral to the hemiparesis. Jerking nystagmus was permanently present in all affected persons. Night blindness, constricted visual fields, and retinitis pigmentosa were noted in one patient, whereas still another exhibited nystagmus and mild ataxia; neither had migraine or deafness. One patient had bilateral posterior subcapsular cataracts.

Nervous System. Hemiplegic migraine, a throbbing, vascular headache preceded by sensory and motor phenomena that persist during and for a brief time after the headache, appeared around the age of 4 to 5 years in three of four patients and recurred three or more times a year. In the other patient, it first appeared at 10 years of age. Prior to a migrainous attack, there was dizziness or lightheadedness or a feeling of tightness in one limb. These symptoms occurred simultaneously or in rapid succession and lasted from 15 to 90 minutes. As well as suffering the headache, patients experienced numbness that began in one hand or foot and spread to half the body. Numbness was followed by severe weakness on the ipsilateral side. This disappeared upon cessation of the headache. The duration of the attacks varied from 12 hours to 5 days. Headache was bilateral in three patients and unilateral in the other patient. During the headache, sensorimotor hemiparesis was evident in four individuals, nausea and vomiting were present in three patients, and ataxia and hemiplegia in only one. The latter patient had permanent mild ataxia of gait.

Auditory System. Hearing loss was first described in the two adults at 4 to 6 years of age. Bilateral sensorineural hearing loss of 70 to 80 dB in the frequency ranges of 750 to 4000 Hz was demonstrated. There was good discrimination bilaterally, no tone decay, and type II Békésy audiograms.

Vestibular System. Vestibular studies were not mentioned.

LABORATORY FINDINGS

Routine blood and urine analyses were normal; studies on cerebrospinal fluid were also normal.

Electroencephalograms made within 72 hours of the attack of migraine showed a slow wave abnormality, which subsequently disappeared.

HEREDITY

Without documentation of additional cases, it is difficult to know whether we are dealing with a new syndrome or with the simultaneous occurrence of two or more disorders in this family, i.e., the Usher syndrome, with hemiplegic migraine and familial nystagmus (see below). If the syndrome is unique, it is probably inherited as an autosomal dominant trait with variable expressivity.

DIAGNOSIS

Retinitis pigmentosa may occur as an isolated finding or may be associated with a plethora of syndromes. Those syndromes in which both deafness and retinitis pigmentosa occur are considered in this section.

Retinitis pigmentosa has also been reported in association with migraine (Friedman, 1951; Connor, 1962). Connor (1962) reviewed the extensive literature on complicated migraine but found no association with deafness. Ohta *et al.* (1967) reported nystagmus and cerebellar manifestations in patients with hemiplegic migraine, but they noted no association with deafness.

Hemiplegic migraine has occurred as an autosomal dominant trait (Clarke, 1910).

TREATMENT

The hemiplegic migraine can be treated with methysergide (Sansert). The retinitis pigmentosa and jerking nystagmus cannot be treated. The deafness can be lessened by means of a hearing aid.

PROGNOSIS

The life span apparently is not shortened. The blindness and deafness are progressive.

SUMMARY

The characteristics of the syndrome include 1) autosomal dominant inheritance with variable expressivity, 2) retinitis pigmentosa, 3) hemiplegic migraine, preceded or accompanied by sensory and motor phenomena, 4) jerking nystagmus, and 5) sensorineural deafness.

REFERENCES

Clarke, J. M., On recurrent motor paralysis in migraine: report of a family in which recurrent hemiplegia accompanied the attacks. *Br. Med. J., 1*:1534–1538, 1910.

Connor, R. C. R., Complicated migraine: a study of permanent neurological and visual defects caused by migraine. *Lancet, 2*:1072–1075, 1962.

Friedman, M. W., Occlusion of central retinal vein in migraine. *Arch. Ophthalmol., 45*:678–682, 1951.

Ohta, M., Araki, S., and Kuroiwa, Y., Familial occurrence of migraine with hemiplegic syndrome and cerebellar manifestations. *Neurology (Minneap.), 17*:813–817, 1967.

Young, G. F., Leon-Barth, C. A., and Green, J., Familial hemiplegic migraine, retinal degeneration, deafness, and nystagmus. *Arch. Neurol., 23*:201–209, 1970.

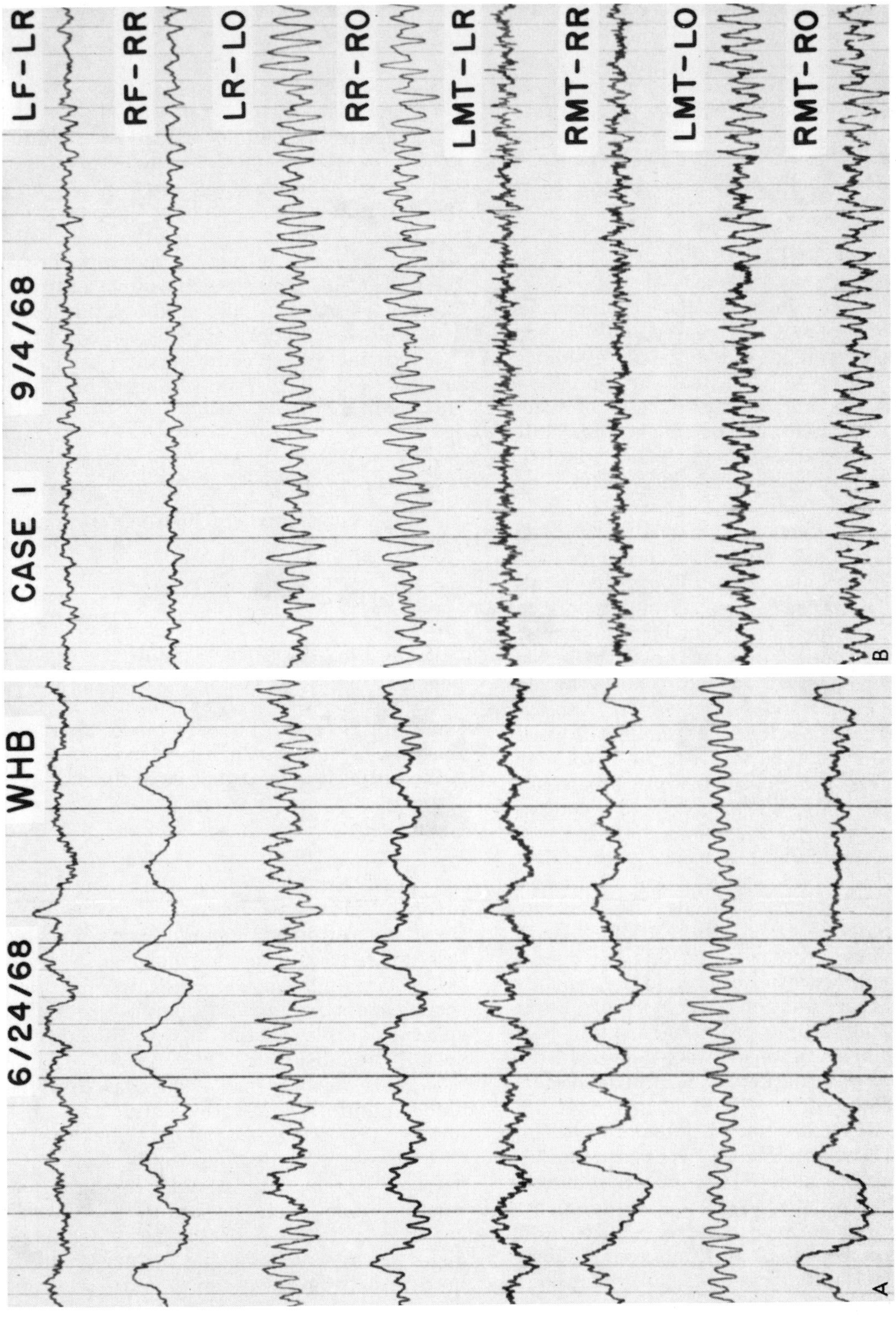

Figure 4-3 Retinitis pigmentosa, nystagmus, hemiplegic migraine, and sensorineural deafness. (A) Electroencephalogram two days after attack of migraine with temporary left hemiplegia. Note right hemispheric slow wave abnormality. (B) Electroencephalogram, taken 10 weeks after a hemiplegic migraine attack, is almost normal. (From G. F. Young et al., Arch. Neurol., 23:201, 1970.)

RETINITIS PIGMENTOSA, PROGRESSIVE QUADRIPARESIS, MENTAL RETARDATION, AND SENSORINEURAL DEAFNESS

Pigmentary degeneration of the retina, progressive quadriparesis, mental retardation, and moderately severe sensorineural hearing loss were described in two male sibs by Gordon, Capute, and Konigsmark (1976).

CLINICAL FINDINGS

Physical Findings. The brothers had short stature with decreased muscle mass in all extremities and dull, expressionless facies (Fig. 4–4*A, B*). Head circumference, body length, and weight were at or below the third percentile. The fingers, especially the middle phalanges, were short, and the fifth fingers showed clinodactyly. The legs exhibited moderate flexion contractures.

Ocular System. Ophthalmologic examination done when the brothers were three and four years old, respectively, showed a diffuse, coarse, granular pigment throughout the retina. The optic discs were pale and small, and the retinal arterioles were decreased in caliber. These changes became progressively more severe with age.

Nervous System. Psychometric tests revealed I.Q.s of 34 and 44. The most striking neurologic findings were progressive spasticity of the legs with flexion contractures of the hips and knees. Reflexes were hyperactive: plantar responses were flexor. Although muscle mass was decreased, strength was rather good. The gait was slow and wide-based, but walking became progressively difficult and finally impossible. There were no abnormal movements; sensory examination was normal. Facial expression became progressively dull. Gag and swallow responses were depressed and drooling was marked. Lid closure became incomplete.

Auditory System. Audiometric testing was somewhat difficult in these mentally retarded brothers. Otologic examinations showed no abnormalities. EEG audiometry revealed moderately severe sensorineural hearing loss at least in the higher frequencies. Other audiometric tests were not done. Neither child developed speech.

Vestibular System. Caloric vestibular tests showed no abnormalities.

LABORATORY FINDINGS

Roentgenograms. Skull roentgenograms showed a small, asymmetric cranium. The middle phalanges were short, and the first metacarpal was hypoplastic.

Other Findings. In one boy the EEG showed excessively slow activity, whereas the EEG of his sib showed no abnormalities. An electroretinographic study of the older boy exhibited subnormal response to light.

Routine blood counts, urinalysis, and tests of electrolytes and cerebrospinal fluid revealed no abnormalities.

PATHOLOGY

No histopathologic findings were presented.

HEREDITY

The parents of these children were remotely related (Fig. 4–4*C*). A maternal aunt had spastic cerebral palsy but no retinopathy. The most likely mode of transmission is autosomal recessive, but X-linked inheritance cannot be excluded.

DIAGNOSIS

In *Usher syndrome*, the motor and mental systems are intact. Other disorders involving retinitis pigmentosa and hearing loss, such as *Cockayne syndrome, Refsum syndrome,* and *Alström syndrome,* have associated abnormalities different from the spastic paraplegia and mental retardation seen in this disorder.

There are several syndromes that include mental retardation and gait disorders. The *Richards-Rundle syndrome* is characterized by deafness and slowly progressive ataxia, but strength remains reasonably good over the years. The Troyer syndrome includes spastic paraplegia and distal muscle wasting that begins in childhood and progresses slowly until walking becomes impossible in the third or fourth decade. Although some patients exhibit mental retardation, they show no evidence

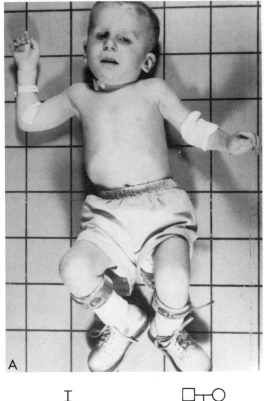

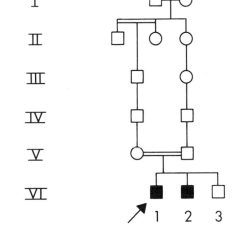

C

Figure 4-4 *Retinitis pigmentosa, progressive quadriparesis, mental retardation, and sensorineural deafness. (A, B)* Two sibs exhibiting short stature, expressionless facies, and low-set, malformed ears. *(C)* Pedigree showing six generations of this consanguineous kindred. (From A. M. Gordon *et al., Johns Hopkins Med. J., 138*: 142–145, 1976.)

of retinitis pigmentosa or optic atrophy (Cross and McKusick, 1967).

Recessive spastic paraplegia with retinal degeneration has been described in one kindred in association with sensorineural deafness, but intelligence was normal (Louis-Bar and Pirot, 1945; Mahloudji and Chuke, 1968).

TREATMENT

Since mental deficiency is rather severe, hearing aids are of limited usefulness.

PROGNOSIS

The disease appears to be very slowly progressive, resulting in complete debility.

SUMMARY

Characteristics of this syndrome include: 1) probable autosomal recessive transmission, 2) progressive retinitis pigmentosa, 3) progressive quadriparesis, 4) marked mental retardation, and 5) moderate sensorineural hearing loss.

REFERENCES

Cross, H. E., and McKusick, V. A., The Troyer syndrome: a recessive form of spastic paraplegia with distal muscle wasting. *Arch. Neurol., 16*:473–485, 1967.

Gordon, A. M., Capute, A. J., and Konigsmark, B. W., Progressive quadriparesis, retinitis pigmentosa, and hearing loss: report of two sibs. Johns Hopkins Med. J., *138*:142–145, 1976.

Louis-Bar, D., and Pirot, G., Sur une paraplégie spasmodique avec dégénérescence maculaire chez deux frères. *Ophthalmologica, 109*:32–43, 1945.

Mahloudji, M., and Chuke, P. O., Familial spastic paraplegia with retinal degeneration. *Johns Hopkins Med. J., 123*:142–144, 1968.

COCKAYNE SYNDROME

This disease, characterized by cachectic dwarfism with senile appearance, mental retardation, retinal degeneration, and moderate sensorineural hearing loss, was described in two sibs by Cockayne (1936). Since then, over 30 cases have been published.

CLINICAL FINDINGS

Physical Findings. At birth, affected persons generally are normal. During the second year of life, growth retardation becomes evident. The hands, feet, and ears, however, are relatively large. Lack of subcutaneous facial fat, combined with microcephaly, sunken eyes, and thin, beaklike nose, imparts a senile appearance.

Ocular System. Nearly all patients have enophthalmos and retinal abnormalities, including progressive optic atrophy and a salt-and-pepper type of speckled pigmentation of the retina, most marked in the macular area. The retinal changes are first seen when the patient is in his second year of life and progress slowly until the patient becomes blind during the second decade. Also present is arteriolar narrowing (Lieberman *et al.*, 1961). The veins are normal. Cataracts develop by adolescence. Corneal scarring, nystagmus, and photophobia are less frequently observed (MacDonald *et al.*, 1960; Paddison *et al.*, 1963; Coles, 1969).

Nervous System. Patients generally have a coarse tremor and unsteady gait complicated by mild flexion contractures of the hips and knees. Reflexes are commonly hyperactive. Plantar responses are flexor.

Although mental activity appears normal during the first year of life, development stops at about a three- or four-year-old level.

Skeletal System. Growth retardation is marked. Kyphosis and flexion contractures of the ankles, knees, and elbows are common. The limbs appear disproportionately long, and the hands and feet seem disproportionately large.

Urogenital System. Often there is cryptorchidism, and, even with descent, the testicles remain small.

Integumentary System. A consistent finding is generalized lack of subcutaneous tissue, resulting in a wizened appearance and sunken eyes. Photosensitivity is a prominent feature. During the second year of life a scaly rash develops on the sun-exposed areas of the body, most prominent over the face and distributed in a butterfly pattern. The rash may spread to involve the rest of the face as well as the hands, wrists, and legs. Scarring and pigmentary changes may occur in the older patient.

Auditory System. Most patients have normal hearing at birth but usually develop a moderate to severe sensorineural hearing loss during childhood (Schönenberg and Frohn, 1969). The hearing loss is somewhat variable in different patients. MacDonald *et al.* (1960) described three affected sibs. In the 5-year-old child, hearing was normal. His 10-year-old brother developed speech at two years of age, but this facility deteriorated progressively. The 7-year-old sib was thought to have normal hearing, but her speech was tremulous and monotonous. The hearing status of the boy reported by Lieberman *et al.* (1961) was not described. However, the child did not talk at five years of age. The 31-year-old patient described by Moossy (1967) was deaf and mute, suggesting an early onset of hearing loss.

Vestibular System. Vestibular testing has not been described.

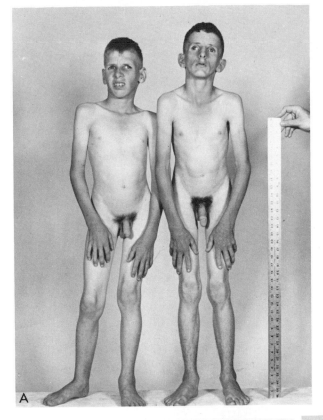

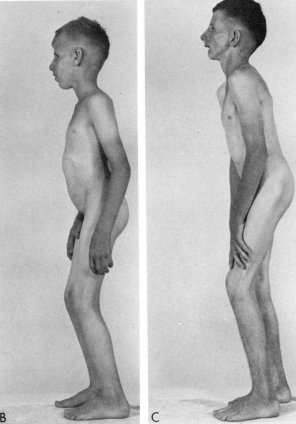

Figure 4-5 Cockayne syndrome. (A, B, and C) Fourteen- and 16-year-old sibs with marked mental and somatic retardation, eye difficulties, and sensorineural deafness. Note wizened appearance, photodermatitis of sun-exposed areas, horse-riding stance, and large hands and feet. (From R. M. Paddison *et al., Derm. Trop.,* 2:196, 1963.)

LABORATORY FINDINGS

Roentgenograms. The calvaria and skull base are quite thick and the facial bones are small. These changes may not be evident in the young child, but they increase in severity with age (MacDonald *et al.*, 1960; Riggs and Seibert, 1972). Irregular calcification along the lateral ventricles has also been described. The spine may show scoliosis and kyphosis.

PATHOLOGY

Neuropathologic studies of the brain have shown microcephaly; widespread mineralization of the cortex, basal ganglia, and cerebellum; and patchy, often severe demyelinization of the subcortical white matter (Moossy, 1967; Rowlatt, 1969; Crome and Kanjilal, 1971).

HEREDITY

There are numerous sibships in which two or more children have been affected. The remaining sibs and both parents have been normal. There is increased parental consanguinity. Equal numbers of males and females have been affected. The syndrome has autosomal recessive inheritance.

DIAGNOSIS

The Cockayne syndrome and progeria both exhibit growth retardation with onset in infancy, lack of subcutaneous tissue, and premature senility. However, patients with the Cockayne syndrome have degenerative retinal lesions, mental deficiency, hearing loss, dermatitis, and ataxia.

Photosensitivity may also be seen in Bloom syndrome, Hartnup disease, xeroderma pigmentosum, or erythropoietic porphyria.

TREATMENT

Little can be done for the visual loss. Although a hearing aid may be considered for the deafness, the mental deficiency precludes much success. The patient should be protected from the sun, since exposure aggravates the dermatitis.

PROGNOSIS

Prognosis is poor, with severe blindness and deafness usually developing. Coordination may deteriorate until the patient is unable to care for himself. During the second or third decade the patient may become bedridden. Death has usually occurred prior to the thirtieth year of life.

SUMMARY

Characteristics of this syndrome include 1) autosomal recessive transmission, 2) visual lesions, including optic atrophy and salt-and-pepper retinal alterations leading to blindness, 3) onset in infancy of growth retardation with lack of subcutaneous fat and skeletal abnormalities including thickened skull and kyphosis, 4) joint contractures, 5) early arrest of mental development, 6) light-sensitive dermatitis involving the face and hands, and 7) moderate to severe sensorineural hearing loss.

REFERENCES

Cockayne, E. A., Dwarfism with retinal atrophy and deafness. *Arch. Dis. Child.*, *11*:1–8, 1936.
Coles, W. H., Ocular manifestations of Cockayne's syndrome. *Am. J. Ophthalmol.*, *62*:762–764, 1969.
Conly, P. W., Tamer, M. A., and Tamer, D., Hyperinsulinemia in Cockayne's syndrome. *South. Med. J.*, *63*:1491, 1970.
Crome, L., and Kanjilal, G. C., Cockayne's syndrome. *J. Neurol. Neurosurg. Psychiatr.*, *34*:171–178, 1971.
Lieberman, W. J., Schimek, R. A., and Synder, C. H., Cockayne's disease. *Am. J. Ophthalmol.*, *52*:116–118, 1961.
MacDonald, W. B., Fitch, K. D., and Lewis, I. C., Cockayne's syndrome. An heredo-familial disorder of growth and development. *Pediatrics, 25*:997–1007, 1960.
Moossy, J., The neuropathology of Cockayne's syndrome. *J. Neuropath. Exp. Neurol., 10*:654–660, 1967.
Paddison, R. M., Moossy, J., Derbes, V. J., and Kloepfer, W., Cockayne's syndrome. *Derm. Trop., 2*:196–203, 1963.
Riggs, W., Jr., and Seibert, J., Cockayne's syndrome; roentgen findings. *Am. J. Roentgenol., 116*:623–633, 1972.
Rowlatt, V., Cockayne's syndrome. Report of a case with necropsy findings. *Acta Neuropath., 14*:52–61, 1969.
Schönenberg, H., and Frohn, K., Das Cockayne-Syndrom. *Mschr. Kinderheilk., 117*:103–108, 1969.

REFSUM SYNDROME

(Heredopathia Atactica Polyneuritiformis)

A syndrome characterized by retinitis pigmentosa, hypertrophic peripheral neuropathy with both motor and sensory losses, ataxia, and, at times, sensorineural hearing loss was first thoroughly described by Refsum (1946) in two unrelated Norwegian families. Over 50 cases have been reported subsequently.

CLINICAL FINDINGS

Physical Findings. The patient usually appears normal until the second decade, when muscle wasting, weakness, and visual deterioration are noted. There is slow progression of the disorder in adult life. The condition may be aggravated by pregnancy (Fryer *et al.*, 1971).

Ocular System. Visual loss is probably one of the first symptoms of the syndrome. Night blindness, first noted at the beginning of the second decade, is slowly progressive, resulting in severe difficulty in the late teens. The visual fields slowly constrict. The pupils react sluggishly. Miosis and hemeralopia are virtually constant findings. Ophthalmologic examination reveals pale discs and mildly increased retinal pigment, most marked in the macula and peripheral retina. The retinal vessels appear narrowed. Posterior cataracts have been noted in about 80 per cent of the cases (Richterich *et al.*, 1965a), and nystagmus and anisocoria are relatively common (Fryer *et al.*, 1971).

Nervous System. Ataxia and weakness are generally noted in childhood or in early adult life, the weakness particularly affecting the legs and later, the arms. Muscle wasting and paralysis are slowly progressive, most marked distally in the extremities. In childhood, numbness to pinprick and touch is noticed in the distal extremities, gradually progressing to impair vibration and position sensation. Tendon reflexes decrease until the patient becomes areflexic. Most patients have abnormal finger-nose test and positive Romberg sign.

In a review of 37 reported patients, Richterich *et al.* (1965a) found the following signs in decreasing order of frequency: anosmia, paresthesias, pain, lack of superficial reflexes, external congenital ophthalmoplegia, and palpable peripheral nerves.

Cardiovascular System. In 20 of 25 reported patients, heart disease was present. Clinical findings included tachycardia, gallop rhythm, systolic murmur, heart enlargement, and cardiac insufficiency (Richterich *et al.*, 1965a). Electrocardiographic abnormalities, such as increased P-Q interval, nodal and auricular extrasystoles, and alteration in the QRS complex, were present in about 35 per cent of the patients.

Skeletal System. About 75 per cent of patients have some type of bone changes, the most common being spondylitis, exostoses of the sternum, kyphoscoliosis, hammer toes, and pes cavus. Occasionally, abnormalities such as shortening of some metacarpal or metatarsal bones or claw hand have been found (Richterich *et al.*, 1965a).

Integumentary System. In about 60 per cent of young patients, a mild ichthyosis has been noted.

Auditory System. Of 44 patients with the Refsum syndrome, Bergsmark and Djupesland (1968) found sensorineural hearing loss in 34 cases. Often the hearing loss is more severe on one side than on the other.

There appears to be mild variation in the degree of deafness in different affected individuals. Hearing loss most often begins in the second or third decade of life and progresses slowly, involving the higher frequencies in particular. Tone decay and speech discrimination tests have been normal.

Vestibular System. Caloric vestibular tests have been normal (Fleming, 1957; Bergsmark and Djupesland, 1968).

PATHOLOGY

There is marked accumulation of lipid in the liver and meninges. Blood vessels of the cerebral cortex are surrounded by numerous lipid-filled macrophages. The larger neurons of the central nervous system are slightly enlarged by accumulation of lipid granules in their cytoplasm. There is also diffuse enlargement of all peripheral nerves. Histologic section shows a marked decrease in the number of fibrils in each nerve. "Onion bulb" formations, due to proliferation of Schwann cells, appear about all nerve fibers, thereby producing the hypertrophic neuropathy. There is also some loss of inferior olivary neurons, which possibly contributes to the ataxia found in many patients (Steinberg et al., 1967; Fardeau and Engel, 1969).

Testicular atrophy occurs with interruption of spermatogenesis but with preservation of supporting cells.

Hallpike (1967), describing the temporal bone abnormalities of a patient with severe hearing loss secondary to the Refsum syndrome, found collapse of Reissner's membrane, degeneration of the stria vascularis, atrophy of the organ of Corti, and loss of spiral ganglion cells.

ETIOLOGY

The disorder results from a metabolic error in the oxidative degradation of phytanic acid, a process that normally proceeds by alpha oxidation followed by successive beta oxidative steps. The enzyme defect results in the accumulation of phytanic acid in the plasma (normal level is less than 2 micrograms per milliliter) to about 100 times the normal level. MacBrinn and O'Brien (1968) found high levels of phytanic acid in peripheral nerves and suggested that the accumulation of phytanate caused demyelination.

HEREDITY

Among the 50 published cases of the Refsum syndrome, all pedigrees are compatible with autosomal recessive transmission (Richterich et al., 1965b). Parental consanguinity was found in over half the cases. Heterozygotes can be identified from fibroblast culture. Prenatal diagnosis should be possible but has not been reported (Steinberg, 1971).

DIAGNOSIS

In *Usher syndrome*, the retinitis pigmentosa and hearing loss are not associated with hypertrophic peripheral neuropathy, as found in Refsum syndrome. Patients with the Dejerine-Sottas syndrome have a slowly progressive polyneuropathy and hypertrophic nerves but no evidence of visual or auditory deficits. The patients described by Kearns and Sayre (1958) and by Jager et al. (1960) with *progressive external ophthalmoplegia, retinal pigmentary degeneration, cardiac conduction defects, and mixed hearing loss* represent a separate entity, since there was no night blindness, pupillary abnormalities, peripheral neuritis, or perineural peripheral changes.

TREATMENT

Eldjarn et al. (1966) and Kark et al. (1971) reported that a diet low in phytanic acid and phytol resulted in decreased plasma phytanic acid concentration and in subjective and objective improvement. Hearing may be improved by use of a hearing aid.

PROGNOSIS

The course is variable. Usually, there is slow progression of the neurologic deficits; complete incapacitation eventually results. Among reported cases, 20 per cent died in the first decade, 30 per cent in the third decade, 20 per cent in the fourth decade, and 10 per cent in the fifth decade of life.

SUMMARY

The syndrome is characterized by: 1) autosomal recessive inheritance, 2) progressive atypical retinitis pigmentosa with constricted visual fields and night blindness, 3) hypertrophic peripheral neuropathy, 4) mild cerebellar ataxia and nystagmus, 5) increased plasma phytanic acid, and 6) progressive sensorineural hearing loss in about half of those affected.

Figure 4-6 Refsum syndrome. (A) Sibs showing muscle wasting of lower legs. (From D. Steinberg et al., Ann. Intern. Med., 66:365, 1967.) (B) Similar changes in patient treated with special diet. (C) Atrophy of hand muscles. (D) Ichthyosis of skin. (B, C, and D courtesy of S. Refsum, Oslo, Norway.) (E) Transverse section of nerve from patient with Refsum syndrome showing decreased numbers of myelinated fibers and proliferation of Schwann sheath. (From M. Fardeau and W. K. Engel, J. Neuropath. Exp. Neurol., 28:278, 1969.)

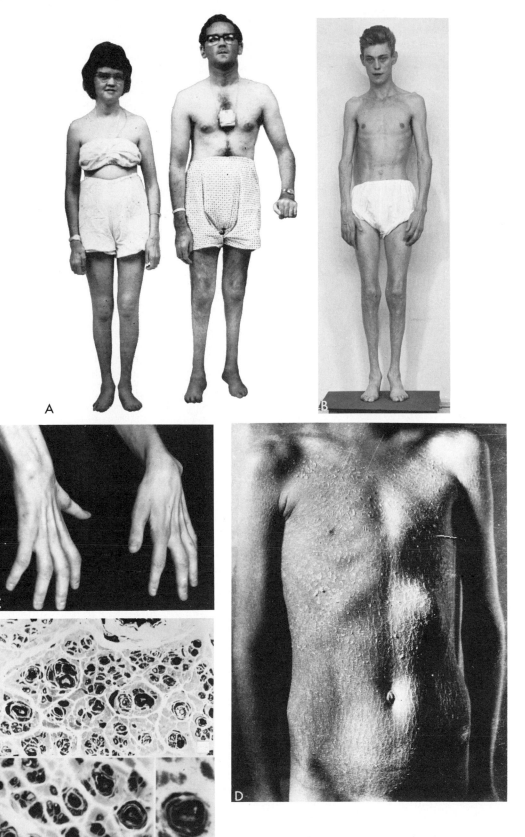

Figure 4-6 See legend on the opposite page

REFERENCES

Bergsmark, J., and Djupesland, G., Heredopathia atactica polyneuritiformis (Refsum's disease). An audiological examination of two patients. *Eur. Neurol., 1*:122–130, 1968.

Eldjarn, L., Try, K., Stokke, O., Munthe-Kaas, A. W., Refsum, S., Steinberg, D., Avigan, J., and Mize, G.: Dietary effects on serum-phytanic acid levels and on clinical manifestations in heredopathia atactica polyneuritiformis. *Lancet, 1*:691–693, 1966.

Fardeau, M., and Engel, W. K., Ultrastructural study of a peripheral nerve biopsy in Refsum's disease. *J. Neuropath. Exp. Neurol., 28*:278–294, 1969.

Fleming, R., Refsum's syndrome. *Neurology (Minneap.), 7*:476–479, 1957.

Fryer, D. G., Winckleman, A. C., Ways, P. O., and Swanson, A. G., Refsum's disease. *Neurology (Minneap.), 21*:162–167, 1971.

Hallpike, C. S., Observations on the structural basis of two rare varieties of hereditary deafness. In *Myotatic, Kinesthetic and Vestibular Mechanisms.* CIBA Foundation Symposium. de Reuch, A. V. S., and Knight, J. (eds.), Boston, Little, Brown and Company, 1967, pp. 285–294.

Jager, B. V., Fred, H. L., Butler, R. B., and Carnes, W. H.: Occurrence of retinal pigmentation, ophthalmoplegia, ataxia, deafness, and heart block. *Am. J. Med., 29*:888–893, 1960.

Kark, A. P., Engel, W. K., Blass, J. P., Steinberg, D., and Walsh, G. O., Heredopathia atactica polyneuritiformis (Refsum's disease): a second trial of dietary therapy in two patients. *Birth Defects, 7*(1):53–55, 1971.

Kearns, T. P., and Sayre, G. P., Retinitis pigmentosa, external ophthalmoplegia, and complete heart block. *Arch. Ophthalmol., 60*:280–289, 1958. (Case 2.)

MacBrinn, M. C., and O'Brien, J. S., Lipid composition of the nervous system in Refsum's disease. *J. Lipid Res., 9*:552–561, 1968.

Refsum, S., Heredopathia atactica polyneuritiformis. *Acta Psychiatr. Neurol. Scand., Suppl. 38*:1–303, 1946.

Richterich, R., Moser, H., and Rossi, E., Refsum's disease (Heredopathia atactica polyneuritiformis). *Humangenetik, 1*:324–332, 1965a.

Richterich, R., Rosin, S., and Rossi, E., Refsum's disease. Formal genetics. *Humangenetik, 1*:333–336, 1965b.

Steinberg, D., The metabolic basis of the Refsum syndrome. *Birth Defects, 7*(1): 42–52, 1971.

Steinberg, D., Vroom, F. Q., Engel, W. K., Cammermeyer, J., Mize, C. E., and Avigan, J., Refsum's disease — a recently characterized lipidosis involving the nervous system. *Ann. Intern. Med., 66*:365–395, 1967.

INVERSE RETINITIS PIGMENTOSA, HYPOGONADISM, AND SENSORINEURAL DEAFNESS

Reinstein and Chalfin (1971) reported a syndrome of inverse retinitis pigmentosa, hypogenitalism, and sensorineural deafness in two female and one male sib.

CLINICAL FINDINGS

Ocular System. Blurring of central vision was first experienced at 20 to 30 years of age. Impairment progressed slowly to a stable end point over the next 5 to 10 years. No impairment of night or color vision was experienced. Alterations in the fundus consisted of a concentration of bone-spicule pigmentation confined to the posterior pole, i.e., surrounding the macula and disc, sometimes in the form of a discrete ring and often with attenuation of retinal vessels and disc pallor. Subadjacent choroidal sclerosis may also be found. Discrete mottled macular lesions were noted in the three sibs.

Dark adaptation thresholds were elevated, electroretinograms were markedly depressed, and visual fields showed dense central scotomas with peripheral depression.

Genital System. In the male sib, secondary sexual characteristics appeared at 14 years of age. At 60 years of age the testes were found to be small and soft. The patient denied impotence.

Neither female sib had spontaneous menarche; menses were achieved only with estrogen therapy. Breast development and pubic hair growth occurred only after hormone therapy.

Auditory System. The male sib noted the onset of a slowly progressive hearing loss from 11 years of age. When over 60 years old, he was found to have a moderately severe sensorineural hearing loss. At about 35 years of age one female sib first experienced hearing impairment, which

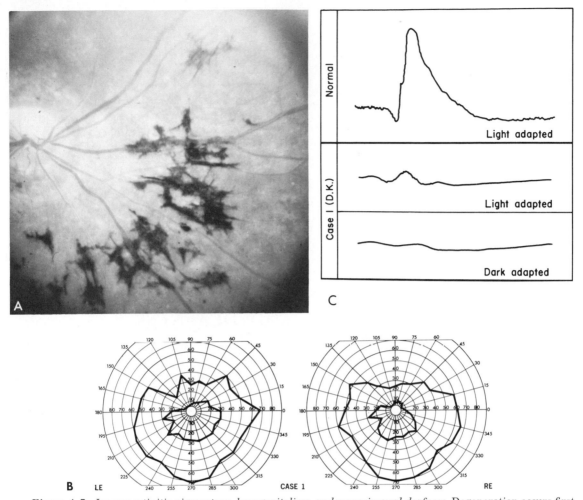

Figure 4-7 *Inverse retinitis pigmentosa, hypogenitalism, and sensorineural deafness.* Degeneration occurs first around macula with loss of central vision—a condition which is the opposite of that seen in the usual form of retinitis pigmentosa. (*A*) Note pigmentary changes, attenuation and sheathing of arterioles, secondary macular degenerative changes as indicated by areas of pigmentation, early secondary optic atrophy, and peripapillary halo. (*B*) Visual fields showing loss of central vision. (*C*) Electroretinograms showing depressed photic curves and extinguished scotopic curves. (From N. M. Reinstein and A. I. Chalfin, *Am. J. Ophthalmol.*, 72:332, 1971.)

slowly progressed to severe sensorineural loss over 2000 Hz. The other female sib initially manifested hearing loss at about 40 years of age and eight years later had a moderate sensorineural deficit, more marked in the higher frequencies.

LABORATORY FINDINGS

No significant findings were reported.

HEREDITY

The three affected sibs were the product of a consanguineous union. The parents and maternal grandparents were both first cousins of Ashkenazic Jewish extraction. Inheritance appears to be autosomal recessive.

DIAGNOSIS

In contrast to the typical peripheral form of retinitis pigmentosa, which can exist as an isolated finding or as part of several syndromes, inverse retinitis pigmentosa is characterized by absence of night blindness, early loss of central vision, and, frequently, preference for dim rather than bright illumination.

TREATMENT

Exogenous hormone treatment is apparently required to initiate pubertal changes.

PROGNOSIS

Impaired vision, usually appearing in the third decade, progressively deteriorates to severe loss over the next decade.

SUMMARY

Characteristics of the syndrome include 1) autosomal recessive inheritance, 2) inverse retinitis pigmentosa, absent night blindness, early loss of central vision, preference for dim illumination, 3) hypogonadism, and 4) sensorineural deafness.

REFERENCE

Reinstein, N. M., and Chalfin, A. I., Inverse retinitis pigmentosa, deafness, and hypogenitalism. *Am. J. Ophthalmol.*, 72:332–341, 1971.

RETINAL CHANGES, MUSCULAR WASTING, MENTAL RETARDATION, AND DEAFNESS

A syndrome including deafness, retinal detachment, muscular dystrophy, and mental retardation appearing in four of seven sibs was described by Small (1968).

CLINICAL FINDINGS

Physical Findings. Each of the affected sibs had wasting of the face, trunk, and limbs, which progressed from childhood (Fig. 4–8A).

Ocular System. The diagnosis of Coats' disease, an exudative or hemorrhagic retinitis, was made in each of the children. The optic fundi showed changes, including mild to moderate tortuosity of retinal vessels, telangiectasia, retinal detachment, and elevation of the peripheral retina by exudate.

Nervous System. All of the affected children were mentally retarded, with I.Q.s ranging from about 35 to 50 in the two children tested. Each of the children had some difficulty walking; clumsiness and weakness were noted at about 1 year of age. Reflexes and coordination were not described.

Musculoskeletal System. The affected children had been weak since infancy. Muscle wasting — particularly of the face, limbs, and trunk — was evident in early childhood, progressing slowly thereafter. The facies

was immobile. All had kyphosis and lordosis.

Auditory System. Hearing defects were noted in each of the affected children. One sib was noted to be deaf since birth, with speech consisting of only a few words. In another child, the hearing loss was not noticed until she was 9 years old. The severity of the hearing loss was not described. No puretone or other audiometric tests were described.

Vestibular System. No vestibular findings were presented.

LABORATORY FINDINGS

The level of creatinine phosphokinase was measured in two patients; it was elevated to 1.2 milliunits (upper normal 0.72) in one and was normal in the other. An electrocardiogram was normal in one patient. In another child there was incomplete right bundle branch block or right ventricular hypertrophy. Electroencephalograms, taken in two cases, showed reduced amplitude. Other laboratory tests were normal.

PATHOLOGY

A gastrocnemius muscle biopsy showed no diagnostic abnormality. Histopathologic

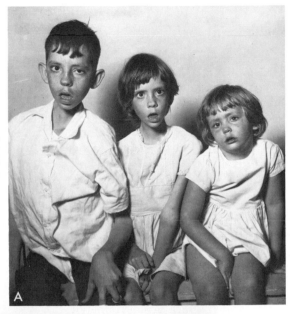

Figure 4-8 Retinal changes, muscular wasting, mental retardation, and deafness. (A) Sibs showing expressionless facies. (B) Marked tortuosity of retinal vessels. (From R. G. Small, Trans. Am. Acad. Ophthalmol. Otolaryngol., 72:225, 1968.)

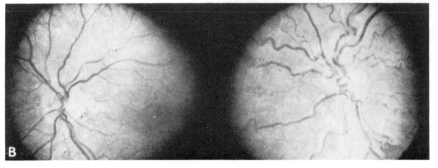

examination of an enucleated eye showed changes consistent with Coats' disease.

HEREDITY

In this family, four of seven sibs had a similar syndrome. The father was examined and found to be normal. The mother was not available for testing, but she was reported to be normal. The parents were not known to be related. From the evidence available it would seem that this syndrome exhibits autosomal recessive inheritance.

DIAGNOSIS

No other known diseases have this combination of retinal disease and exudative retinitis. In classic Coats' disease there is no associated hearing loss or mental deficiency.

TREATMENT

Patients should be referred to an ophthalmologist for treatment of hemorrhagic retinitis as indicated.

PROGNOSIS

Prognosis is poor due to progressive eye changes and mental retardation.

SUMMARY

Characteristics of this syndrome include: 1) autosomal recessive inheritance, 2) retinal changes, including tortuous vessels and exudative retinitis, 3) moderate to severe mental retardation, 4) muscle weakness and wasting involving the face, trunk, and extremities, 5) mild but progressive ataxia, and 6) moderate to severe hearing loss.

REFERENCE

Small, R. G., Coats' disease and muscular dystrophy. *Trans. Am. Acad. Ophthalmol. Otolaryngol.,* 72:225–231, 1968.

CRYPTOPHTHALMIA SYNDROME AND MIXED DEAFNESS

First described by Zehender (1872), the cryptophthalmia syndrome consists of extension of the skin of the forehead to completely cover one or both eyes, total or partial soft tissue syndactyly of fingers and/or toes, coloboma of the nasal alae, abnormal hairline, various urogenital abnormalities, and mixed deafness.

About 60 cases have been reported under a variety of names. Especially good reviews are those of Sugar (1968), Ide and Wollschlaeger (1969), François (1969) and Schönenberg (1973).

CLINICAL FINDINGS

Physical Findings. Usually, the cranium and the face are asymmetric.

Ocular System. In about 65 per cent of the cases, the cryptophthalmos is bilateral (Schönenberg, 1973). The eyebrows may be completely or partially missing (Zinn, 1955). The globes can be seen and felt beneath the skin, which extends from the forehead to cover the eyes. Exposure to strong light may induce reflex wrinkling of the skin resulting from contraction of the orbicularis muscles. In the case of unilateral cryptophthalmos, the opposite eye may exhibit upper-lid coloboma, symblepharon, microphthalmia, or epibulbar dermoid (Sugar, 1968). A tongue of hair often extends from the forehead into the area normally occupied by the eye.

Nasal System. Abnormality of the nose is seen in about 50 per cent of the patients. In most cases, a bulbous tip and coloboma of the nasal alae with a groove extending to the nasal tip are noted. The alar defect may be unilateral or bilateral, and often there is associated nasal asymmetry.

Genital System. Malformation of the genitals have included small penis, cryptorchidism, chordee, hypospadias, and hypertrophy of the clitoris with vaginal aplasia or hypoplastic fused labia and bicornuate uterus (Gupta and Saxena, 1966; Ide and Wollschlaeger, 1969).

Nervous System. Some patients have exhibited calcification of the falx cerebri. Ide and Wollschlaeger (1969) found the foramen magnum to be heart-shaped with incomplete closure of the exoccipital portion of the occipital bone. Meningoencephalocele has been described in about 10 per cent (Zinn, 1955). A small percentage of patients has been found to be mentally retarded (Ide and Wollschlaeger, 1969).

Integumentary System. Soft tissue syndactyly of variable degree of the fingers and/or toes has been present in about 35 per cent of the cases (Sugar, 1968).

Skeletal System. There may be hypoplasia of the parietal bone with increased digital markings, and flattening of the orbital and temporal regions (Schönenberg, 1973). Spina bifida occulta has been noted in at least 10 per cent of affected persons, and often wide separation of the symphysis pubis has been found (Zehender, 1872; Fraser, 1962; Ide and Wollschlaeger, 1969).

Oral Findings. Cleft lip and/or cleft palate and ankyloglossia have been noted in about 10 per cent of the cases. Laryngeal stenosis occurs in about 10 per cent.

Miscellaneous Findings. Anal atresia, umbilical hernia, and unilateral renal aplasia have been evident in 10 per cent (Fraser, 1962; Gupta and Saxena, 1962; Steidl, 1962; Viallefont *et al.*, 1965; François, 1969).

Auditory System. The pinnae are small, poorly modeled, lowset, or posteriorly rotated in at least 30 per cent of the cases. Not uncommonly, the skin of the upper part of the helix is continuous with that of the scalp. The external auditory canals are often narrowed or completely stenotic in the outer third to outer half (Chiari, 1883; Thorp, 1945; Gupta and Saxena, 1962; Otradovec and Janovsky, 1962; Fraser, 1963; Viallefont *et al.*, 1965; Ehlers, 1966; François, 1969; Ide and Wollschlaeger, 1969; Schönenberg, 1973). This narrowing or stenosis may occur bilaterally, even though the cryptophthalmos is unilateral (Schönenberg, 1973). Ide and Wollschlaeger (1969) found normal internal auditory canals. Ossicles have been noted to be malformed, resulting in mixed, mostly conductive hearing loss (Ide and Wollschlaeger, 1969).

Vestibular System. No studies have been reported.

LABORATORY FINDINGS

Roentgenograms. Roentgenographic studies have shown flattening of the orbital

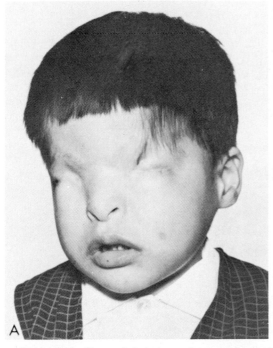

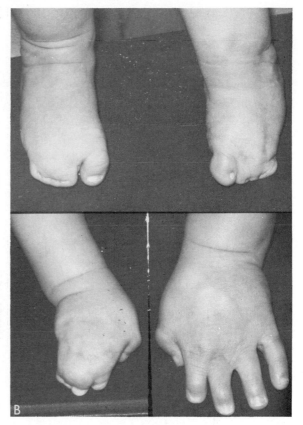

Figure 4–9 *Cryptophthalmia syndrome and mixed deafness.* *(A)* Cryptophthalmia in a Greenlandic boy of normal intelligence. He had unilateral renal aplasia and hypospadias. (From M. Warburg, *Birth Defects,* 7(3):136, 1971.) *(B)* Variable soft tissue syndactyly of fingers and toes. (From N. D. Dinno *et al., Clin. Pediatr.,* *13*:219, 1974.)

and temporal regions, hypoplasia of the parietal bone with increased digital markings, and widening of the symphysis pubis.

HEREDITY

The syndrome is inherited in an autosomal recessive pattern. Parental consanguinity has been present in at least 15 per cent.

DIAGNOSIS

This disorder is so striking that other conditions would not be considered.

TREATMENT

Surgical correction of the cryptophthalmos has been uniformly of no avail. The cutaneous syndactyly, if severe, may be corrected by plastic surgery. Neither has surgical correction of the stenotic ear canals been carried out nor has treatment of the ossicular defects been attempted.

SUMMARY

Cryptophthalmia syndrome is characterized by: 1) autosomal recessive inheritance, 2) unilateral or more often bilateral extension of skin of the forehead to completely cover the eye or eyes, 3) variable soft tissue syndactyly of the fingers and/or toes, 4) coloboma of the nasal alae, 5) various urogenital anomalies, and 6) mixed deafness and atresia of the external auditory canals.

REFERENCES

Chiari, H., Congenitales Ankylo- et Symblepharon. *Prag. Z. Heilk., 4*:143–154, 1883.

Ehlers, N., Cryptophthalmos with orbito-palpebral cyst and microphthalmos. *Acta Ophthalmol. (Kbh.), 44*:84–94, 1966.

François, J., Syndrome malformatif avec cryptophtalmie. *Acta Genet. Med. (Roma), 18*:18–50, 1969.

Fraser, G. R., Our genetical load. *Ann. Hum. Genet., 25*:387–415, 1962.

Gupta, S. P., and Saxena, R. C., Cryptophthalmos. *Br. J. Ophthalmol., 46*:629–632, 1962.

Guttman, A., Einseitiger Kryptophthalmos. *Zbl. Prakt. Augenheilk., 33*:264, 1909.

Ide, C. H., and Wollschlaeger, P. B., Multiple congenital abnormalities associated with crypt-ophthalmia. *Arch. Ophthalmol., 81*:640–644, 1969.

Otradovec, J., and Janovsky, M., Cryptophthalmos. *Cs. Oftal., 18*:128–138, 1962.

Schönenberg, H., Kryptophthalmos-Syndrom. *Klin. Pediätr., 185*:165–171, 1973.

Steidl, P., Un cas de cryptophtalmie. *Union Méd. Can., 91*:159–161, 1962.

Sugar, H. S., The cryptophthalmos-syndactyly syndrome. *Am. J. Ophthalmol., 66*:897–899, 1968.

Thorp, A. T., Bilateral cryptophthalmos and syndactylism. *N.C. Med. J., 6*:484, 1945.

Viallefont, H., Boudet, C., Balmes, J., and Costeau, J., Un cas de cryptophtalmie. *Bull. Soc. Ophtalmol. Franç., 65*:329–332, 1965.

Zehender, W., Eine Missgeburt mit hautüberwachsenen Augen oder Kryptophthalmos. *Klin. Mbl. Augenheilk., 10*:225–234, 1872.

Zinn, S., Kryptophthalmia. *Am. J. Ophthalmol., 40*:219–223, 1955.

MYOPIA, CATARACT, SADDLE NOSE, AND SENSORINEURAL HEARING LOSS

(Marshall Syndrome)

Seven members in four generations of a family studied by Marshall (1958) had a syndrome that included saddle-nose defect, congenital and juvenile cataracts, myopia, and sensorineural hearing loss. Another kindred was reported by Ruppert, Buerk, and Pfordrescher (1970). Zellweger, Smith, and Grutzner (1974) studied the same syndrome in a mother and in several of her children. The cases of Keith *et al.* (1972) are less certain examples.

CLINICAL FINDINGS

Physical Findings. The facies produced by the markedly small nose with sunken nasal bridge, anteverted nostrils, and hypoplastic midface is striking.

Ocular System. Failing vision usually occurs in the second decade of life, but in one patient of Ruppert *et al.* and in one patient of Marshall it occurred within the first six months. Posterior polar cortical and subcapsular opacities that spontaneously resorbed were noted in the second, third, and fourth decades by Marshall and in the first decade by Ruppert *et al.* Although the mother reported by Zellweger *et al.* had cataracts since 15 years of age, her children had not yet developed cataracts at 7 to 11 years of age. Severe myopia (10 diopters or more) was also evident from birth, as was fluid vitreous.

Retinal detachment occurred in one patient of Marshall and in the father of Ruppert's proband at 14 years of age.

Auditory System. In the kindred stud-ied by Marshall, affected family members reported some hearing loss in childhood. This loss progressed, and eventually hearing aids were required. Audiometric tests were reported as showing about 50 dB mixed or mostly sensorineural hearing loss in several members.

Ruppert *et al.* found severe deafness as early as 9 months of age in one child; at 6 years it did not appear to be progressive. A moderate high-tone sensorineural loss was noted in the father.

Zellweger *et al.* reported a 30 to 60 dB sensorineural hearing loss in the affected members of his kindred.

Vestibular System. Ruppert *et al.* reported normal vestibular findings.

LABORATORY FINDINGS

Roentgenograms. Roentgenographic studies have shown hypoplastic nasal bones, hypoplastic maxilla, absent frontal sinuses, and thickening of the outer table of the skull. O'Donnell *et al.* (1976) noted intracranial calcifications, beaked or bullet-shaped vertebrae in children, markedly concave vertebral margins in adults, small irregular pelvis with delayed closure of pubic and ischial bones, coxa valga, mild bowing of the radius and ulna, and somewhat irregular epiphyses of the extremities.

HEREDITY

The disorder, occurring in several generations, is clearly dominant. However,

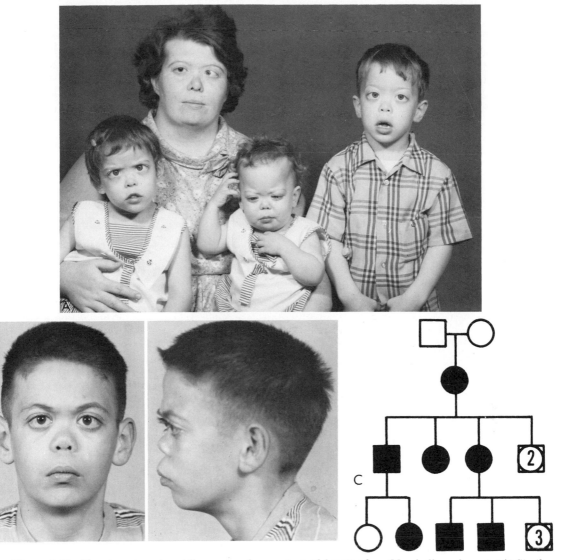

Figure 4–10 *Myopia, cataract, saddle nose, and sensorineural hearing loss* (Marshall syndrome). (*A*) Similar facies in a mother and three of her affected children. (From H. Zellweger *et al., J. Pediatr., 84*:868, 1975.) (*B*) Details of facies: small nose, depressed nasal bridge, and anteverted nostrils. Note that both eyes may be seen from the side. (From D. Marshall, *Am. J. Ophthalmol., 45*:143, 1958.) (*C*) Pedigree of affected kindred, modified from report of D. Marshall.

since there have been no examples of male-to-male transmission, X-linkage cannot yet be excluded.

DIAGNOSIS

Saddle-nose defect may be seen in congenital syphilis, acrodysostosis, and chondrodysplasia punctata. Myopia may occur as an isolated finding, as an autosomal dominant or recessive trait, or as a compo-

nent of numerous syndromes such as X-linked myopia and external ophthalmoplegia, *autosomal dominant spondyloepiphyseal dysplasia, Alport syndrome, or hereditary progressive arthroophthalmopathy* (Waardenburg *et al.,* 1961; McKusick, 1971).

TREATMENT

The cataracts should be removed and hearing aids should be employed. Maxillo-

facial surgery can correct the midface hypoplasia if such a correction is deemed cosme-
tically desirable by the patient.

PROGNOSIS

The deafness is progressive.

SUMMARY

Characteristics of this syndrome include: 1) autosomal dominant transmission,
2) severe myopia, 3) congenital and juvenile
cataracts, 4) saddle-nose defect, 5) various
skeletal abnormalities, and 6) early-onset
progressive moderate sensorineural hearing
loss.

REFERENCES

Keith, C. G., Dobbs, R. H., Shaw, D. G., and Cottrall, K., Abnormal facies, myopia, and short
    stature. *Arch. Dis. Child., 47*:787–793, 1972.
McKusick, V. A., *Mendelian Inheritance in Man,* 3rd Ed. Baltimore, Md., Johns Hopkins Press,
    1971.
Marshall, D., Ectodermal dysplasia. Report of kindred with ocular abnormalities and hearing
    defect. *Am. J. Ophthalmol., 45*:143–156, 1958.
O'Donnell, J. J., Sirkin, S., and Hall, B. D., Generalized osseous abnormalities in Marshall's
    syndrome. *Birth Defects,* in press.
Ruppert, E. S., Buerk, E., and Pfordrescher, M. F., Hereditary hearing loss with saddle-nose and
    myopia. *Arch. Otolaryngol., 92*:95–98, 1970.
Waardenburg, P. J. M., Franceschetti, A., and Klein, D., *Genetics and Ophthalmology.* Spring-
    field, Ill., Charles C Thomas, Publisher, 1961.
Zellweger, H., Smith, J. K., and Grutzner, P., The Marshall syndrome: report of a new family. *J.
    Pediatr., 84*:868–871, 1974.

MYOPIA, BLUE SCLERAE, MARFANOID HABITUS, AND SENSORINEURAL DEAFNESS

Walker (1971) described a syndrome of
loose-jointedness, arachnodactyly, keratoconus, myopia, and sensorineural deafness
in three or possibly four generations.

CLINICAL FINDINGS

Ocular System. Keratoconus and myopia with rupture posteriorly in Descemet's
membrane were noted in the proposita (Fig.
4–11*D*). Blue sclerae and myopia were
present in all affected.
Musculoskeletal System. Striking arachnodactyly and loose-jointedness were
noted at birth in all affected. The nails were
longitudinally grooved. The joint hypermobility was most marked in the fingers,
thumbs, wrists, and elbows. Genu recurvatum was present in at least two affected
persons, but scoliosis was not evident in
any of the kindred. Pectus excavatum was
present in some (Fig. 4–11*A* to *D*).
Auditory System. Audiograms done at
7 to 9 years of age showed a mild sensorineural hearing loss. This progressed to se-

vere loss, being more marked at higher
frequencies in both children. The father
was not deaf. The father's mother did not
experience hearing loss until she was 60
years old.
Vestibular System. Studies were not
described.

LABORATORY FINDINGS

No studies were reported.

HEREDITY

The syndrome, present with variable
expressivity in three or possibly four generations, has autosomal dominant inheritance.

DIAGNOSIS

Joint hypermobility can be inherited as
an isolated dominant trait or as part of
numerous syndromes. Arachnodactyly, joint
hypermobility, and dominant inheritance

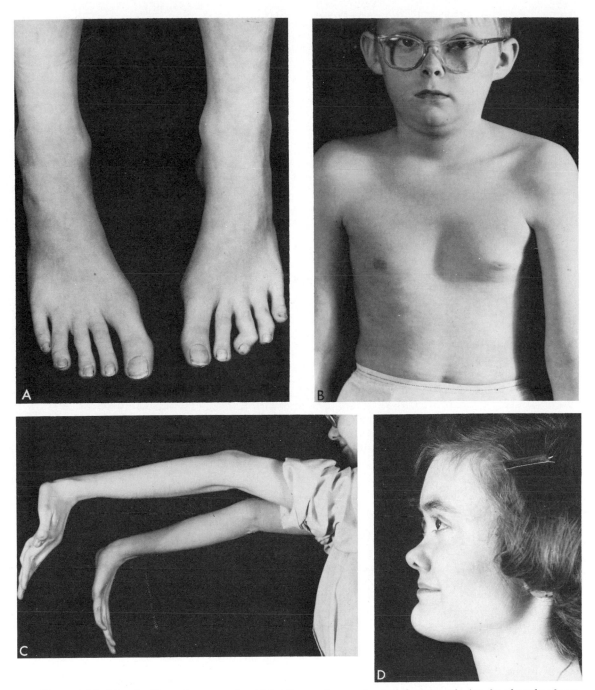

Figure 4–11 *Myopia, blue sclerae, marfanoid habitus, and sensorineural deafness.* (A) Arachnodactyly of toes. (B) Pectus excavatum in 11-year-old male. (C) Nineteen-year-old sib exhibiting hyperextension of elbows, wrists, and fingers. (D) Note keratoconus in lateral view. (A–D from B. A. Walker, *Birth Defects*, 7(4):137, 1971.)

are present in Marfan syndrome; however, no dislocation of lenses or cardiovascular anomalies should rule out that disorder. One must exclude the Ehlers-Danlos syndrome and the autosomal recessively inherited syndrome of *keratoconus, blue sclerae, loose ligaments, and conduction deafness.*

TREATMENT

The hearing loss may be minimized by use of a hearing aid.

PROGNOSIS

The deafness is progressive.

SUMMARY

Characteristics of this syndrome include: 1) autosomal dominant inheritance, 2) myopia, blue sclerae, and occasionally keratoconus, 3) arachnodactyly and loose-jointedness, and 4) progressive sensorineural deafness that is more marked in the higher frequencies.

REFERENCES

Walker, B. A., A syndrome of nerve deafness, eye anomalies, and marfanoid habitus with autosomal dominant inheritance. *Birth Defects,* 7(4):137–139, 1971.

MYOPIA, PERIPHERAL NEUROPATHY, SKELETAL ABNORMALITIES, AND SENSORINEURAL DEAFNESS

A syndrome characterized by myopia, hearing loss, shooting pains, joint stiffness, and mental symptoms was described in 15 members of a family by Flynn and Aird in 1965. Bilateral sensorineural hearing loss and myopia developed in the first decade of life. Ataxia, peripheral shooting pains, joint symptoms, and cerebral changes followed in the second and third decades.

CLINICAL FINDINGS

Physical Findings. Affected persons had moderate kyphosis and were thin with poor muscular development (Fig. 4–12*A*).

Ocular System. Eye defects included severe myopia (90 per cent), bilateral cataracts (50 per cent), atypical retinitis pigmentosa (20 per cent), and total blindness (5 per cent). Visual difficulties (especially myopia), beginning in the second decade, progressed in the third decade to restricted visual fields and night blindness, resulting finally in severe visual loss.

Nervous System. Shooting pains in the limbs and face with progressive sensory loss, decreased reflexes, muscle wasting, and weakness began at about 20 years of age and progressed slowly thereafter.

Atypical seizures consisting of episodes of expressive aphasia without the demonstrable defects of comprehension were noted in several patients.

Skeletal System. Many patients had kyphoscoliosis that followed the muscle wasting and peripheral neuritis.

Integumentary System. Atrophy of the skin and subcutaneous tissue was found in 85 per cent of the cases. The skin over the ankles and feet tended to break down easily, resulting in chronic ulcers. Baldness was a late manifestation.

Auditory System. Bilateral sensorineural hearing loss was variable in different affected persons, beginning in the first decade and progressing either slowly or moderately rapidly to severe deafness by the second to sixth decades. Hearing loss was present in all of 15 cases reviewed by the authors. No further hearing tests were noted.

Vestibular System. No vestibular findings were described.

LABORATORY FINDINGS

Roentgenographic examination showed generalized emphysema, kyphoscoliosis, and generalized osteoporosis as well as multiple cystic areas measuring up to 3 cm. in diameter in the pelvis above the acetabulae (Fig. 4–12*C*).

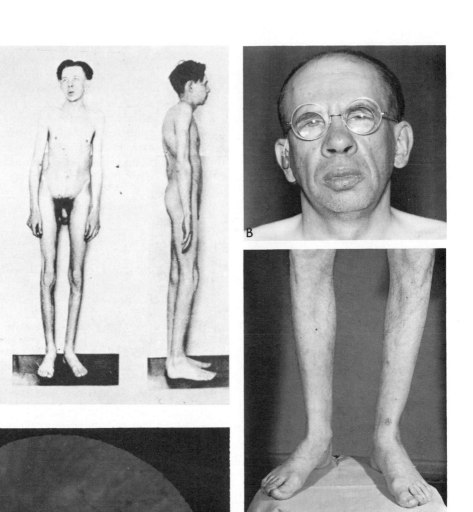

Figure 4-12 *Myopia, peripheral neuropathy, skeletal abnormalities, and sensorineural deafness. (A)* A 24-year-old showing kyphoscoliosis and muscle wasting. (From P. Flynn and R. B. Aird, *J. Neurol. Sci.*, *2*:161, 1965.) *(B)* Same patient at 51 years of age. He had become progressively kyphotic, his features had coarsened, his musculature had remained poorly developed, and his vision and hearing had become progressively worse. (Courtesy of P. Flynn, San Francisco.) *(C)* Note muscular atrophy of lower legs. The skin is atrophic and subject to indolent ulcers. (Courtesy of P. Flynn, San Francisco.) *(D)* Fundus showing atypical retinitis pigmentosa. (Courtesy of P. Flynn, San Francisco.) *(E)* Pedigree of family showing 15 affected persons in five generations of this kindred. (Modified from P. Flynn and R. B. Aird.)

Electroencephalographic studies showed generalized dysrhythmia compatible with a convulsive disorder.

Routine blood and urine examinations were normal. Serum calcium and phosphorus levels were normal. Liver and kidney function tests were normal. Spinal fluid protein was elevated in a few patients.

PATHOLOGY

Autopsies performed on five patients showed brain atrophy with ischemia in three cases. In another case the thyroid was enlarged. Diffuse bilateral adrenal hypertrophy associated with pituitary basophilic hyperplasia was found in one case. In two other cases the adrenals were atrophic. Bilateral cataracts and retinitis pigmentosa were found.

Skin biopsies showed hyperkeratosis with absence of rete ridges. Sweat glands and hair follicles were sparse. Nerve biopsy showed changes indicative of a peripheral neuropathy.

HEREDITY

In five generations of this family there were 15 persons affected with the syndrome. The pedigree demonstrated autosomal dominant transmission of the syndrome with variable expressivity.

DIAGNOSIS

Various syndromes must be excluded. Werner syndrome is characterized by sclerodermatoid alterations that appear in the second decade accompanied by premature aging, bilateral cataracts, osteoporosis, arteriosclerosis, ulcers of the lower legs, and autosomal recessive inheritance. The *Refsum syndrome* with its progressive retinitis pigmentosa, sensorineural hearing loss, and peripheral neuropathy also exhibits similarities. However, in the Refsum syndrome, there is no severe skin atrophy or myopia; it is inherited as an autosomal recessive condition, and there is elevated serum phytanic acid. The *Usher syndrome* is characterized by progressive retinitis pigmentosa and sensorineural hearing loss, is transmitted recessively, and lacks the skin involvement or myopia found in the syndrome considered here.

TREATMENT

Only a few of the effects of the syndrome can be treated. The myopia can be corrected by glasses, and the hearing loss can be minimized by a hearing aid.

PROGNOSIS

Although the rate of progression varied, the hearing and visual loss caused severe disability early in life. The peripheral neuropathy was slowly progressive and may have been a factor in some of the patients' developing pneumonia, thereby shortening the life span.

SUMMARY

Characteristics of this disease include: 1) dominant transmission with variable expressivity, 2) eye defects including myopia, cataracts, and retinitis pigmentosa, 3) peripheral neuropathy with shooting pains, sensory loss, and weakness, 4) skeletal abnormalities including kyphoscoliosis, 5) central nervous system involvement including peculiar seizures and abnormal EEG findings, and 6) progressive sensorineural hearing loss.

REFERENCE

Flynn, P., and Aird, R. B., A neuroectodermal syndrome of dominant inheritance. *J. Neurol. Sci.*, 2:161–182, 1965.

MYOPIA AND CONGENITAL SENSORINEURAL HEARING LOSS

The combination of congenital sensorineural hearing loss, myopia, and low intelligence was described in a sibship by Eldridge, Berlin, Money, and McKusick (1968), who studied an Amish family in which four of seven sibs had this syndrome.

CLINICAL FINDINGS

Physical Findings. Each of the four affected children was well developed with normal stature.

Ocular System. Visual tests in three of the sibs exhibited myopia of about 15 diopters.

Nervous System. Psychometric testing showed retardation; this condition may have resulted from sensory deprivation rather than from neurologic disturbance.

Auditory System. Hearing loss in each of the affected children was noted in early childhood. There was no evident progression of the hearing loss. Otologic examinations revealed normal external auditory canals and tympanic membranes. Pure-tone audiometric tests showed a 30 to 100 dB sensorineural hearing loss, which was more marked in the higher frequencies. A SISI test carried out on one child was positive, suggesting a cochlear locus for the hearing loss. Other audiologic tests were not done.

Vestibular System. Caloric vestibular tests showed normal vestibular function.

LABORATORY FINDINGS

Analyses of blood, urine, and cerebrospinal fluid as well as a radiologic survey showed no abnormalities. In a 13-year-old girl an electroencephalogram showed slightly more slow activity than normal.

HEREDITY

The pedigree of Eldridge *et al.* showed four affected in a sibship of seven. The parents were normal; there was no history of hearing or visual defect in either family. The parents were distantly related, thus making autosomal recessive transmission most likely.

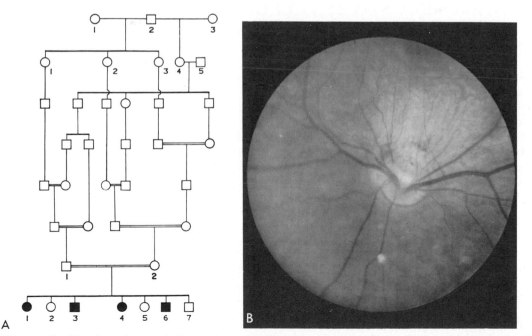

Figure 4–13 *Myopia and congenital sensorineural hearing loss. (A)* Pedigree of inbred Amish family showing four affected persons. *(B)* Fundus showing temporal pallor and prominent choroidal vascular pattern associated with severe myopia. (From R. Eldridge *et al., Arch. Otolaryngol., 88*:49, 1968.)

DIAGNOSIS

A family was described by Ohlsson (1963) in which three boys in a sibship of seven had sensorineural deafness and severe myopia. Six of the seven sibs, including the three with deafness and myopia, had albuminuria or hematuria, as did the mother. Audiometric tests of the three male sibs showed a sensorineural hearing loss of 50 to 60 dB. Each affected sib had myopia of 20 to 22 diopters. Intelligence in one was stated to be somewhat low. Although Ohlsson concluded that the syndrome in this family was different from the *Alport syndrome* because of the milder course of the renal disease and the severe myopia, we believe that Ohlsson's kindred probably had a variant of Alport syndrome. Myopia of mild degree has been described in Alport syndrome by Sturtz and Burke (1956).

TREATMENT

Affected persons can be aided by glasses for the extreme myopia and by a hearing aid for the severe hearing loss.

PROGNOSIS

There is no evidence of progression either of the myopia or of the hearing loss.

SUMMARY

Characteristics of the syndrome include: 1) autosomal recessive transmission, 2) congenital severe myopia, 3) mild intellectual impairment in some affected persons, and 4) congenital moderate to severe nonprogressive sensorineural hearing loss.

REFERENCES

Eldridge, R., Berlin, C. I., Money, J. W., and McKusick, V. A., Cochlear deafness, myopia, and intellectual impairment in an Amish family. *Arch. Otolaryngol., 88*:49–54, 1968.

Ohlsson, L., Congenital renal disease, deafness, and myopia in one family. *Acta Med. Scand., 174*:77–84, 1963.

Sturtz, G. S., and Burke, E. C., Hereditary hematuria, nephropathia, and deafness. *N. Engl. J. Med., 254*:1123–1126, 1956.

MYOPIA, SECONDARY TELECANTHUS (HYPERTELORISM), AND CONGENITAL SENSORINEURAL DEAFNESS

Holmes and Schepens (1972) reported a sister and brother with severe eye abnormalities, telecanthus, and congenital sensorineural deafness. The same children were reported by Murdoch and Mengel (1971) and by Özer (1974).

CLINICAL FINDINGS

Physical Findings. Head circumference was large. The brow was prominent with a broad, flat nasal bridge. The anterior fontanelle measured 2×2 cm. at almost 3 years of age. Height ranged from the 10th to the 25th percentile.

Ocular System. The sister had congenital myopia in excess of 10 diopters, posterior staphyloma, incompletely developed filtration angle, extensive choroidal atrophy, posterior subcapsular cataracts, iris stroma hypoplasia, and congenital pupillary membrane.

The brother had congenital myopia of 25 diopters, pupillary remnants, nasal synechiae, incompletely developed filtration angle, and coloboma of the iris on the right. Retinal detachment occurred at about 4 years of age followed by cataract development a year later. At 6 1/2 years of age retinal detachment occurred in the other eye. In both children, the inferior lacrimal punctae were laterally displaced. Inner canthal, interpupillary, and outer canthal distances were all greater than normal. There was antimongoloid obliquity of the palpebral fissures.

Nervous System. Intelligence was normal in the girl. The boy was hyperactive and somewhat mentally retarded.

Auditory System. Both sibs had severe congenital sensorineural deafness. No other data were presented.

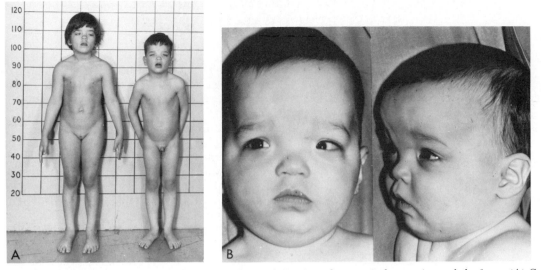

Figure 4-14 *Myopia, secondary telecanthus (hypertelorism), and congenital sensorineural deafness. (A)* Congenitally deaf sibs with severe eye abnormalities and telecanthus. Note flat nasal bridge. (From F. L. Özer, *Birth Defects, 10*(4):168, 1974.) *(B)* Male sib at 7 months of age. Note large head circumference, prominent frontal bone, and ocular hypertelorism. (From L. B. Holmes and C. L. Schepens, *J. Pediatr., 81*:552, 1972.)

Vestibular System. No vestibular tests were described.

Other Systems. The boy had umbilical hernia, inguinal hernia, and intussusception. Ureteral reflex and dilatation were also described.

LABORATORY FINDINGS

Albuminuria was found in both children. The boy had generalized aminoaciduria.

HEREDITY

The syndrome appears to have autosomal recessive inheritance.

DIAGNOSIS

Myopia has been described in a number of disorders discussed in this section, but the combination of myopia and other symptoms described here appears unique. Although patients with *Waardenburg syndrome* have increased inner canthal distances and displacement of the lacrimal punctae, the rest of the stigmata as well as the inheritance pattern are different.

TREATMENT

The many eye problems present in the syndrome require ophthalmologic consultation.

PROGNOSIS

Retinal detachment occurred in the male sib. Cataracts were present in both sibs. It is not known whether renal complications supervened.

SUMMARY

The syndrome is characterized by: 1) autosomal recessive inheritance, 2) secondary telecanthus (hypertelorism) and prominent brow, 3) myopia, choroidal atrophy, cataract, iris stroma hypoplasia, and possibly retinal detachment, and 4) congenital profound sensorineural deafness.

REFERENCES

Holmes, L. B., and Schepens, C. L., Syndrome of facial anomalies, telecanthus, and deafness. *J. Pediatr., 81*:552-555, 1972.

Murdoch, J. L., and Mengel, M. C., An unusual eye-ear syndrome with renal abnormality. *Birth Defects, 7*(4):136, 1971.

Özer, F. L., A possible "new" syndrome with eye and renal anomalies. *Birth Defects, 10*(4):168, 1974.

OPTIC ATROPHY, POLYNEUROPATHY, AND SENSORINEURAL DEAFNESS

(Rosenberg-Chutorian Syndrome)

A syndrome characterized by polyneuropathy, optic atrophy, and sensorineural hearing loss in two brothers and their nephew was described by Rosenberg and Chutorian (1967). Sibs having somewhat similar anomalies were reported by Iwashita et al. (1970). A less well-documented case is that of Taylor (1912). The sibs described by Jéquier and Deonna (1973) are discussed under Diagnosis.

CLINICAL FINDINGS

Physical Findings. Affected persons had normal height and build, except for muscular atrophy restricted to the extremities (Fig. 4–15A, B).

Ocular System. In the patients reported by Rosenberg and Chutorian, visual loss was first noted in both older patients at about 20 years of age. This loss began with nyctalopia, which was followed by gradual reduction in daytime visual acuity. Ophthalmologic examination of the brothers at 29 and 32 years of age showed optic atrophy—more marked temporally—but no retinitis pigmentosa. Corrected visual acuity in one brother was 20/100 bilaterally; in the other brother it was 20/400. Only gross hand movements were perceived. Visual field studies showed bilateral, concentric constriction in one brother. Examination of the 3-year-old nephew showed normal vision and no optic atrophy.

The patients reported by Iwashita et al., in contrast to those reported by Rosenberg and Chutorian, developed muscular wasting about five years before loss of vision and hearing.

Nervous System. In the patients described by Rosenberg and Chutorian, motor development was delayed, with walking beginning at about 2 years of age. Gait began to deteriorate between 5 and 10 years of age with atrophy of leg muscles; support by canes was finally required. Intelligence was normal. Neurologic examination of the adults showed severe distal weakness and atrophy of all extremities, including the intrinsic hand and foot muscles (Fig. 4–15A, B). Facial, neck, and trunk muscles were spared. Deep tendon reflexes were depressed or absent in the legs. There was marked depression of touch and position sense in the distal extremities as well as a decrease in nerve conduction velocities, with evidence of denervation. The 3-year-old boy exhibited a somewhat awkward gait and absent deep tendon reflexes. Strength and sensation were normal. The patients of Iwashita et al. showed disturbance of gait and coordination, sensory impairment, and positive Romberg sign.

Auditory System. In the cases of Rosenberg and Chutorian, hearing loss was noted in infancy and progressed to severe deafness by 5 to 6 years of age. Speech was slow in onset and remained rudimentary. Audiometric testing in the 29- and 32-year-old male sibs showed a bilateral sensorineural hearing loss of 60 to 90 dB. The 3-year-old responded only to loud noises. No other audiometric tests were described. In the sibs described by Iwashita et al. severe sensorineural hearing loss was noted at about 15 years of age.

Vestibular System. No vestibular tests were described.

LABORATORY FINDINGS

Roentgenographic, electroencephalographic, electroretinographic, and electrocardiographic studies were normal. Electromyographic studies revealed a mild to moderate reduction in nerve conduction rates in the three patients described by Rosenberg and Chutorian. In the sibs of Iwashita et al., scoliosis and normal motor nerve conduction rates were described.

Blood and urine tests, including levels of serum creatinine phosphokinase, and cerebrospinal fluid were also normal.

PATHOLOGY

Gastrocnemius muscle biopsy in the two older patients of Rosenberg and Chutorian showed severe neural atrophy. In the younger patient, the muscle appeared normal, but sural nerve biopsy revealed demyelination with preservation of axons. Ultrastructural studies were nonspecific (Ohta, 1970).

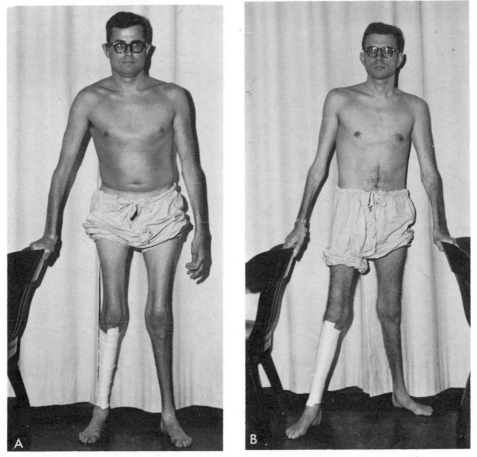

Figure 4–15 Optic atrophy, polyneuropathy, and sensorineural deafness (Rosenberg-Chutorian syndrome). (A, B) Sibs exhibiting muscle atrophy (most marked distally) of extremities, and sparing the facial, neck, and trunk musculature. To stand, the affected individuals require a broad base and support. (From R. N. Rosenberg and A. Chutorian, *Neurology (Minneap.)*, 17:827, 1967.)

HEREDITY

In the kindred of Rosenberg and Chutorian, a similar course occurred in the two brothers; early signs were seen in their nephew. Inheritance appeared to be X-linked recessive. However, in the brother-sister sib pair of Iwashita *et al.*, autosomal recessive inheritance appeared more likely. These two conditions probably represent different disorders.

DIAGNOSIS

Charcot-Marie-Tooth syndrome, a genetic heterogeneity, is characterized by progressive muscular atrophy beginning in the feet and legs (Dyck and Lambert, 1968). The peroneal muscles are involved first, the tibialis anticus, extensor longus digitorum

or gastrocnemius later. With time, the hands and arms may become involved. Pes cavus and hammer toes are frequent (Allen, 1939). Although optic atrophy is uncommon in Charcot-Marie-Tooth syndrome, it has been documented.

Peroneal muscular atrophy has been seen in association with cataracts and hearing loss (Campbell, 1900). It may also occur in *sensory radicular neuropathy*, a dominantly inherited syndrome consisting of marked peripheral sensory changes, trophic foot ulceration, and sensorineural deafness (Campbell and Hoffman, 1964). Dejerine and Thomas (1901) described atrophy of the extremities, palpable nerves, and sensorineural deafness in a brother and sister. Conceivably, these patients are examples of the syndrome under discussion.

Leber disease (hereditary optic atrophy), a genetic heterogeneity, must also be considered, since it shows onset in early adulthood and may be associated with ataxia, pyramidal tract and posterior column disease. Occasionally, there is an associated hearing deficit (Wilson, 1963). In the kindred documented by Veit (1940), however, the association between deafness and Leber optic atrophy appears to be one of chance.

The disorder in sisters reported by Jéquier and Deonna (1973) probably represents a separate syndrome. Both exhibited bilateral rapidly progressive severe sensorineural deafness and vestibular dysfunction at the age of 8 to 10 years, followed almost immediately by rapidly progressive visual impairment due to optic atrophy. A few years later there were loss of postural sense, pallesthesia, and tendon reflexes. Scheuermann disease of the spine was also found in both sibs. Inheritance was probably autosomal recessive.

TREATMENT

A hearing aid may be of value during the first few years of life.

PROGNOSIS

Prognosis for vision and hearing is poor because of the progressive nature of the syndrome.

SUMMARY

The characteristics of this syndrome include: 1) X-linked or autosomal recessive transmission, 2) progressive visual loss with optic atrophy beginning at about 20 years of age, 3) progressive peripheral polyneuropathy beginning in early childhood, and 4) progressive sensorineural hearing loss leading to severe deafness by 6 years of age.

REFERENCES

Allen, W., Relation of hereditary pattern to clinical severity as illustrated by peroneal atrophy. *Arch. Intern. Med., 63*:1123–1131, 1939.

Campbell, A., and Hoffman, H., Sensory radicular neuropathy associated with muscle wasting in two cases. *Brain, 87*:67–74, 1964.

Campbell, G., Two cases of muscular atrophy of the peroneal type. *J. Nerv. Ment. Dis., 27*:274–280, 1900.

Dejerine, J., and Thomas, A., Un cas de névrite interstitielle hypertrophique et progressive de l'enfance, suive d'autopsie. *Rev. Neurol. (Paris), 9*:557–559, 1901.

Dyck, P. J., and Lambert, E. H., Lower motor and primary sensory neuron diseases with peroneal muscular atrophy. *Arch. Neurol., 18*:603–625, 1968.

Hoyt, W. F., Charcot-Marie-Tooth disease with primary optic atrophy. *Arch. Ophthalmol., 64*:925–928, 1960.

Iwashita, H., Inoue, N., Araki, S., and Kuroiwa, Y., Optic atrophy, neural deafness, and distal neurogenic amyotrophy. *Arch. Neurol., 22*:357–364, 1970.

Jéquier, M., and Deonna, T., Surdité, atrophie optique, et ataxie sensitive progressives chez deux soeurs. *Schweiz. Arch. Neurol. Neurochir. Psychiatr., 112*:219–227, 1973.

Milhorat, A. T., Progressive muscular atrophy of peroneal type associated with atrophy of the optic nerves. *Arch. Neurol. Psychiatr., 50*:279–287, 1943.

Ohta, M., Electron microscopic observations of sural nerve in familial opticoacoustic nerve degeneration with polyneuropathy. *Acta Neuropathol. (Berl.), 15*:114–127, 1970.

Rosenberg, R. N., and Chutorian, A., Familial opticoacoustic nerve degeneration and polyneuropathy. *Neurology (Minneap.), 17*:827–832, 1967.

Schneider, D. E., and Abeles, M. M., Charcot-Marie-Tooth disease with primary optic atrophy; report of two cases occurring in brothers. *J. Nerv. Ment. Dis., 85*:541–547, 1937.

Taylor, J., Peroneal atrophy. *Proc. R. Soc. Med., 6* (Part 2):50–51, 1912.

Veit, G., Über eine Familie mit Leberscher Opticusatrophie und Taubstummheit. *Z. Mensch. Vererb. Konstit.-lehre, 24*:620–647, 1940.

Wilson, J., Leber's hereditary optic atrophy. *Brain, 86*:347–362, 1963.

OPTIC ATROPHY, JUVENILE DIABETES, AND SENSORINEURAL HEARING LOSS

Several families have been described in which sibs had a syndrome comprising optic atrophy, progressive sensorineural hearing loss, and diabetes mellitus (Barjon *et al.*, 1964; Rose *et al.*, 1966; Herrera Pombo *et al.*, 1971; Moore, 1971; Stevens and Macfayden, 1972). During the first decade of life, both hearing and visual losses were noted. By the second and third decades there was severe loss of hearing and sight. Diabetes mellitus was of early onset, was usually mild, and generally became manifest in the first or, less often, in the second decade.

CLINICAL FINDINGS

Physical Findings. Generally, physical examinations showed normal stature. Some children were slightly obese (Wolfram, 1938).

Ocular System. Visual loss was noted most often during the first decade of life, and less often during the second decade. The loss generally progressed slowly, resulting in severe deficit in the third decade (Rose *et al.*, 1966).

Ophthalmologic examination demonstrated bilateral optic atrophy—in most cases before the sixteenth year of life. Rarely did the optic atrophy antedate the onset of the diabetes mellitus. Several patients have manifested a mild pigment disturbance of the fundus (Stevens and Macfayden, 1972).

Nervous System. Examination of the 34-year-old patient described by Tunbridge and Paley (1956) showed a lurching, drunken gait but no other neurologic changes (see below). Two of the five cases described by Rose *et al.* had nystagmus and one had low intelligence. No other neurologic abnormalities have been described.

Endocrine System. The mild diabetes mellitus is of early onset. Weight loss and polyuria become manifest between 2 and 18 years of age—in most persons prior to the age of 11 years. Ikkos *et al.* (1970) and Moore (1971) also noted diabetes insipidus. This association was also pointed out in a number of case reports reviewed by Stevens and Macfayden (1972).

Auditory System. Hearing difficulty has been noted as early as in the first few years of life (Shaw and Duncan, 1958; Herrera Pombo *et al.*, 1971). The deafness becomes progressively worse, resulting finally in bilateral symmetrical moderate to severe sensorineural hearing loss in the second decade (Ikkos *et al.*, 1970; Cordier *et al.*, 1970; Moore, 1971; Stevens and Macfayden, 1972; Sauer *et al.*, 1972). There may be some variation in age of onset and severity of hearing loss; it is more marked at higher frequencies. The sibs described by Tun-

bridge and Paley (1956) noted hearing loss beginning in the second decade. This progressed to severe sensorineural hearing loss by the time they reached their 30s. Other types of audiometric tests have not been described.

Vestibular System. Vestibular tests on 10- and 13-year-old brothers showed diminished vestibular reaction (Barjon *et al.*, 1964).

LABORATORY FINDINGS

Roentgenograms of the skull have been normal. Electroencephalograms were considered abnormal in three of five cases (Rose *et al.*, 1966). These investigators also found spinal fluid protein to be increased in one case. Analyses of serum electrolytes and other blood tests showed no abnormalities.

HEREDITY

If we are careful in selection of cases and accept the sibships described by Tunbridge and Paley (1956), Shaw and Duncan (1958), Barjon *et al.* (1964), and Herrera Pombo *et al.* (1971), we see that a rather discrete syndrome emerges. In each of the families in which individuals have exhibited this syndrome, the parents were normal. Consanguinity has been described (Herrera Pombo *et al.*, 1971). There are several isolated cases (Demailly *et al.*, 1969; Moore, 1971). From the available data, it appears that the syndrome has autosomal recessive inheritance. It is difficult to classify the kindred reported by Sauer *et al.* (1973), since some components of the syndrome were seen in members in three generations.

DIAGNOSIS

Stevens and Macfayden (1972) cited numerous cases of the binary combination of diabetes mellitus and optic atrophy in sibs. Although those investigators did not mention associated deafness, we know that the hearing loss in the syndrome is high-tone sensorineural and that the patient is often unaware of the deficit. Therefore, it is not unlikely that many of these cases are examples of this syndrome. Although Tunbridge and Paley (1956) suggested that the family described by Wolfram (1938) and by Wagener (1938) has this syndrome, we feel that it is best not to accept this family as having the syndrome under discussion, since some members developed additional neurologic problems suggestive of Friedreich's ataxia. In none of the other families were spinocerebellar signs evident. The *Alström syndrome,* with diabetes mellitus, progressive sensorineural hearing loss, transient obesity, and retinitis pigmentosa, can be distinguished from the present syndrome because of the retinitis pigmentosa and cortical cataracts, which are associated with Alström syndrome. Patients with the Laurence-Moon and Bardet-Biedl syndrome show other signs, including mental deficiency, hypogonadism, and polydactyly.

TREATMENT

Medical therapy for the diabetes mellitus has been quite effective. In obese patients, the condition was treated by diet. In others, low doses of insulin were found effective. Little can be done for the optic atrophy, although the sensorineural hearing loss can be minimized by a hearing aid.

PROGNOSIS

Although patients develop a severe visual and hearing loss by middle age, their life span is probably normal.

SUMMARY

This syndrome is characterized by: 1) autosomal recessive transmission, 2) onset in childhood of progressive visual loss due to optic atrophy, 3) diabetes mellitus with onset in the first or second decade, and 4) onset in childhood of progressive sensorineural hearing loss.

REFERENCES

Barjon, P., Lestradet, H., and Labauge, R., Atrophie optique primitive et surdité neurogène dans le diabète juvénile. *Presse Méd., 72*:983–986, 1964.

Cordier, J., Reny, A., and Raspiller, A., Atrophie optique familiale et diabète juvénile. *Rev. Otoneuroophtalmol., 42*:269–280, 1970.

Demailly, P., Dérot, M., and Rougerie, J., Atrophie optique primitive chez l'enfant diabétique. *Bull. Soc. Franc. Ophtalmol., 82*:29–40, 1969.

Herrera Pombo, J. L., Hawkins, F., Arrieta, F., and Rodriguez-Miñon, J. L., El sindrome genético diabétes mellitus, atrófia óptica y otras manifestaciones. *Rev. Clin. Esp., 122*:13–18, 1971.

Ikkos, D. G., Fraser, G. R., Matsouki-Gavra, E., and Petrochilos, M., Association of juvenile diabetes mellitus, primary optic atrophy, and perceptive hearing loss in three sibs, with additional idiopathic diabetes mellitus insipidus in one case. *Acta Endocrinol. (Kbh.), 65*:95–102, 1970.

Moore, J. R., Juvenile diabetes mellitus insipidus and neurological abnormalities. *Proc. R. Soc. Med., 64*:730, 1971.

Rose, F. C., Fraser, G. R., Friedman, A. I., and Kohner, E. M., The association of juvenile diabetes mellitus and optic atrophy: clinical and genetic aspects. *Q. J. Med., 35*:385–405, 1966.

Sauer, H., Chüden, H., Gottesbüren, H., Schmitz-Valckenberg, P., and Seitz, D., Familiäres Vorkommen von Diabetes mellitus, primären Opticusatrophie und Innenohrschwerhörigkeit. *Dtsch. Med. Wschr., 98*:243–255, 1973.

Shaw, D. A., and Duncan, L. J. P., Optic atrophy and nerve deafness in diabetes mellitus. *J. Neurol. Neurosurg. Psychiatr., 21*:47–49, 1958.

Stevens, P. R., and Macfayden, W. A. L., Familial incidence of juvenile diabetes mellitus, progressive optic atrophy, and neurogenic deafness. *Br. J. Ophthalmol., 56*:496–500, 1972.

Tunbridge, R. E., and Paley, R. G., Primary optic atrophy in diabetes mellitus. *Diabetes, 5*:295–296, 1956.

Wolfram, D. J., and Wagener, H. P., Diabetes mellitus and simple optic atrophy among siblings: report of four cases. *Proc. Mayo Clin., 13*:715–718, 1938.

PROGRESSIVE OPTIC ATROPHY AND CONGENITAL SENSORINEURAL DEAFNESS

Konigsmark, Knox, Hussels, and Moses (1974) reported a syndrome of congenital severe sensorineural deafness and progressive midlife visual failure due to optic atrophy. Somewhat similar cases were described by Gernet (1964) and by Michal, Ptasinska-Urbanska, and Mitkiewicz-Bochenek (1968).

CLINICAL FINDINGS

Ocular System. Visual loss was noted in each of the patients described by Konigsmark *et al.;* however, it was first experienced in middle to later life. The patients described by Michal *et al.*, in contrast, experienced severe visual loss within the first six years of life. In both kindreds optic atrophy was documented. In the family described by Konigsmark *et al.*, the 9-year-old son of the proband had no visual difficulties, but he did show evidence of moderate optic atrophy on examination (Fig. 4–16). It is assumed that eye changes begin at an early age and are slowly progressive. Color blindness was noted in both kindreds.

Nervous System. Neurologic examination revealed normal cranial nerve function except for the deafness and optic atrophy. Strength was normal in all extremities and sensation was intact in all modalities. Tendon reflexes were symmetric and normal, with flexor plantar responses. Coordination tests, including the finger tap, the finger-to-nose, and hand rotation showed normal responses. Gait was normal except for some loss of balance in one patient.

Auditory System. Severe congenital bilateral sensorineural hearing loss, most marked in the mid-frequencies, was noted. In the son of the proband the deficit was greater than 90 dB in all frequencies. In other affected relatives there was some mild residual low-frequency hearing. In the kindred documented by Michal *et al.* all affected persons were deaf-mutes.

Vestibular System. Vestibular testing indicated no spontaneous or positional nystagmus. The optokinetic responses were normal, and the caloric vestibular tests were bilaterally active and normal in both kindreds.

LABORATORY FINDINGS

Temporal bone tomograms were normal.

Laboratory tests indicated that with the exception of elevated cerebrospinal fluid protein in one patient, C.S.F. protein was within normal limits in all other patients (Konigsmark *et al.*, 1974). Stimulation of various peripheral nerves showed normal conduction velocity and latency times with no evidence of a lower motor neuron abnormality.

HEREDITY

The syndrome was transmitted in an autosomal dominant manner through several generations in the kindreds described by Konigsmark *et al.* and by Michal *et al.*

DIAGNOSIS

It is probable that the two kindreds described here represent a genetic heterogeneity, since the onset of visual difficulties occurred in mid-life in one, and in childhood in the other. Additional cases are necessary to establish this point.

Several syndromes include hearing loss and optic atrophy. In the syndrome of *optic atrophy, ataxia, and progressive sensorineural hearing loss*, the hearing deficit is only moderate and slowly progressive. In the syndrome considered here, there was no evidence of ataxia, and the deafness was congenital. The syndrome of *optic atrophy, polyneuropathy, and sensorineural hearing loss* is transmitted in an autosomal recessive manner and includes a slowly progressive distal weakness. In *optic atrophy, juvenile diabetes, and sensorineural hearing loss*, the hearing deficit progresses slowly over the first three decades of life, eventually resulting in severe deafness; in the present syndrome the deafness is congenital. *Opticocochleodentate degeneration* clearly differs from the present syndrome because of its recessive transmission, infantile onset

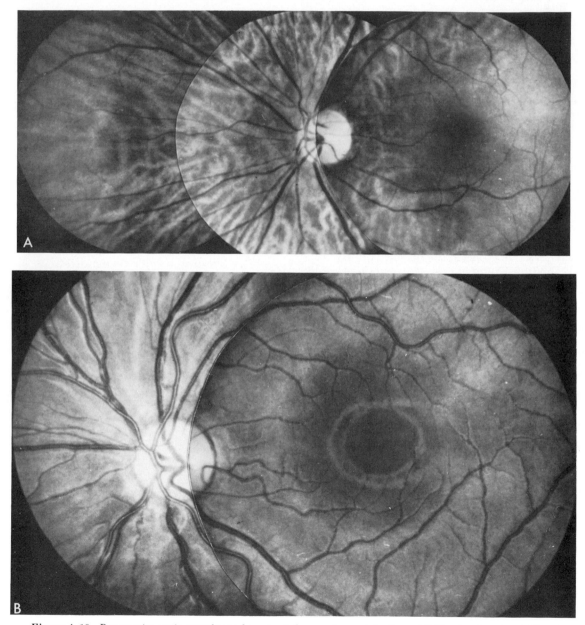

Figure 4–16 *Progressive optic atrophy and congenital sensorineural deafness. (A)* Fundus showing optic nerve atrophy, normal macular reflex, and retinal periphery. *(B)* Fundus with optic nerve atrophy. *(A and B from* B. W. Konigsmark *et al., Arch. Ophthalmol., 91*:99, 1974.)

of progressive spastic quadriplegia, and progressive hearing and mental deterioration. Leber's optic atrophy, certainly a genetic heterogeneity, is occasionally associated with neural deafness (Bhaduri, 1945; Wilson, 1963; de Weerdt and Went, 1971).

TREATMENT

Because of the severity of the congenital deafness a hearing aid is generally useless.

PROGNOSIS

Vision decreases progressively from midlife. The deafness is congenital, severe, and nonprogressive.

SUMMARY:

Characteristics of this syndrome include: 1) autosomal dominant transmission, 2) progressive optic atrophy, and 3) congenital severe sensorineural deafness.

REFERENCES

Bhaduri, B. N., Hereditary optic atrophy (Leber's disease). *Calcutta Med. J., 42*:1–4, 1945.
de Weerdt, C. J., and Went, L. N., *Acta Neurol. Scand., 47*:541–554, 1971.
Gernet, H., Hereditäre Opticusatrophie in Kombination mit Taubheit. *Ber. Dtsch. Ophthalmol. Ges., 65*:545–547, 1963.
Konigsmark, B. W., Knox, D. L., Hussels, I. E., and Moses, H., Dominant congenital deafness and progressive optic atrophy: report of a family through four generations. *Arch. Ophthalmol., 91*:99–103, 1974.
Michal, S., Ptasinska-Urbanska, M., and Mitkiewicz-Bochenek, W., Atrophie optique hérédofamiliale dominante associée à la surdi-mutité. *Ann. Ocul. (Paris), 201*:431–435, 1968.
Wilson, J., Leber's hereditary optic atrophy: some clinical and aetiological considerations. *Brain, 86*:347–362, 1963.

OPTIC ATROPHY, ATAXIA, AND PROGRESSIVE SENSORINEURAL HEARING LOSS

A syndrome characterized by progressive optic atrophy, progressive sensorineural hearing loss, and ataxia occurring in a father and in six of his nine children was described by Sylvester in 1958. Since transmission was autosomal dominant, this syndrome clearly was not Friedreich's ataxia.

CLINICAL FINDINGS

Visual System. The onset of visual loss was between 2½ and 9 years of age; the loss was progressive. Visual fields measured in two sibs showed peripheral constriction with no central scotoma. Light reflexes were normal.

Nervous System. The sibs were mentally dull and were either irritable or apathetic. Four of the six children showed nystagmus, which was horizontal in two, rotatory in one, and multidirectional in another. Three children showed weakness of the extremities, and four had an unsteady gait. The father's gait was normal except

for shortening of one leg, which was the result of having had poliomyelitis. General muscle tone was poor in two sibs, increased in the legs in two sibs, and normal in the remaining two. Four children showed muscle wasting involving the deltoid muscles, scapular muscles, and intrinsic hand muscles. In three children there was fibrillation involving the deltoids, spinalis muscles, or quadriceps. Deep tendon reflexes were increased in one child and diminished in three, particularly in the knees and ankles. Three children had extensor plantar responses.

Skeletal System. Postural abnormalities included dorsal kyphosis, lordosis, scoliosis, pes cavus, and claw hand.

Auditory System. The sensorineural hearing loss was somewhat variable, being mild in three sibs, moderate in another, and severe in two others. Although the father was severely deaf, there was no proof that the hearing loss was progressive. No further audiometric findings were described.

Vestibular System. No vestibular findings were noted.

LABORATORY FINDINGS

Electrocardiographic, electromyographic, and cerebrospinal fluid studies were normal. Other routine laboratory examinations were also normal.

PATHOLOGY

Histologic sections of the brain from one patient showed marked loss of myelinated fibers in the dorsal and ventral spinocerebellar tracts and in the posterior funiculus. Sensory testing had not been done in this child. The corticospinal tracts and optic nerve were also demyelinated. Sections of the cerebellum were not available.

Muscle biopsy was normal.

HEREDITY

Since the disorder appeared in a father and in six (three males, three females) of his nine children, autosomal dominant inheritance is likely.

DIAGNOSIS

Optic atrophy and hearing loss occur in *progressive optic atrophy and congenital sensorineural deafness;* in *optic atrophy, juvenile diabetes, and sensorineural hearing loss;* and in *optic atrophy, polyneuropathy, and sensorineural deafness.* In the first two disorders, transmission is autosomal recessive; in the second, juvenile diabetes supervenes. In the last disorder, inheritance is autosomal recessive, and a polyneuropathy that includes sensory loss is evident. Friedreich's ataxia, which has autosomal recessive transmission, shows no visual or hearing loss.

TREATMENT

Little therapy other than a hearing aid for the auditory loss can be given.

PROGNOSIS

There was marked variation in the age of onset of symptoms. In the father, the slow progression of the disorder resulted in severe hearing loss and poor vision in middle age. The age of onset in his children ranged from 2½ to 9 years of age, with death occurring between 8 months and 4 years after onset.

SUMMARY

The major characteristics include: 1) autosomal dominant transmission with variable age of onset, 2) progressive visual loss due to optic atrophy beginning in childhood, 3) a variable degree of ataxia, particularly involving the legs, 4) weakness and muscle wasting, particularly involving the shoulder girdle and hands, and 5) moderate to severe progressive sensorineural hearing loss beginning in childhood.

REFERENCE

Sylvester, P. E., Some unusual findings in a family with Friedreich's ataxia. *Arch. Dis. Child.,* 33:217–221, 1958.

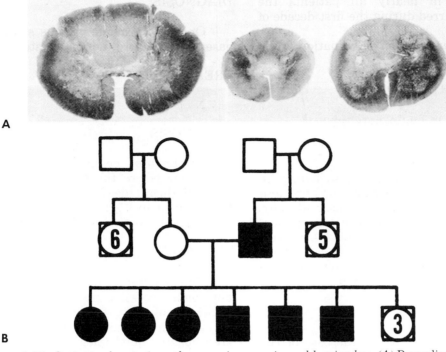

Figure 4-17 *Optic atrophy, ataxia, and progressive sensorineural hearing loss.* (A) Demyelination of posterior columns; dorsal and ventral spinocerebellar tracts in sections of cord at cervical, thoracic, and sacral levels (×5). (B) Pedigree showing affected father and six of his nine children. (A and B from P. E. Sylvester, *Arch. Dis. Child.*, 33:217, 1958.)

OPTICOCOCHLEODENTATE DEGENERATION

A syndrome characterized by progressive visual and sensorineural hearing loss and progressive spastic quadriplegia was reported in two male sibs by Muller and Zeman in 1965. Similar cases were described earlier by Meyer (1949), Levy (1951), and Hasaerts (1957). The case of Nyssen and van Bogaert (1934) is less certain to be an example.

CLINICAL FINDINGS

Ocular System. Vision in nearly all patients was normal until about 1 year of age. Optic atrophy and visual loss without retinal degeneration were noted at about 2½ years, with blindness at about 3 years of age in nearly all cases.

Nervous System. In general, the affected children developed normally until about 6 months of age when quivering, lack of use of the legs, or failure to lift the head was noted. A slowly progressive, spastic quadriplegia, more marked in the lower extremities, developed. By 3 years of age, flexion contractures were noted in the legs and marked rotoscoliosis was observed. In most cases, reflexes were hyperactive. Muscle tone varied from hypotonic to spastic.

Mental deterioration was progressive, resulting in complete dementia in most patients, although intelligence was normal in the cases studied by Nyssen and van Bogaert. Microcephaly was noted in several patients. Speech was either slow and scanning, or in most cases never developed.

Auditory System. Hearing was considered normal during the first year of life. Because the mental deterioration in the children was so severe, it was impossible to determine whether they could hear. The age at which hearing loss became evident

IRIS DYSPLASIA, OCULAR HYPERTELORISM, PSYCHOMOTOR RETARDATION, AND SENSORINEURAL DEAFNESS

DeHauwere, Leroy, Adriaenssens, and van Heule (1973) described a syndrome of mesodermal dysgenesis of the iris, telecanthus, sensorineural deafness, psychomotor retardation, and hypotonia in two generations. A similar disorder was reported by van Noorden and Baller (1963).

CLINICAL FINDINGS

Physical Findings. Height was reduced below the third percentile with head circumference at or below the tenth percentile.

Ocular System. In all patients hypoplasia of the iris stroma, abnormally prominent line of Schwalbe, adhesions between the iris and posterior surface of the cornea, and pear-shaped pupils (Rieger's anomaly) have been found. Ocular hypertelorism and strabismus were marked.

Nervous System. Psychomotor retardation was a common feature. In the children, milestones were reached late. The adult had an I.Q. of 75.

Musculoskeletal System. Hypotonia and hyperlaxity of joints with dislocation of the hips were documented in all patients.

Auditory System. Mild sensorineural deafness was noted in each patient.

Vestibular System. Vestibular studies were not mentioned.

LABORATORY FINDINGS

Radiologic studies showed retarded bone age, ocular hypertelorism, coxa valga, and hip dislocation. Pneumoencephalographic studies revealed dilated ventricles.

Routine laboratory studies of urine, serum, and cerebrospinal fluid were unremarkable as were electroencephalographic, electromyographic, and nerve conduction studies.

HEREDITY

The disorder is inherited as a dominant trait. X-linkage cannot be excluded since there has been no male-to-male transmission.

DIAGNOSIS

One must exclude Rieger's syndrome, which comprises autosomal dominant inheritance of Rieger anomaly, maxillary hypoplasia, and hypodontia (Gorlin *et al.*, 1976).

TREATMENT

Esotropia and glaucoma, if present, should be corrected.

PROGNOSIS

Prognosis depends largely on the degree of psychomotor retardation, since none of the other components effect severe disability.

SUMMARY

Characteristics of this syndrome include: 1) autosomal dominant inheritance, 2) Rieger's mesodermal dysgenesis of the iris, 3) hypertelorism, 4) psychomotor retardation, 5) hypotonia with joint hypermobility, 6) dilated cerebral ventricles, and 7) mild sensorineural deafness.

REFERENCES

DeHauwere, R. C., Leroy, J. G., Adriaenssens, K., and van Heule, R., Iris dysplasia, orbital hypertelorism, and psychomotor retardation: a dominantly inherited developmental syndrome. *J. Pediatr., 82*:679–681, 1973.

Gorlin, R. J., Pindborg, J. J., and Cohen, M. M., Jr., *Syndromes of the Head and Neck,* 2nd Ed., New York, McGraw-Hill Book Company, 1976.

Van Noorden, G. K., and Baller, S. R., The chamber angle in split pupil. *Arch. Ophthalmol., 70*:598–602, 1963.

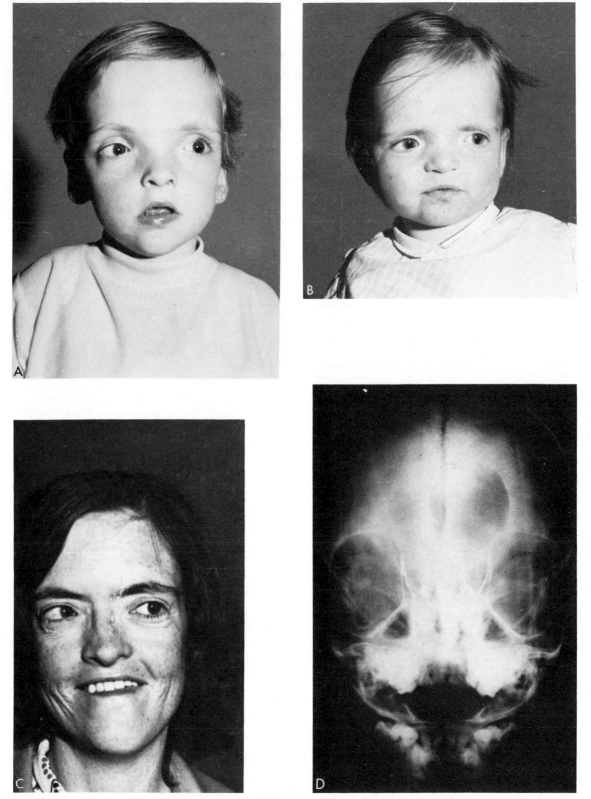

Figure 4-19 *Iris dysplasia, ocular hypertelorism, psychomotor retardation, and sensorineural deafness.* *(A–C)* Note irregular pupils and orbital hypertelorism in a mother and her two children. A similarly affected child had died. *(D)* Pneumoencephalogram showing hypertelorism, dilated and asymmetric lateral ventricle, and indication of a fifth ventricle. (From R. C. DeHauwere *et al., J. Pediatr.,* 82:679, 1973.)

CONGENITAL CORNEAL DYSTROPHY AND PROGRESSIVE SENSORINEURAL HEARING LOSS
(Harboyan Syndrome)

The combination of congenital corneal dystrophy and progressive sensorineural hearing loss was described in two of ten sibs from a first-cousin mating and in one of ten sibs from another first-cousin mating by the same father (Harboyan *et al.*, 1971).

CLINICAL FINDINGS

Ocular System. Whitish opacities of the cornea with decreased vision were evident from birth. Ophthalmologic examination of the three patients, ranging in age from 12 to 50 years, showed similar changes. The corneal epithelium was roughened but did not stain. The stroma was thickened, edematous, and homogeneously white (Fig. 4–20*A*). Vision was decreased to 20/200 bilaterally in the 12-year-old boy, to counting fingers at less than one meter in the 28- and 50-year-old men, and to counting fingers at less than one meter in the 28- and 50-year-old women. The younger woman exhibited increased intraocular pressure, whereas the older woman noted deterioration in vision after menopause. These observations suggest some progression of visual loss.

Auditory System. Hearing loss was first noticed in patients at the age of 10 to 25 years; the loss slowly progressed. An audiogram of the 12-year-old boy showed a 20 to 50 dB bilateral sensorineural hearing loss, worse in higher frequencies. The hearing loss in his two half-sisters was from 40 to 70 dB. Speech discrimination was 90 per cent to 100 per cent, and SISI and tone-decay tests were negative.

Vestibular System. Caloric vestibular tests were normal in all three patients.

LABORATORY FINDINGS

Routine laboratory tests, including levels of urinary mucopolysaccharides, were normal.

HEREDITY

The normal parents and the existence of parental consanguinity clearly indicate that the syndrome has autosomal recessive inheritance.

DIAGNOSIS

Congenital corneal dystrophy may be an isolated finding that is inherited as an autosomal recessive trait (Maumenee, 1960). Corneal clouding is a feature of several of the *mucopolysaccharidoses (Hurler, Scheie, and Maroteaux-Lamy syndromes).* The clinical features of these conditions, however, are quite distinctive. In congenital glaucoma, one finds corneal haziness, photophobia, enlargement of the cornea, increased intraocular pressure, and lacrimation. In Cogan syndrome, one notes photophobia and injection of the eyes; the keratitis is deep in the stroma. Tinnitus, severe vertigo, and ultimately marked deafness and loss of labyrinthine function are also associated with Cogan's syndrome. Congenital syphilitic keratitis must also be excluded.

In Fehr's autosomal recessive corneal dystrophy, the corneal changes become evident during the first decade of life; in the present syndrome the dystrophy is congenital (François, 1966). We are aware of only one example of the association of Fehr's corneal dystrophy with congenital neural deafness. The patient was the offspring of a consanguineous union (Moro and Ameidi, 1957).

Other possible examples of Harboyan syndrome are the sibs reported by Scialfa *et al.* (1975). The parents were consanguineous. However, they differed in having mental retardation and clinodactyly of the fifth fingers.

TREATMENT

Corneal transplants and treatment for the glaucoma are clearly indicated. A hearing aid should be employed.

PROGNOSIS

The loss of vision and hearing is slowly progressive.

SUMMARY

Major features of this syndrome include: 1) autosomal recessive transmission, 2) congenital corneal dystrophy with slow progression, and 3) childhood onset of slowly progressive sensorineural hearing loss.

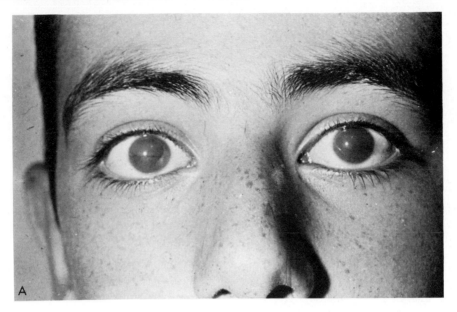

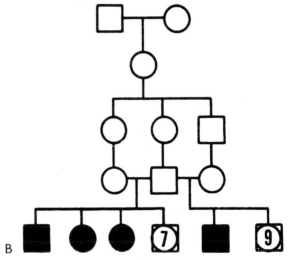

Figure 4-20 *Congenital corneal dystrophy and progressive sensorineural hearing loss. (A)* Note homogeneous white opacification of corneas in 12-year-old male. *(B)* Modified pedigree showing parental consanguinity. *(A* and *B* from G. Harboyan *et al., Arch. Ophthalmol., 85:27, 1971.)*

REFERENCES

François, J., Heredofamilial corneal dystrophies. *Trans. Ophthalmol. Soc. U.K., 86*:367–416, 1966.

Harboyan, G., Mamo, J., der Kaloustian, V., and Karam, F., Congenital corneal dystrophy. Progressive sensorineural deafness in a family. *Arch. Ophthalmol., 85*:27–32, 1971.

Maumenee, A. E., Congenital hereditary corneal dystrophy. *Am. J. Ophthalmol., 50*:1114–1123, 1960.

Moro, F., and Ameidi, B., Distrófia corneale screziata (o di Fehr) associata a sordita e balbuzie. *Ann. Ottalmol. Clin. Ocul., 83*:30–52, 1957.

Scialfa, A., Mollica, F., and Pavone, L., Dystrophie congénitale héréditaire de la cornéa associée à des anomalies extraoculaire diverses. *Ophthalmologica, 171*:410–418, 1975.

FAMILIAL CORNEAL DEGENERATION, ABNORMAL CALCIUM METABOLISM, AND HEARING LOSS

A syndrome comprising ribbonlike degeneration of the cornea, hearing loss, and abnormal calcium metabolism occurring in three of five brothers was described by Hallermann and Doering (1964).

CLINICAL FINDINGS

Physical Findings. The sibs were apparently normal in stature. A general physical examination was not mentioned, however.

Ocular System. The three brothers exhibited the senile type of primary ribbonlike degeneration of the cornea. Although the authors did not describe the age of onset of the degeneration, they did mention that this abnormality was not found in the patients' offspring, none of whom had reached the age of 45.

Auditory System. The three brothers, ranging from 65 to 69 years of age, exhibited a hearing deficit, the severity of which was not indicated. Age of onset or possible progression of hearing loss was not mentioned.

LABORATORY FINDINGS

Metabolic studies showed a normal plasma concentration of calcium. However, the mean transit time of calcium in the metabolically active pool studied with calcium-47 was significantly prolonged. They found that the totally available active calcium was increased, whereas its turnover was sluggish and reduced.

No other laboratory findings were described.

HEREDITY

Three of five sibs had the syndrome. Although the father was not examined, the paternal uncle probably also had the same disorder, according to the authors. Children of the affected persons did not exhibit signs of the syndrome, although they may have been too young to display any. Examination and metabolic studies of the parents of the affected individuals would have been valuable. It is possible that the syndrome is autosomal dominant with incomplete penetrance, but it is just as likely that it is autosomal recessive.

The authors mentioned another family in which both parents had hearing deficit. Of the ten children of this family, one had ribbonlike corneal degeneration and hearing loss, whereas six others had hearing loss but no corneal involvement. Three were normal. No metabolic studies were done on this family. The authors suggested that members of this family had the same syndrome.

DIAGNOSIS

Ribbonlike degeneration of the cornea has been described in a father and son. However, no hearing loss was mentioned (Glees, 1950).

TREATMENT

The patient should be referred to an ophthalmologist for treatment of the band keratopathy if this is deemed necessary.

PROGNOSIS

Apparently, this disease appears in the later decades of life and is slowly progressive.

SUMMARY

Characteristics of this syndrome include: 1) possible autosomal dominant transmission with variable expressivity, 2) ribbonlike degeneration of the cornea with onset in the later decades, 3) abnormal calcium metabolism characterized by prolonged transit time of calcium in the metabolically active pool, and 4) hearing loss, otherwise undefined.

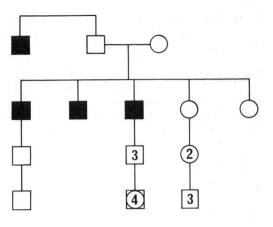

Figure 4-21 *Familial corneal degeneration, abnormal calcium metabolism, and hearing loss.* Modified pedigree of kindred described by Hallermann and Doering. (From W. Hallermann and P. Doering, *Ber. Deutsch. Ophthal. Ges.*, 65: 285, 1963.)

REFERENCES

Glees, M., Über familiäres Auftreten der primären bandförmigen Hornhautdegeneration. *Klin. Mbl. Augenheilk.*, *116*:185–187, 1950.

Hallermann, W., and Doering, P., Primäre bandförmige Hornhautdegeneration, Schwerhörigkeit und gestörter Calciumumsatz — ein hereditärer Symptomenkomplex. *Ber. Dtsch. Ophthalmol. Ges.*, *65*:285–288, 1963.

NORRIE SYNDROME

(Oculoacousticocerebral Degeneration)

A syndrome characterized by lens opacities, atrophic irises, and proliferating retrolental mass was probably first described by Fernandez-Santos (1905), although Clarke (1898) may have noted it earlier. Norrie (1927) reported two affected families in his article on causes of blindness in children. Subsequently, about 30 families have been described (Brini *et al.*, 1972). Extensive study of these and other families in Scandinavia was undertaken by Warburg (1966).

CLINICAL FINDINGS

Ocular System. Ocular alterations change dramatically with age (Holmes, 1971). The eyes are normal at birth, but during the first few days or weeks a yellowish retinal pigment appears in both eyes. At that time, ophthalmologic examination shows a white, vascularized mass behind a clear lens. Fradkin (1971) found anisocoria, shallow anterior chambers, retrolental vascular membrane, and vitreous hemorrhage. During preschool years cataract develops, the cornea becomes opaque, and the eyes begin to shrink. By school age corneal changes are present in most cases, although in some persons iris atrophy and synechiae are evident. By ten years of age, the eye changes cease. Because of pain, enucleation is occasionally required (Warburg, 1966).

Nervous System. Among 30 patients on whom information concerning mental status was available, about a third showed severe mental deficiency, a third exhibited mild retardation, and a third were normal. In the more severe cases, deterioration began in the third or fourth year of life; in milder cases, deterioration was much slower, some requiring institutionalization in the fifth or sixth decade (Forssman, 1960; Warburg, 1966; Lomičková and Raška, 1970).

Auditory System. In Warburg's study (1966) of 35 affected persons in 6 families, 11 had hearing deficit. Because of severe mental retardation, hearing loss could not be ascertained in several patients. Auditory impairment that is progressive develops in the second or third decade. Of 13 persons whose hearing was evaluated, a mild to severe hearing loss was found in 6. Audiograms showed a 20 to 100 dB, usually symmetric, sensorineural hearing loss (Fig. 4-22B, C).

Vestibular System. Vestibular tests

were not performed by Warburg (1966) because several patients had nystagmus and some had enucleation.

LABORATORY FINDINGS

Electroencephalograms in individuals with severe oligophrenia have shown marked diffuse abnormalities with distinct spikes.

Urine and serum amino acid chromatography, serum and cerebrospinal fluid immunoelectrophoresis, and cerebrospinal fluid protein have been normal.

PATHOLOGY

Examination of the eye has shown the vitreous cavity to be filled with collagenous fibers and vascular scar tissue with proliferation of retinal pigment epithelium. The inner layer of the retina has been absent except for undifferentiated glial tissue. The eyeball usually has been small and the cornea dome-shaped. A vascular membrane has covered the anterior surface of the iris. The choroid has been edematous and has contained engorged blood vessels. The lens has been cataractous. Section of the optic nerve has shown myelinated fibers in the periphery with only connective tissue in the remainder of the nerve (Warburg, 1968; Townes and Roca, 1973).

The optic tracts have been small or threadlike, consisting mostly of glia, and the lateral geniculate bodies have been about half the normal size with a concomitant decrease in ganglion cells. The surface area, including the medial surface of an occipital lobe, has been smaller than normal. The cerebral cortex has shown only slight irregularity in the arrangement of nerve cells with incomplete stratification.

HEREDITY

In many families described, the syndrome occurred in several generations. Only males were affected and an affected man had only unaffected sons and daughters. Several affected men had affected grandsons through their daughters. All pedigrees published are compatible with X-linked transmission. The female carriers show no ocular or hearing defects. Homozygous females may have been described by Clarke (1898). Linkage studies have not been rewarding (Nance et al., 1969).

DIAGNOSIS

Retinoblastoma has been diagnosed erroneously in several patients with this disorder. This condition can be ruled out by noting the other eye findings in Norrie syndrome. Patients with juvenile retinoschisis have much better vision than patients with Norrie syndrome. Falciform and retinal detachment, toxoplasmosis, retrolental fibroplasia, and trauma with massive retinal fibrosis must be excluded. Metastatic ophthalmia (almost always monocular) and X-linked congenital cataract as well as ophthalmia neonatorum and X-linked microphthalmia may require differentiation (Hansen, 1968).

TREATMENT

The eye pain that occurs occasionally is relieved by enucleation. A hearing aid may be effective for the hearing loss if severe mental retardation does not preclude its use.

PROGNOSIS

All affected persons become blind. There has been moderate to severe sensorineural hearing loss, which does not appear to be progressive. The oligophrenia is progressive, with affected children appearing mentally normal for only the first one or two years of life. Several patients with acute psychosis have died in mental institutions.

SUMMARY

The major characteristics of this syndrome include: 1) X-linked recessive transmission, 2) eye changes, including retinal glial proliferation, cataract, and microphthalmia, 3) mild to severe mental deficiency in about two thirds of the cases, and 4) mild to severe sensorineural hearing loss in about one third of the patients.

REFERENCES

Brini, A., Sacrez, P., and Levy, J. P., Maladie de Norrie. *Ann. Ocul., 205*:1–16, 1972.
Clarke, E., "Pseudoglioma" in both eyes. *Trans. Ophthalmol. Soc. U.K., 18*:136–138, 1898.

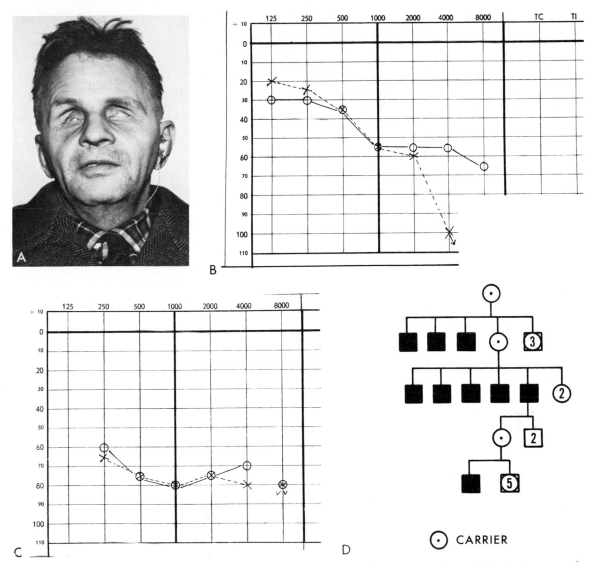

Figure 4-22 *Norrie syndrome.* (A) Eyes are deep-set and phthisic. The corneas are hazy. (B, C) Audiograms of patients with Norrie syndrome, showing moderate to severe bilateral hearing loss. (D) Pedigree of affected family showing X-linked inheritance. (A–D from M. Warburg, *Acta Ophthalmol. (Kbh.), Suppl. 89*:1–147, 1966.)

Fernandez-Santos, J., Total congenital detachment of the retina in two brothers. *Arch. Ophthalmol., 34*:338–340, 1905.

Forssman, H., Mental deficiency and pseudoglioma, a syndrome inherited as an X-linked recessive. *Am. J. Ment. Def., 64*:984–987, 1960.

Fradkin, A. H., Norrie's disease: congenital progressive oculo-acoustico-cerebral degeneration. *Am. J. Ophthalmol., 72*:947–948, 1971.

Hansen, A. C., Norrie's disease. *Am. J. Ophthalmol., 66*:328–332, 1968.

Holmes, L. B., Norrie's disease: an X-linked syndrome of retinal malformation, mental retardation, and deafness. *J. Pediatr., 70*:89–92, 1971.

Lomičková, H., and Raška, B., Norriesche Krankheit. *Mschr. Kinderheilk., 118*:272, 1970.

Nance, W. E., Hara, S., Hansen, A., Elliott, J., Lewis, M., and Chowen, B., Genetic linkage studies in a Negro kindred with Norrie's disease. *Am. J. Hum. Genet., 21*:423–429, 1969.

Norrie, G., Causes of blindness in children. *Acta Ophthalmol. (Kbh.), 5*:357–386, 1927.

Townes, P. L., and Roca, P. D., Norrie's disease (hereditary oculo-acoustico-cerebral degeneration). Report of a United States family. *Am. J. Ophthalmol., 76*:797–803, 1973.

Warburg, M., Norrie's disease. A new hereditary bilateral pseudotumor of the retina. *Acta Ophthalmol. (Kbh.) 39*:757–772, 1961.

Warburg, M., Norrie's disease, a congenital progressive oculo-acoustico-cerebral degeneration. *Acta Ophthalmol. (Kbh.), Suppl. 89*:1–147, 1966.

Warburg, M., Norrie's disease. *J. Ment. Def. Res., 12*:247–251, 1968.

Whitnall, S. E., and Norman, R. E., Microphthalmia and the visual pathways. *Br. J. Ophthalmol., 24*:229–244, 1940.

KERATOCONUS, BLUE SCLERAE, LOOSE LIGAMENTS, AND CONDUCTION DEAFNESS

A syndrome including keratoconus, blue sclerae, middle-ear conduction defects, and spondylolisthesis was reported in sibs by Greenfield, Romano, Stein, and Goodman (1973). They analyzed eleven similar reported cases and tabulated the findings. Only these authors and Behr (1913) noted hearing loss. We believe that Lamba *et al.* (1971) documented another example. It is possible that some of the above-mentioned patients have lysyl hydroxylase deficiency.

CLINICAL FINDINGS

Physical Findings. Changes are limited to the eyes, joints, and ears. Patients are of normal stature and body proportions.

Ocular System. All patients had blue sclerae and nearly all had keratoconus or keratoglobus, i.e., cone-shaped cornea or globe, respectively. In Bowman's and Descemet's membranes tears were always present.

Gradual and progressive visual impairment began after puberty with perforation of the thinned cornea (a *sine qua non* of keratoconus and keratoglobus) and traumatic cataract. Corneal fragility was present in several cases cited by Greenfield *et al.* Horizontal nystagmus with severe bilateral vernal conjunctivitis was evident. Intraocular pressure was normal.

Musculoskeletal System. Scoliosis and spondylolisthesis were found in both sibs by Greenfield *et al.* (1973). Various other inconsistent alterations were noted: "champagne glass" pelvic configuration, wide "female type" pelvis in a male sib, hypoplasia of styloid of one ulna, and hypoplasia of the lesser trochanter of one femur.

Hyperextensible joints were present in about 80 per cent of the published cases. Increased tendency to fracture was not part of the syndrome. Pes cavus and umbilical hernia were noted by Lamba *et al.* (1971).

Auditory System. In one patient of Greenfield *et al.*, progressive unilateral hearing loss began at 10 years of age, followed by deafness on the other side at 27 years of age. At 30 years, diagnosis of bilateral otosclerosis was established. Audiometry disclosed air/bone thresholds of 45–60/15–20 dB. In the other sib, progressive bilateral hearing loss began at 14 years of age. Air/bone thresholds were 60/30 dB bilaterally. Behr (1913) studied two brothers with keratoconus, blue sclerae, and repeated dislocations. One had bilateral hearing loss that was not otherwise characterized. Lamba *et al.* (1971) described bilateral conduction deafness.

Vestibular System. Vestibular tests were not mentioned.

Other Findings. Dermatoglyphic abnormalities of very low ridge count, low a-b ridge count, and low maximal "atd" angles were found, but their significance is doubtful.

LABORATORY FINDINGS

No abnormal findings were noted.

HEREDITY

The disorder is clearly inherited as an autosomal recessive trait. Parental consanguinity has been demonstrated in seven of nine kindreds.

DIAGNOSIS

The syndrome of *myopia, blue sclerae, marfanoid habitus, and sensorineural deafness,* inherited as a dominant condition, must be excluded. Blue sclerae can occur in a number of connective tissue disorders: *osteogenesis imperfecta,* Ehlers-Danlos syndrome, and Marfan syndrome. This abnormality may also be seen in Hallermann-Streiff syndrome and in incontinentia pigmenti. However, there should be no difficulty in excluding these conditions on clinical grounds.

Although keratoconus is usually an isolated finding, there are several kindreds in which transmission has been in either an autosomal dominant or an autosomal recessive (less likely) manner (McKusick, 1975). Keratoconus has also been reported in association with oculodentoosseous dysplasia, and occasionally with Ehlers-Danlos syndrome, osteogenesis imperfecta, and Rieger's syndrome.

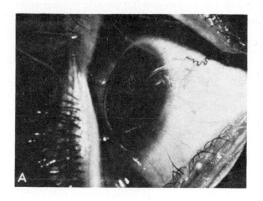

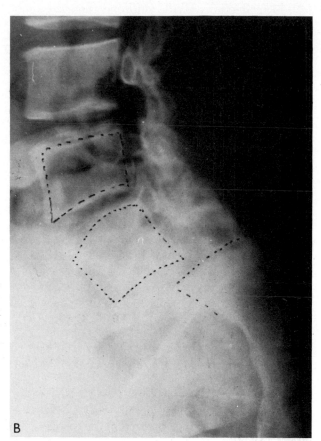

Figure 4-23 *Keratoconus, blue sclerae, loose ligaments, and conduction deafness.* (A) Note keratoglobus. (B) Lateral view of spine showing spondylolisthesis. (C) Family pedigree. (From G. Greenfield *et al.*, *Clin. Genet.*, 4:8, 1973.)

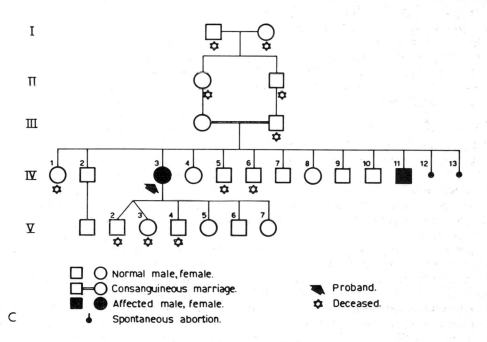

TREATMENT

Stapedectomy will improve hearing Contact lenses can be effectively employed for the keratoconus or keratoglobus.

PROGNOSIS

The outlook for these patients is generally good. The syndrome is not life-threatening, and although the deafness is progressive, it can be minimized with stapedectomy. The keratoconus may cause rupture of the cornea with resultant complications.

SUMMARY

The characteristics of the syndrome include: 1) autosomal recessive inheritance, 2) keratoconus or keratoglobus with thin, fragile cornea, 3) blue sclerae, 4) loose ligaments, and 5) conduction deafness.

REFERENCES

Behr, C., Beitrage zur Aetiologie des Keratokonus. *Klin. Mbl. Augenheilk., 51*:281–286, 1913.

Greenfield, G., Romano, A., Stein, R., and Goodman, R. M., Blue sclerae and keratoconus: key features of a distinct heritable disorder of connective tissue. *Clin. Genet., 4*:8–16, 1973.

Lamba, P. A., Shukla, K. N., and Ganapathy, K., Blue sclerae with keratoglobus. *Orient. Arch. Ophthalmol., 9*:123–126, 1971.

McKusick, V. A., *Mendelian Inheritance in Man,* 4th Ed. Baltimore, Johns Hopkins Press, 1975.

PROGRESSIVE EXTERNAL OPHTHALMOPLEGIA, RETINAL PIGMENTARY DEGENERATION, CARDIAC CONDUCTION DEFECTS, AND MIXED HEARING LOSS

Kearns and Sayre (1958) first described a syndrome of "retinitis pigmentosa, external ophthalmoplegia, and complete heart block" in two unrelated patients. Subsequently, Kearns (1965, 1966) added an additional nine patients, six with the "complete" and three with the "incomplete" syndrome, i.e., lacking cardiomyopathy. Additional cases were reported by Jager, Fred, Butler and Carnes (1960), Drachman (1968), Danta *et al.* (1975) and Gadoth (1976).

CLINICAL FINDINGS

Physical Findings. If the onset of the syndrome is early, patients tend to be short and slightly built.

Ocular System. Ptosis and progressive external ophthalmoplegia are usually the first apparent signs of the disorder—in most cases appearing in the second decade. Retinal pigmentary degeneration and optic atrophy appear soon thereafter. Although some patients find ptosis to be a major disability, most are able to compensate by tilting the head backward. Proptosis, which has been found in several cases, probably results from weak ocular muscles. The retinal pigmentary degeneration is characterized by a scattering of fine pigment, occasionally in small clumps, throughout the retina, essentially sparing the area around the disc. The typical "bone spicule" pattern is not present. The retinal arteries are not narrowed, but the retina is thinned. Visual acuity is often impaired.

Nervous and Muscular Systems. Bulbar weakness is manifested by dysphonia, dysphagia, and hoarseness. The voice is weak and the speech is "nasal" with incomplete closure of the epiglottis. Facial weakness, manifested both in the opening and closing of the eyelids, has been noted in most cases. Proximal limb girdle myopathy has been found in several patients. Some have exhibited distal weakness and sensory loss, suggesting a peripheral neuropathy. Cerebellar ataxia, corticospinal tract signs (positive Babinski, hyperreflexia, or areflexia), and organic mental changes have been inconstant findings.

Cardiac System. Cardiac conduction defects have been present in most patients. Bundle branch block may progress to atrioventricular blocks of varying degrees. Some patients exhibit Stokes-Adams syncopal episodes related to shifting cardiac rhythms.

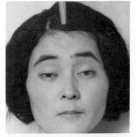

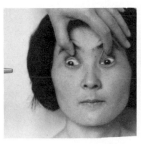 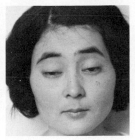 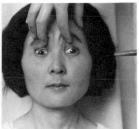

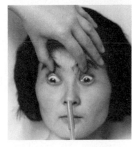

Figure 4–24 Progressive external ophthalmoplegia, retinal pigmentary degeneration, cardiac conduction defects, and mixed hearing loss. *(A)* Maximal deviation of eye in four main directions of gaze. Marked limitation is shown. *(B)* Moderate wasting and weakness in the shoulder and pelvic girdle muscles and in the proximal muscles of the arm and legs.

A

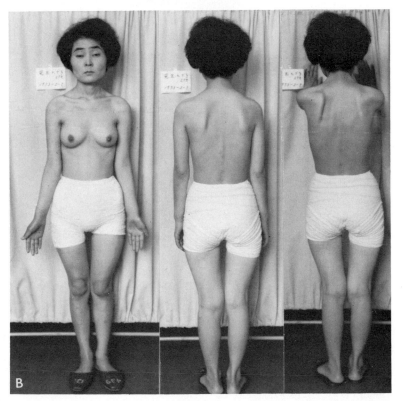

B

Illustration continued on the following page

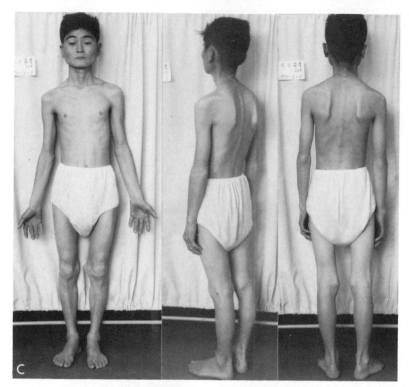

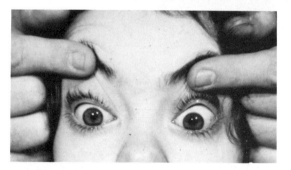

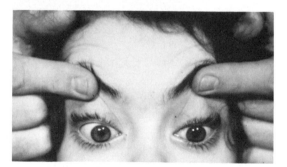

Eye movement to right   Eye movement to left

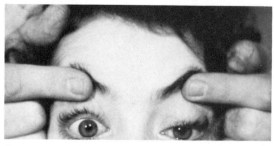

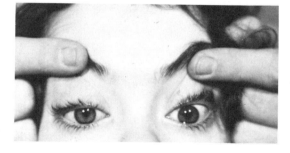

D

Eye movement upward   Eye movement downward

Figure 4–24   *(C)* Moderate weakness and atrophy of the sternocleidomastoid muscle. In the supine position, patient was unable to lift his head. The shoulder, pelvic girdle muscles, and proximal limb muscles showed moderate wasting and weakness. *(D)* Patient attempting to maintain extreme positions of gaze. (A, B, C, and D from K. Tamura *et al.*, *Brain*, 97:665, 1974.)

Illustration continued on the opposite page

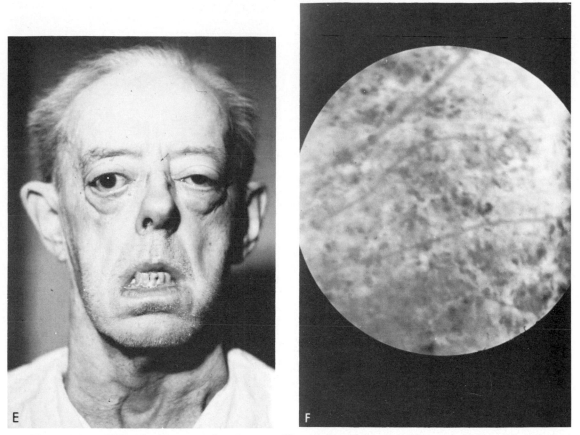

Figure 4-24 *(E)* Patient (72 years of age) at rest. Note ptosis of left eye and extreme atrophy of face. Patient also had generalized weakness and atrophy of all muscles and loss of sensory modalities distally in limbs, ventricular hypertrophy, and heart block. *(F)* Fundus showing areas of retinal pigmentary degeneration. *(E* and *F* from D. A. Drachman, *Arch. Neurol., 18*:654, 1968.)

Endocrine System. Several patients have had delayed sexual development.

Auditory System. Hearing loss has been of a mixed type in most patients, although only sensorineural deafness was documented in a few. Loss was most pronounced in the higher frequencies. Békésy and SISI tests revealed recruitment phenomena at high frequencies but not at lower ones, suggesting a cochlear or brain-stem lesion.

Vestibular System. Caloric testing revealed markedly diminished or absent responses to vestibular stimulation.

LABORATORY FINDINGS

Electroretinography has shown diminished responses. Electroencephalographic changes have been nonspecific, ranging from severe diffuse parietal and occipital slowing with spike and wave complexes to mild bifrontal slowing. Electromyographic and biopsy findings suggest myopathy.

All patients have elevated cerebrospinal protein levels.

Serum phytanic acid, SGOT, CPK, and LDH are not elevated. None had abetalipoproteinemia, malabsorption, or acanthocytosis. Some patients have exhibited diminished steroid excretion.

PATHOLOGY

Ocular muscle biopsies have shown increased endomysial and perimysial connective tissue, variation in fiber size, and some central nucleation. No enlarged muscle fibers, sarcolemmic nuclei, or inflammatory infiltrate were found.

HEREDITY

All have been isolated examples. See below for further discussion.

DIAGNOSIS

Progressive external ophthalmoplegia with or without ptosis may occur as an isolated finding, or it may be found in association with a dozen or more syndromal combinations, some of which may be spurious. These have been elegantly reviewed by Drachman (1968). *Refsum syndrome* may be excluded by the finding of normal levels of serum phytanic acid.

There are a number of cases that defy precise classification. Olson *et al.* (1972), DiMauro *et al.* (1973), and Morgan-Hughes and Mair (1973) reported patients with signs and symptoms described in this syndrome. Increased glycogen storage and giant mitochondria with paracrystalline inclusions were found. All were isolated cases. However, Tamura *et al.* (1974) described three affected sibs whose parents were consanguineous. Probably, we are dealing with etiologic heterogeneity.

TREATMENT

The patient should be referred to a cardiologist for management of his heart conduction defect. Plastic surgery may be required for correction of the ptosis.

PROGNOSIS

The various facets of the syndrome are progressive; in most cases the condition has not resulted in markedly shortened lifespan.

SUMMARY

The characteristics of the syndrome include: 1) progressive external ophthalmoplegia, 2) retinal pigmentary degeneration, 3) ptosis of eyelids, 4) optic atrophy, 5) proptosis in some individuals, 6) bulbar weakness (dysphonia, dysphagia, hoarseness), 7) proximal muscle weakness, 8) cerebellar ataxia and corticospinal tract signs occasionally, 9) cardiac conduction defects, 10) delayed sexual development, 11) mixed hearing loss, and 12) vestibular abnormalities.

REFERENCES

Danta, G., Hilton, R. C., and Lynch, P. G., Chronic progressive external ophthalmoplegia. *Brain, 98*:473–492, 1975.

DiMauro, S., Schotland, D. L., Bonella, E., Lee, C., Gambetti, P., and Rowland, L. P., Progressive ophthalmoplegia, glycogen storage and abnormal mitochondria. *Arch. Neurol., 29*:170–179, 1973.

Drachman, D. A., Ophthalmoplegia plus. The neurodegenerative disorders associated with progressive external ophthalmoplegia. *Arch. Neurol., 18*:654–674, 1968.

Gadoth, N., Kearns' syndrome (chronic external progressive ophthalmoplegia, retinitis pigmentosa, and cardiac conduction abnormalities). *Birth Defects* (in press).

Jager, B. V., Fred, H. L., Butler, R. B., and Carnes, W. H., Occurrence of retinal pigmentation, ophthalmoplegia, ataxia, deafness, and heart block. *Am. J. Med., 29*:888–893, 1960.

Kearns, T. P., External ophthalmoplegia, pigmentary degeneration of the retina, and cardiomyopathy: a newly recognized syndrome. *Trans. Am. Ophthalmol. Soc., 63*:559–625, 1965.

Kearns, T. P., Neuro-ophthalmology. *Arch. Ophthalmol., 76*:729–755, 1966.

Kearns, T. P., and Sayre, G. P., Retinitis pigmentosa, external ophthalmoplegia, and complete heart block. *Arch. Ophthalmol., 60*:280–289, 1958.

Metz, H., and Cohen, M., Progressive external ophthalmoplegia. *Ann. Ophthalmol., 5*:775–778, 1973.

Morgan-Hughes, J. A., and Mair, W. G., Atypical muscle mitochondria in oculoskeletal myopathy. *Brain, 96*:215–224, 1973 (Case 2).

Olson, W., Engel, W. K., Walsh, G. O., and Einaugler, R., Oculocraniosomatic neuromuscular disease with "ragged red fibers," histochemical and ultrastructural changes in limb muscles of a group of patients with idiopathic progressive external ophthalmoplegia. *Arch. Neurol., 26*: 193–211, 1972 (Cases 1, 2).

Tamura, K., Santa, T., and Kuroiwa, Y., Familial oculocranioskeletal neuromuscular disease with abnormal muscle mitochondria. *Brain, 97*:665–672, 1974.

Chapter 5

GENETIC HEARING LOSS ASSOCIATED WITH MUSCULOSKELETAL DISEASE

There are numerous genetic diseases that exhibit hearing loss and musculoskeletal abnormalities. The skeletal diseases range from bone abnormalities that are limited to only a few bones such as mandibulofacial dysostosis and orofaciodigital II syndrome to generalized skeletal disorders such as Paget disease, craniometaphyseal dysplasia, and sclerosteosis. Several syndromes are very rare, with only a single kindred recorded as being affected, as in deafness and tibial dysgenesis. In some syndromes the hearing deficit is conductive, in others it is sensorineural or mixed.

OTOPALATODIGITAL (OPD) SYNDROME

The OPD syndrome is characterized by conductive deafness, growth retardation, cleft palate, pugilistic facies, and generalized bone dysplasia. Several groups from the University of Minnesota (Dudding, Gorlin, and Langer, 1967; Langer, 1967; Buran and Duvall, 1967) have described the clinical and roentgenographic findings of three affected sibs. An earlier case is that of Taybi (1962). Extensive radiologic study of a large kindred was carried out by Poznanski et al. (1973).

CLINICAL FINDINGS

Physical Findings. The infant is of normal size at birth but develops more slowly than normal during childhood, falling below the tenth percentile in weight and height. The facies is characterized by an overhanging brow with large supraorbital ridges, flat midface, prominent occiput, antimongoloid obliquity of palpebral fissures, ocular hypertelorism, and broad, flat nasal bridge. The total effect is a pugilistic appearance (Fig. 5–1*A, B*). The palate is usually cleft.

There may be subluxation of the radial and femoral heads. The terminal phalanges are wide, and the fifth fingers are short with clinodactyly. The halluces are abbreviated, and the toes are broad and curved, resembling those of a tree frog. Often, there is webbing between the toes (Fig. 5–1*C*).

Nervous System. All patients have been mildly retarded, with I.Q.s ranging from 75 to 90.

Auditory System. Each of the affected children was thought to have hearing loss from infancy. Audiometric tests in three sibs showed a 30 to 90 dB bilateral conductive deafness (Buran and Duvall, 1967). Unilateral tympanotomy was performed on two of the sibs; in each case thickened ossicles were found. In one sib, the long process of the incus was thickened, forming an unstable incudostapedial joint. The stapedial head was widened, and the anterior crus did not reach the footplate. In the other sib, neither crus of the stapes reached the footplate.

Vestibular System. Vestibular tests were not described.

LABORATORY FINDINGS

Roentgenograms. The supraorbital ridges are prominent. Frontal and occipital bossing and thickening give the skull a mushroom appearance. The base of the anterior fossa is also thickened. The facial bones as well as the maxillary and sphenoid sinuses are small. The nasion-sella-basion angle is markedly reduced.

Frequently, there is posterior dislocation of the radial head. The hands show clinodactyly of the fifth finger due to shortening of the radial side of the middle phalanx. The distal phalanges of the first through fourth fingers are short and broad. Other anomalies include accessory ossification center of the second metacarpal and a teardrop-shaped lesser multangular. Females may have greater multangular-navicular fusion.

Abnormalities of the legs include lateral bowing of the femurs and the lower half of the tibias. The phalanges of the toes are short. The second and third metatarsals are oar-shaped, due to fusion with cuneiform bones. The fifth metatarsal may be prominent with an extra ossification center (Langer, 1967; Gall *et al.*, 1972).

PATHOLOGY

Histological sections of the stapes removed in one patient revealed normal but poorly modeled bone (Buran and Duvall, 1969).

HEREDITY

The syndrome is transmitted in an X-linked recessive manner; female heterozygotes exhibit prominent lateral supraorbital ridges and minor skeletal alterations (Gorlin *et al.*, 1973; Poznanski *et al.*, 1973).

DIAGNOSIS

Patients with Larsen syndrome have a somewhat similar facies, cleft palate, and joint dislocations. However, differentiation can be made on the basis of radiologic findings (multiple carpal bones, juxtacalcaneal bone, etc.) and autosomal recessive or dominant inheritance (Gorlin *et al.*, 1976).

TREATMENT

The cleft palate may be repaired surgically. Hearing loss can be treated by a hearing aid and by tympanotomy with a prosthesis replacing the abnormal ossicles.

SUMMARY

Characteristics of this syndrome include: 1) X-linked recessive inheritance, 2) pugilistic facies, including broad nasal root, hypertelorism, frontal and occipital bossing, and small mandible, 3) cleft palate, 4) growth retardation, 5) abnormalities of hands and feet, including widely spaced first and second digits and shortened halluces, 6) a wide variety of skeletal abnormalities, 7) mild mental retardation, and 8) moderate conductive hearing loss.

REFERENCES

Buran, D. J., and Duvall, A. J., The oto-palato-digital (OPD) syndrome. *Arch. Otolaryngol.,* 85:394–399, 1967.

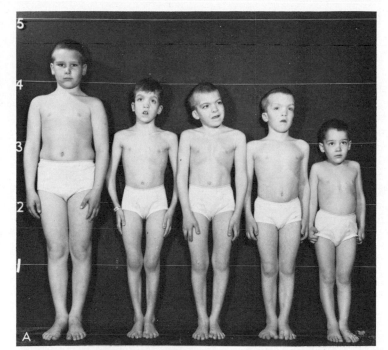

Figure 5-1 *Otopalatodigital (OPD) syndrome.* *(A)* Three affected sibs flanked by their two normal male sibs. *(B)* Broad nasal base gives patients a pugilistic appearance. *(C)* Feet of three sibs showing short halluces and exaggerated separation between first and second toes, syndactyly, and clinodactyly of lesser toes. *(A–C* from B. A. Dudding *et al., Am. J. Dis. Child., 113*:214, 1967.)

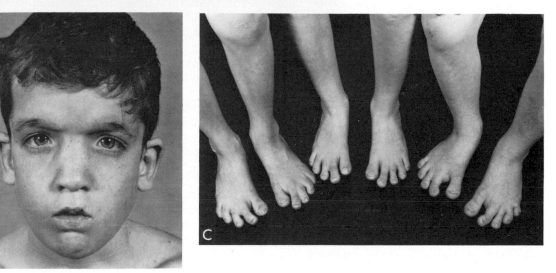

Dudding, B. A., Gorlin, R. J., and Langer, L. O., The oto-palato-digital syndrome. *Am. J. Dis. Child., 113*:214–221, 1967.

Gall, J. C., Jr., Stern, A. M., Poznanski, A. K., Garn, S. M., Weinstein, E. D., and Hayward, J. R., Oto-palato-digital syndrome. Comparison of clinical and radiographic manifestations in males and females. *Am. J. Hum. Genet., 24*:24–36, 1972.

Gorlin, R. J., Pindborg, J. J., and Cohen, M. M., Jr., *Syndromes of the Head and Neck,* 2nd Ed. New York, McGraw-Hill Book Company, 1976.

Gorlin, R. J., Poznanski, A. K., and Hendon, I., The oto-palato-digital (OPD) syndrome in females. Heterozygotic expression of an X-linked trait. *Oral Surg., 35*:218–224, 1973.

Langer, L. O., The roentgenographic features of the oto-palato-digital (OPD) syndrome. *Am. J. Roentgenol., 100*:63–70, 1967.

Poznanski, A. K., Macpherson, R., Gorlin, R., Garn, S., Nagy, J., Gall, J., Stern, A., and Dijkman, D., The hand in the oto-palato-digital syndrome. *Ann. Radiol., 16*:203–209, 1973.

Taybi, H., Generalized skeletal dysplasia with multiple anomalies. *Am. J. Roentgenol., 88*:450–457, 1962.

OROFACIODIGITAL II SYNDROME
(Mohr Syndrome)

This syndrome, characterized by cleft lip and lobulated nodular tongue, broad nasal root, hypoplasia of the body of the mandible, polydactyly and syndactyly, and conductive hearing loss, was described by Mohr (1941) and Claussen (1946) in four of seven sibs and by Rimoin and Edgerton (1967) in three of four sibs. Rimoin and Edgerton separated the orofaciodigital syndrome into two distinct genetic entities—one inherited in an X-linked dominant manner (OFD I) and the other inherited in an autosomal recessive mode (OFD II). Gorlin, Pindborg, and Cohen (1976) have reviewed all published cases.

CLINICAL FINDINGS

Physical Findings. The facies characteristically shows marked hypoplasia of the zygomatic arch, maxilla, and body of the mandible. The nasal bridge is broad and flattened. Often there is a midline cleft of the upper lip; sometimes there is cleft palate as well as cleft of the tongue (Fig. 5-2 A, B). Fatty hamartomas and general ankyloglossia have been described.

Bilateral manual ulnar hexadactyly and bilateral polysyndactyly of the halluces are common. In a few cases there have been five fingers with ulnar deviation of the fifth finger, syndactyly of the third and fourth fingers with extra bones in the web or hexadactyly of only one hand (Gorlin et al., 1976).

Nervous System. In several cases mental retardation has been reported. Various anomalies have included microcephaly, porencephaly, internal hydrocephaly, muscular hypotonia, and poor coordination (Gustavson et al., 1971).

Auditory System. One of the three affected sibs described by Rimoin and Edgerton (1967) was stillborn. The remaining two had moderate bilateral conductive hearing loss. Other audiometric hearing tests were not described. In one sib tympanotomy revealed congenital malformation of the incus with failure of articulation with the stapes. The long process of the incus had the appearance of a blunted sausage and the lenticular process was absent. A sister also had moderate conductive hearing loss. Tympanotomy was not performed. Goldstein and Medina (1974) reported 40 per cent conductive hearing loss in both sibs.

Vestibular System. Vestibular tests were not described.

LABORATORY FINDINGS

Roentgenograms showed hypoplasia of the zygomatic arches and body of the mandible. The remainder of the bony changes, which were limited essentially to the hands and feet, were those of syndactyly and polydactyly discussed earlier (Fig. 5-2C).

HEREDITY

In the family described by Mohr (1941) and Claussen (1946), four brothers were affected. Rimoin and Edgerton (1967) noted three of four affected sibs (Fig. 5-2D). Goldstein and Medina (1974) found two of three sibs to have the syndrome. Several other examples of the syndrome in sibs have been published (Gorlin et al., 1976). Since the parents have been normal in all cases, autosomal recessive inheritance is apparent.

DIAGNOSIS

OFD I syndrome is characterized by nasal alar hypoplasia, transient facial milia, coarse and thin hair, normal hearing, and X-linked dominant inheritance, which is lethal in the male (Gorlin et al., 1976).

TREATMENT

The cleft lip, palate, and tongue may be surgically repaired. The polydactylous digits may be removed. The hearing loss may be treated surgically with insertion of a prosthesis to replace the abnormal ossicles. A hearing aid may also be employed.

PROGNOSIS

The deafness is congenital and does not appear to progress. Although most affected persons have a normal life span, several infants have died of respiratory infection (Gorlin et al., 1976).

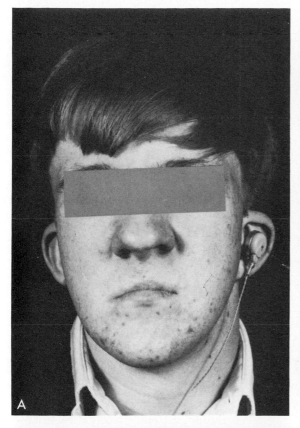

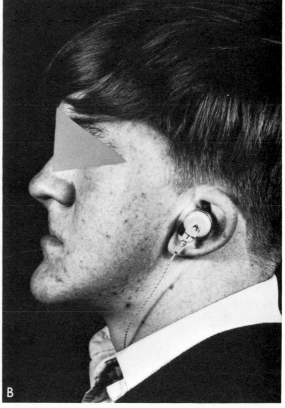

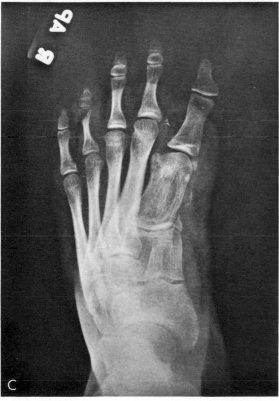

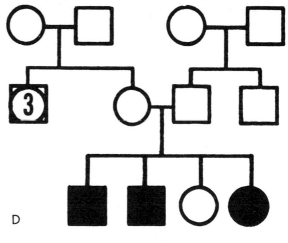

Figure 5-2 *Orofaciodigital II syndrome (Mohr syndrome).* (*A, B*) Note maxillary hypoplasia, broad nasal root, and bifid tip. Median upper lip cleft was surgically removed in infancy. (From D. L. Rimoin and M. T. Edgerton, *J. Pediatr., 71*:94, 1967.) (*C*) Broad cuboidal, first metatarsal, navicular and extra cuneiform bone. (*D*) Modified pedigree from Rimoin and Edgerton.

SUMMARY

OFD II syndrome is characterized by: 1) autosomal recessive inheritance, 2) facial deformities with hypoplastic mandibular body, flat nasal ridge, and widely spaced medial canthi, 3) digital abnormalities, including polydactyly, syndactyly, and brachydactyly, 4) lobulated tongue, and 5) conductive hearing loss secondary to ossicular malformations.

REFERENCES

Claussen, O., Et arvelig syndrom omfattende tungemissdannelse og polydaktyli. *Nord. Med.,* 30:1147–1151, 1946.

Goldstein, E., and Medina, J. L., Mohr syndrome or oral-facial-digital II: report of two cases. *J. Am. Dent. Assoc., 89*:377–382, 1974.

Gorlin, R. J., Pindborg, J. J., and Cohen, M. M., Jr., *Syndromes of the Head and Neck,* 2nd Ed. New York, McGraw-Hill Book Company, 1976.

Gustavson, K. H., Kreuger, A., and Petersson, P. O., Syndrome characterized by lingual malformation, polydactyly, tachypnea, and psychomotor retardation (Mohr syndrome). *Clin. Genet., 2*:261–266, 1971.

Mohr, O. L., A hereditary sublethal syndrome in man. *Nor. Vidensk.-Akad. Oslo I. Mat. Natur. Klasse, 14*:3–18, 1941.

Rimoin, D. L., and Edgerton, M. T., Genetic and clinical heterogeneity in the oral-facial-digital syndrome. *J. Pediatr., 71*:94–102, 1967.

DYSPLASIA OF THE CAPITAL FEMORAL EPIPHYSES, SEVERE MYOPIA, AND SENSORINEURAL DEAFNESS

Pfeiffer, Jünemann, Polster, and Bauer (1973) described a syndrome consisting of severe myopia, epiphyseal dysplasia of the femoral heads, and sensorineural deafness in three brothers.

CLINICAL FINDINGS

Physical Findings. Height was normal.

Musculoskeletal System. Mild pectus excavatum and hypermobility of joints, manifested by genua valga and recurvata, were noted in all three brothers. One brother had inguinal hernias.

Ocular System. Myopia of about 10 diopters became evident at 5 years of age in each brother. Fundus examination showed supertraction of the retina on the nasal side of the disc, atrophy of the pigmentary epithelium, diminution of the choroid nasally, and scattered diffuse peripheral pigmentation.

Auditory System. A symmetrical, sensorineural deafness with abrupt high-tone loss above 3000 to 4000 Hz was noted in all brothers. Speech reception threshold was at 30 to 35 dB. Speech discrimination showed a 20 per cent loss.

Vestibular System. No vestibular testing was described.

LABORATORY FINDINGS

Radiographic study of each boy showed flattened, irregularly shaped femoral heads with fragmentation. The distal metaphyses of the radius and ulna were irregular. There were two accessory centers of ossification in the carpus. Two brothers (identical twins) showed atypical ossification of the talus.

Electroretinograms were normal.

HEREDITY

The disorder appears to be inherited in an autosomal recessive manner. The parents were consanguineous.

DIAGNOSIS

This combination of symptoms is unique; severe myopia and sensorineural deafness, however, do occur in a number of syndromes: *hereditary arthro-ophthalmopathy, Marshall syndrome, spondyloepiphyseal dysplasia congenita,* and others. Asep-

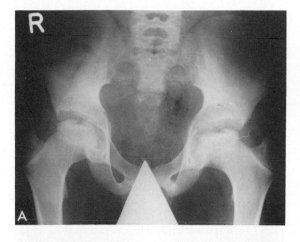

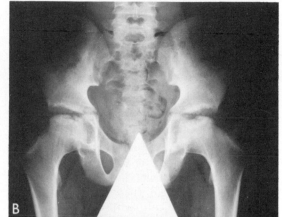

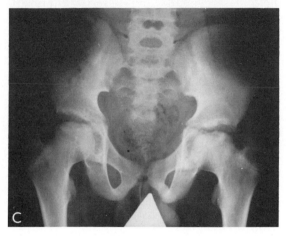

Figure 5-3 *Dysplasia of the capital femoral epiphyses, severe myopia, and sensorineural deafness.* *(A–C)* Radiographs of male patient taken at 10, 11, and 12 years of age and showing regression of epiphyseal deformity. *(A–C* from R. A. Pfeiffer *et al., Clin. Genet.,* 4:141, 1973.)

tic necrosis of the femoral heads (Perthes disease) must be excluded. A dominantly inherited Perthes-like dysplasia associated with brachydactyly was described by Robinson *et al.* (1968). Multiple epiphyseal dysplasia (Hunt *et al.,* 1967) must be excluded.

PROGNOSIS

There was progressive improvement of the epiphyseal dysplasia. The hearing loss did not appear to be progressive.

TREATMENT

No therapy, other than glasses, was necessary.

SUMMARY

Characteristics of this syndrome include: (1) autosomal recessive inheritance, (2) epiphyseal dysplasia, especially of the femoral capital epiphyses, (3) severe myopia, and (4) sensorineural hearing loss.

REFERENCES

Hunt, D. D., Ponseti, I. V., Pedrini-Mille, A., and Pedrini, V., Multiple epiphyseal dysplasia in two siblings. *J. Bone Joint Surg., 49A*:1611–1627, 1967.

Pfeiffer, R. A., Jünemann, G., Polster, J., and Bauer, H., Epiphyseal dysplasia of the femoral head, severe myopia, and perceptive hearing loss in three brothers. *Clin. Genet., 4*:141–144, 1973.

Robinson, G. C., Wood, B. J., Miller, J. R., and Baillie, J., Hereditary brachydactyly and hip disease. *J. Pediatr., 72*:539–543, 1968.

ABSENCE OF TIBIA AND CONGENITAL DEAFNESS

In 1931, Carraro described a syndrome characterized by absence of one or both tibias and severe congenital hearing loss in four of six sibs.

CLINICAL FINDINGS

Physical Findings. The affected sibs were normal except for abbreviation of one or both of their lower legs. Two sibs had marked shortening of the right leg and mild shortening of the left, whereas another sib had marked shortening of the left leg and moderate shortening of the right lower leg.

Auditory System. Each of the four sibs was congenitally deaf. No further audiometric testing was mentioned.

Vestibular System. No vestibular findings were described.

LABORATORY FINDINGS

Roentgenograms of the lower legs in one boy showed a striking shortening and a mild thickening of both tibias. The fibulas were of normal length and appeared to project above the knee joint. Roentgenograms of the remaining three sibs showed somewhat similar findings with a variable degree of bowing of the fibula.

HEREDITY

This syndrome involved four of six sibs. Both parents as well as the remaining two sibs were normal. Since there was no history of hearing loss or bony deformities in either family, autosomal recessive inheritance is probable.

DIAGNOSIS

A syndrome of multiple bony anomalies (aplasia of tibias, heptadactyly of toes and/or fingers), prognathism, and hypodontia was described by Reber (1968) and by Pashayan *et al.* (1971). Pfeiffer and Roeskau (1971) indicated that this represented a genetic heterogeneity and delineated four different syndromes, none of which had associated deafness. All showed autosomal dominant inheritance.

TREATMENT

Referral to orthopedic surgeon is indicated.

PROGNOSIS

The hearing loss is congenital and severe.

SUMMARY

This syndrome is characterized by: 1) autosomal recessive transmission, 2) congenital absence of one or both tibias and shortened, malformed fibulas, and 3) severe congenital hearing loss.

REFERENCES

Carraro, A., Assenza congenita della tibia e sordomutismo nel quattro fratelli. *Chir. Organi. Mov.,* *16*:429–438, 1931.

Pashayan, H., Fraser, F. C., McIntyre, J., and Dunbar, J., Bilateral aplasia of the tibia, polydactyly and absent thumbs in a father and daughter. *J. Bone Joint Surg., 53B*:495–499, 1971.

Pfeiffer, R. A., and Roeskau, M., Agenesie der Tibia, Fibulaverdoppelung und spiegelbildische Polydaktylie (Diplopodie) bei Mutter und Kind. *Z. Kinderheilk., 111*:38–50, 1971.

Reber, M., Un syndrome osseux peu commun associant une heptadactylie et une aplasie des tibias. *J. Génét. Hum., 16*:15–39, 1968.

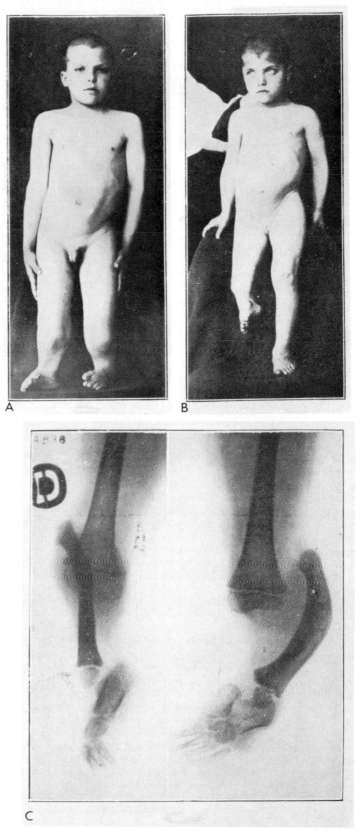

Figure 5-4 Absence of tibia and congenital deafness. (A, B) Two of four affected sibs showing asymmetric alteration of lower extremities. (C) Radiograph showing displaced, curved fibula, talipes equinovarus, and apparently displaced talus. (A and B from A. Carraro, *Chir. Organi Mov.*, *16*:429, 1931.)

BROAD TERMINAL PHALANGES, ABNORMAL FACIES, AND SENSORINEURAL DEAFNESS

Keipert, Fitzgerald, and Danks (1973) described two brothers with severe sensorineural hearing loss, unusual facies, and broad terminal phalanges.

CLINICAL FINDINGS

Physical Findings. The facies was marked by ocular hypertelorism, a large nose with a high bridge, large rounded columella, and prominent nasal alae. The upper lip protruded, had a cupid's bow configuration, and laterally overlapped the rather straight lower lip.

Musculoskeletal System. The head circumference was large. The distal phalanges of the thumbs, first, second, and third fingers, and all toes were markedly broad. The fifth fingers were short and clinodactylous. The toes were rotated medially. A third fontanelle was present during infancy.

Nervous System. One sib was severely mentally retarded.

Auditory System. In one brother there was severe sensorineural hearing loss in one ear but normal hearing in the other ear. The other sib exhibited moderately severe bilateral high-tone sensorineural deafness.

Vestibular System. No studies were reported.

LABORATORY FINDINGS

Radiographically, one sib had bifid terminal phalanges in both index fingers. In the halluces of both brothers, the proximal phalanges were short, and the terminal phalanges were markedly abbreviated with large, rounded epiphyses.

Dermatoglyphic studies showed an increase in digital whorls.

HEREDITY

Autosomal or X-linked recessive inheritance is likely.

DIAGNOSIS

Broad thumbs and halluces are seen in Rubinstein-Taybi syndrome (Rubinstein, 1968), in the frontodigital syndrome of Marshall and Smith (1970), in a disorder of unusual facies, cleft palate, mental retardation, and limb abnormalities (Palant *et al.*, 1971) and in Pfeiffer syndrome (Gorlin *et al.*, 1976). However, these other conditions differ markedly on clinical grounds from the syndrome under consideration here.

TREATMENT

A hearing aid is indicated if the patient is not too mentally retarded.

PROGNOSIS

Prognosis depends on the degree of mental retardation.

SUMMARY

The characteristics of this syndrome include: 1) recessive inheritance — either autosomal or X-linked, 2) broad terminal phalanges of fingers and toes, 3) unusual facies, and 4) sensorineural hearing loss.

REFERENCES

Gorlin, R. J., Pindborg, J. J., and Cohen, M. M., Jr., *Syndromes of the Head and Neck.* 2nd Ed. New York, McGraw-Hill Book Company, 1976.

Keipert, J. A., Fitzgerald, M. G., and Danks, K. M., A new syndrome of broad terminal phalanges and facial abnormalities. *Aust. Paediatr. J., 9*:10–13, 1973.

Marshall, R. E., and Smith, D. W., Frontodigital syndrome: a dominant inherited disorder with normal intelligence. *J. Pediatr., 77*:129–133, 1970.

Palant, D. I., Feingold, M., and Berkman, F. M. D., Unusual facies, cleft palate, mental retardation and limb abnormalities in siblings — a new syndrome. *J. Pediatr., 78*:686–689, 1971.

Rubinstein, J. H., The broad thumbs syndromes. *Birth Defects, 5*(2):25–41, 1969.

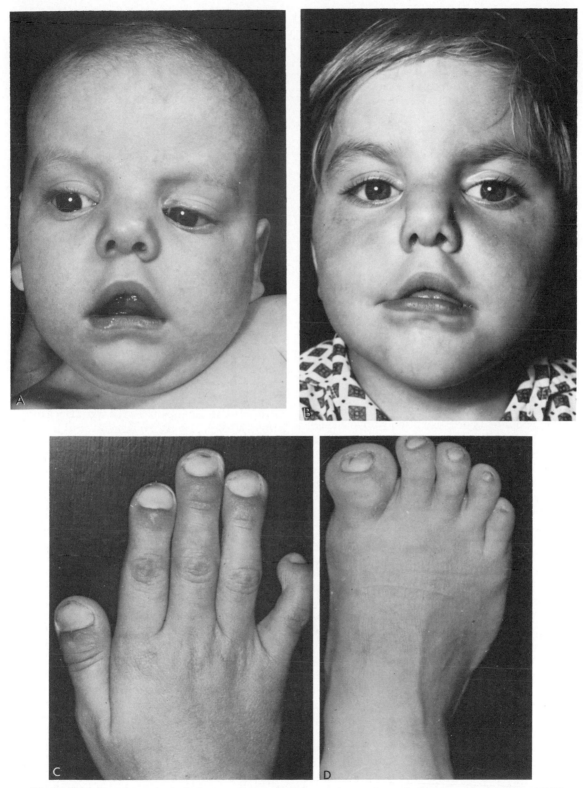

Figure 5–5 *Broad terminal phalanges, abnormal facies, and sensorineural deafness. (A, B)* Sibs exhibiting cupid's bow mouth and unusual nasal form. Younger sib also had ptosis of left lid and mild hydrocephalus. *(C, D)* Right hand of older boy showing broad terminal phalanx of thumb and first three fingers as well as clinodactyly of fifth finger. Right foot of same child showing broad terminal phalanges and medial rotation of toes. *(A–D* from J. A. Keipert *et al., Aust. Paediatr. J.,* 9:10, 1973.)

DOMINANT CRANIOMETAPHYSEAL DYSPLASIA

Craniometaphyseal dysplasia is characterized by hyperostosis of the cranial and facial bones and splaying of the metaphyseal ends of long bones. There are two heritable forms: dominant and recessive. We shall consider each in turn. Numerous reports have described associated hearing loss. The disorder has been reported under a variety of terms; most often it has erroneously been called "Pyle's disease." Early cases are those of Brown and Harper (1946) and Mitchell and Macleod (1952).

CLINICAL FINDINGS

Physical Findings. Although expressivity is somewhat variable, in most cases the facies is quite characteristic. Usually within the first year of life the root of the nose begins to broaden and an elevated wing of bone extends to the zygoma bilaterally. Increasing bony hyperostosis often narrows the nasal lumen, leading to obstruction and resultant open mouth.

Skeletal System. The skeletal abnormalities have been discussed above under *Physical Findings* and will be discussed below under *Laboratory Findings.*

Ocular System. Ocular hypertelorism is a constant finding. Nystagmus is common. There may be visual loss due to optic atrophy, suggesting bony encroachment upon the optic foramina (Mori and Holt, 1956; Saunders, 1957; Walker, 1966; Rimoin *et al.,* 1969).

Nervous System. Although most patients are neurologically normal except for hearing loss, several have had peripheral facial nerve paralysis, headache, or vertigo. Occasional patients exhibit depressed facial sensation, which suggests fifth nerve involvement. Some patients have seizures or long tract signs (Walker, 1966; Holt, 1966; Spranger *et al.,* 1967; Rimoin *et al.,* 1969; Kietzer and Paparella, 1969; Gladney and Monteleone, 1970; Cooper, 1974).

Auditory System. Varying degrees of hearing loss have been found in nearly all cases. Not uncommonly, it is the presenting symptom (Saunders, 1957). The hearing loss begins in childhood and is slowly progressive until there is moderate to severe (30 to 90 dB) deafness in the third or fourth decade. In two of three cases SISI tests that were initially negative became positive at about 12 years of age (Gladney and Monteleone, 1970). Although the loss is largely conductive, in many cases it has a sensorineural component (Saunders, 1957; Kietzer and Paparella, 1969; Gladney and Monteleone, 1970).

Vestibular System. Vestibular tests have been normal (Paulsen *et al.,* 1967).

LABORATORY FINDINGS

Roentgenograms. The calvaria exhibits frontal and occipital hyperostosis and/or sclerosis. The skull base is usually dense with obliteration of the paranasal sinuses and lack of pneumatization of the mastoids. Ocular hypertelorism is marked. During the first six years of life the long bones begin to have a club-shaped metaphyseal flare that is far milder than that seen in Pyle's disease (metaphyseal dysplasia) and may be minimal during early childhood. Diaphyseal sclerosis occurs in the infant and young child, but it disappears with age (Beckman, 1954; Walker, 1966). The short tubular bones exhibit the same changes as those noted in the long bones. The sternal halves of the clavicles may be somewhat widened. The pelvis and lateral spine are normal. In several documented cases the internal auditory meatuses have been narrowed (Rimoin *et al.,* 1969) and polytomograms have shown deposit of bone in the region of the cochlea (Gladney and Monteleone, 1970).

PATHOLOGY

Failure of resorption of the secondary spongiosa probably produces the splayed metaphyses and thickening of the skull and facial bones. The cranial nerve foramina, probably narrowed by bony encroachment, lead to deafness and, in some cases, visual loss, nystagmus, and facial nerve palsy. Generally, hearing loss is mixed. Since narrowing of the internal auditory meatus has been identified in radiographs, encroachment on the auditory nerve probably produces the sensorineural component (Miller *et al.,* 1969). The origin of the conductive component in most cases is probably due to ankylosis of the stapedial footplate or to bony overgrowth of the ossicles with re-

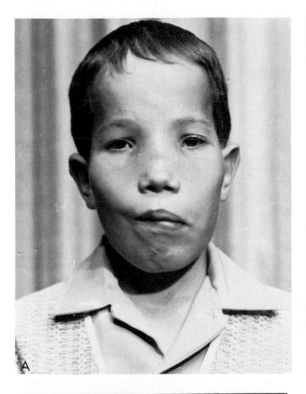

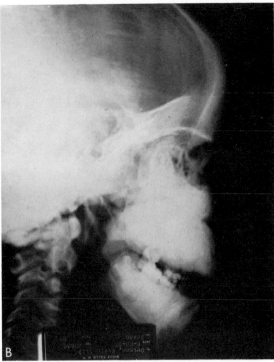

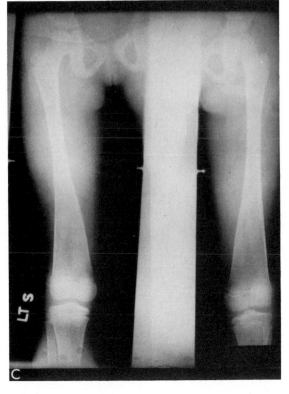

Figure 5–6 *Dominant craniometaphyseal dysplasia.* (A) Facial features showing hypertelorism, broad nasal bridge, enlarged paranasal area, and left facial paralysis. (B) Radiograph showing cranial sclerosis and deposit of bone in paranasal area, thus eliminating maxillary sinuses. (C) Radiograph of femora showing lack of metaphyseal modeling. (C from J. H. Gladney and P. L. Monteleone, *Arch. Otolaryngol.,* 92:147, 1970.)

sultant immobilization (Kietzer and Paparella, 1969).

HEREDITY

The appearance of the disorder in several successive generations as well as male-to-male transmission clearly demonstrates autosomal dominant inheritance (Brown and Harper, 1946; Spranger *et al.,* 1965; Rimoin *et al.,* 1969).

DIAGNOSIS

Hyperostosis of the skull is also seen in *recessive craniometaphyseal dysplasia, craniodiaphyseal dysplasia, congenital hyperphosphatasia,* Schwarz-Lélek syndrome, *Paget's disease, osteopetrosis, Van Buchem's disease, frontometaphyseal dysplasia,* dysosteosclerosis, and *sclerosteosis.* The long bone abnormalities in Pyle's disease (metaphyseal dysplasia) should easily be distinguished from those in craniometaphyseal dysplasia (Gorlin *et al.,* 1970). The transient diaphyseal sclerosis seen in infancy in craniometaphyseal dysplasia may appear similar to that seen in *Engelmann's disease.*

Splaying of long bone metaphyses is also found in patients with *osteopetrosis,* bone marrow hyperplasia, bone marrow infiltration as in Gaucher's disease or leukemias, some deficiency states such as healing scurvy and healing rickets, or toxic states such as lead poisoning. Cranial hyperostosis is found in none of these states.

TREATMENT

A hearing aid may lessen the deafness. Stapedectomy should be considered for persons with predominantly conductive hearing loss.

PROGNOSIS

Hearing may be decreased soon after birth and may show little change thereafter. In most cases, however, it is slowly progressive until adolescence. A similar variation in severity and progression is found in visual loss and facial palsy.

SUMMARY

Characteristics of this syndrome include: 1) autosomal dominant transmission, 2) cranial sclerosis with narrowing of cranial nerve foramina resulting, in some cases, in cranial nerve palsies, 3) metaphyseal dysplasia affecting long bones, and 4) mixed hearing loss in about half the cases.

REFERENCES

Beckmann, R., Zur Pathogenese der Marmorknochenkrankheit (Albers-Schönberg). *Med. Monatsschr., 8*:158–164, 1954.

Brown, A., and Harper, R., Craniofacial dysostosis. The significance of ocular hypertelorism. *Q. J. Med., 15*:171–182, 1946.

Cooper, J. C., Craniometaphyseal dysplasia. *J. Oral Surg., 12*:196–204, 1974.

Gladney, J. H., and Monteleone, P. L., Metaphyseal dysplasia. Genetic and otolaryngologic aspects. *Arch. Otolaryngol., 92*:147–153, 1970.

Gorlin, R. J., Spranger, J., and Koszalka, M. F., Genetic craniotubular bone dysplasias and hyperostoses: a critical analysis. *Birth Defects, 5*(4):79–95, 1969.

Holt, J. F., The evolution of cranio-metaphyseal dysplasia. *Ann. Radiol. (Paris), 9*:209–224, 1966.

Kietzer, G., and Paparella, M. M., Otolaryngological disorders in craniometaphyseal dysplasia. *Laryngoscope, 79*:921–941, 1969.

Miller, A. L., Lehman, R. H., and Geretti, R., Unusual audiological findings in cranial-metaphyseal dysplasia. *Arch. Otolaryngol., 89*:861–864, 1969.

Mitchell, R. G., and Macleod, W., Leontiasis ossea due to Albers-Schönberg's disease. *Br. J. Radiol., 25*:442–445, 1952.

Mori, P. A., and Holt, J. F., Cranial manifestations of familial metaphyseal dysplasia. *Radiology, 66*:335–343, 1956.

Paulsen, K., Spranger, J., and Lehmann, W., Otorhinologische Gesichtspunkte bei der kraniometaphysären Dysplasie (Pyle-Syndrom). *Z. Laryngol. Rhin. Otol., 46*:916–927, 1967.

Rimoin, D. L., Woodruff, S. L., and Holman, B. L., Craniometaphyseal dysplasia (Pyle's disease): autosomal dominant inheritance in a large kindred. *Birth Defects, 5*(4):96–104, 1969.

Saunders, W. H., Conductive deafness due to Pyle's disease. *Laryngoscope, 67*:147–154, 1957 (same cases as Mori and Holt).

Spranger, J., Paulsen, K., and Lehmann, W., Die kraniometaphysäre Dysplasie (Pyle). *Z. Kinderheilk., 93*:64–79, 1965 (same cases as Paulsen *et al.,* 1967).

Walker, N., Pyle's disease or cranio-metaphyseal dysplasia. *Ann. Radiol. (Paris), 9*:197–207, 1966.

RECESSIVE CRANIOMETAPHYSEAL DYSPLASIA

Clinically and pathologically this disorder is somewhat more severe than dominant craniometaphyseal dysplasia. Within the first few years of life, there is a noticeable change in facial features marked by ocular hypertelorism and broad nasal bridge. A history of cranial nerve alteration is common.

CLINICAL FINDINGS

Physical Findings. The facial features are somewhat grotesque with glabellar and paranasal prominence and/or severe mandibular prognathism. Nasal obstruction is usually complete, requiring a permanently open mouth.

It is interesting to note that the female sib described by Millard *et al.* (1967) and Ross and Altman (1967) had marked involvement of the mandible, whereas her brother did not. Both had severe bony deposition in the nasal area.

Skeletal System. The bony abnormalities have been described above under *Physical Findings* and below under *Laboratory Findings.*

Ocular System. Marked ocular hypertelorism is a constant feature. Blindness at 7 months of age due to optic atrophy was described in their Case 4 by Jackson *et al.* (1954). Graf's (1965) patient developed a moderate visual loss, more marked on one side. Progressive visual disturbances, not otherwise characterized, were noted by Sommer (1954). No optic atrophy was found.

Nervous System. Graf's (1965) patient developed unilateral facial paresis. Case 5 of Jackson *et al.* (1954), who was also described by Thoma and Goldman (1960), at 21 years of age also developed this form of paralysis. Mental retardation was noted in Case 4 by Jackson *et al.*

Auditory System. Many of these patients had deafness. Severe hearing loss was noted in their Case 5 by Jackson *et al.* (1954) and by Sommer (1954) in his patient by the age of 10 to 15 years. The patient described by Graf (1965) was shown to have hearing loss by 6 years of age. Audiometry demonstrated a 90 dB hearing loss by air conduction and a 20 to 50 dB hearing loss by bone conduction. These findings suggested that predominantly conductive hearing loss was probably due to ankylosis of the footplate of the stapes.

Vestibular System. No vestibular tests have been described.

LABORATORY FINDINGS

Roentgenograms. Cranial and facial bone abnormalities are numerous. These include hyperostosis of the calvaria, widening of the cranial cortex, sclerosis of the basal skull, ocular hypertelorism, absent paranasal sinuses, bony encroachment on cranial nerve foramina, delayed eruption of permanent teeth, and mandibular prognathism (Sommer, 1954; Lièvre and Fischgold, 1956).

The long bones show widening of the metaphyses, most severe in the distal femur, similar to that seen in the dominant form of the disorder. Sclerosis is marked; its severity is between that exhibited in dominant craniometaphyseal dysplasia and that of craniodiaphyseal dysplasia.

Other Findings. Laboratory studies have shown no abnormalities in blood, serum, urine, or spinal fluid.

HEREDITY

This disorder has autosomal recessive inheritance. Affected sibs with normal parents were described by Lehmann (1957) and Millard *et al.* (1967). Parental consanguinity was evident in the cases of Lièvre and Fischgold (1956) and Graf (1965).

DIAGNOSIS

The radiologic findings resemble those seen in the dominant form of the disorder. Craniometaphyseal dysplasia of either dominant or recessive form should not be confused with metaphyseal dysplasia (Pyle disease). This disorder, having autosomal recessive inheritance, is associated with rather severe generalized bone changes; however, facial and cranial bones are not affected (Gorlin *et al.*, 1970).

TREATMENT

The bone dysplasia may be treated by surgical contouring (Millard *et al.*, 1967). A hearing aid can be employed. Replacement of the ossicles with a prosthesis has met with varying success.

PROGNOSIS

The bony alterations appear to be slowly progressive. Overgrowth of the cranial foramina may result in cranial nerve paralysis.

SUMMARY

The major features of this disorder include: 1) autosomal recessive transmission, 2) characteristic leonine facies, 3) typical radiologic findings, including hyperostosis of cranial vault and base of skull, widening of metaphyses of long bones with Erlenmeyer-flask deformity, 4) cranial nerve paralyses, and 5) mixed but largely conductive hearing loss.

REFERENCES

Gorlin, R. J., Koszalka, M. F., and Spranger, J., Pyle's disease. Familial metaphyseal dysplasia. A presentation of two cases and argument for its separation from craniometaphyseal dysplasia. *J. Bone Joint Surg., 52A*:347–354, 1970.

Graf, K., Die Bedeutung des Pyle-Syndroms (Leontiasis ossea) für die Oto-Rhino-Laryngologie. *Z. Laryngol. Rhin. Otol., 44*:438–445, 1965.

Jackson, W. P. U., Albright, F., Drewry, G., Hanelin, J., and Rubin, M. I., Metaphyseal dysplasia, epiphyseal dysplasia, diaphyseal dysplasia, and related constitutions. *Arch. Intern. Med., 94*:871–885, 1954 (cases 4, 5).

Lehmann, E. C., Familial osteodystrophy of the skull and face. *J. Bone Joint Surg., 39B*:313–315, 1957.

Lièvre, J. A., and Fischgold, H., Leontiasis ossea chez l'enfant (ostéopétrose partielle probable). *Presse Méd., 64*:763–765, 1956.

Millard, D. R., Maisels, D. O., Batstone, J. H. F., and Yates, B. W., Craniofacial surgery in craniometaphyseal dysplasia. *Am. J. Surg., 113*:615–621, 1967 (same cases as Ross and Altman, 1967).

Ross, M. W., and Altman, D. H., Familial metaphyseal dysplasia. Review of the clinical and radiological features of Pyle's disease. *Clin. Pediatr., 6*:143–149, 1967.

Sommer, F., Eine besondere Form einer generalisierten Hyperostose mit Leontiasis ossea faciei et cranii. *Radiol. Clin., 23*:65–75, 1954.

Thoma, K. H., and Goldman, H. M., *Oral Pathology,* 5th Ed. St. Louis, C. V. Mosby Company, 1960, pp. 627–634.

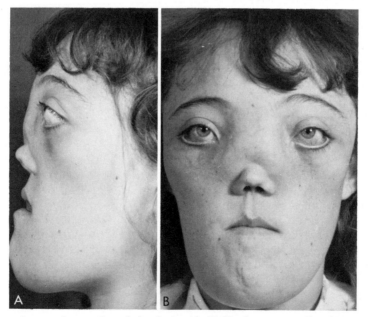

Figure 5–7 *Recessive craniometaphyseal dysplasia. (A, B)* Head appears rather large with extremely broad and flat nasal body. Paranasal masses and mandibular prognathism are due to bony involvement. (*A* and *B* from D. R. Millard Jr. *et al., Am. J. Surg., 113*:615, 1967.)

CRANIODIAPHYSEAL DYSPLASIA

Gorlin, Spranger, and Koszalka (1969) employed the term "craniodiaphyseal dysplasia" to designate a very severe bone disorder characterized by massive generalized hyperostosis and sclerosis, involving especially the skull and facial bones (de Souza, 1927; Halliday, 1949; Stransky *et al.*, 1962; Macpherson, 1974). The patient described by Gemmell (1935) may have had a mild form of the disease.

CLINICAL FINDINGS

Physical Findings. The facial and cranial thickening, distortion, and enlargement are severe in this disorder. Nasal obstruction and recurrent upper respiratory infection appear within the first few years or even first few months of life. Marked bony thickening, ocular hypertelorism, nasal flattening, and severe dental malocclusion generally follow. Bilateral choanal stenosis can be demonstrated within the first few years; a patient must keep his mouth open to breathe.

Growth is retarded and early death is common.

Skeletal System. Bony alterations have been described in part above under *Physical Findings* and below under *Laboratory Findings.*

Ocular System. All patients have severe ocular hypertelorism, lacrimal duct obstruction resulting from bony overgrowth, and diminished visual acuity or blindness due to optic atrophy (de Souza, 1927; Gemmell, 1935; Halliday, 1949; Joseph *et al.*, 1958).

Nervous System. Developmental milestones are delayed. Compression of cranial nerves results from bony overgrowth. This relentless process results in headache, progressive mental retardation, and seizures (Gemmell, 1935; Halliday, 1949; Stransky *et al.*, 1962). Increased intracranial pressure has been demonstrated (Macpherson, 1974). Lack of sexual maturity, perhaps due to impingement on the pituitary gland, has been observed (de Souza, 1927; Stransky *et al.*, 1962).

Auditory System. Deafness has been noted in all cases. In some, the deafness was congenital (Stransky *et al.*, 1962). The deafness was described as mixed by Gemmell (1935) and as sensorineural by Halliday (1949).

Vestibular System. No studies have been reported.

LABORATORY FINDINGS

Radiographically, the skull and facial bones as well as the mandible are severely sclerotic and hyperostotic. The paranasal sinuses and mastoids do not develop (Fig. 5–8B). There is moderate thickening and marked sclerosis of the ribs and clavicles. The long tubular bones do not exhibit metaphyseal flare but rather have a "policeman's nightstick" shape and show diaphyseal endostosis. The short tubular bones of the hands and feet—especially the first metapodial—exhibit cylindrization. Bone age may be retarded.

Joseph *et al.* (1958), Stransky *et al.* (1962), and Macpherson (1974) found elevated levels of serum alkaline phosphatase but normal levels of calcium and phosphorus.

HEREDITY

All of the cases cited above, with the exception of the male and female sibs described by de Souza (1927), have been isolated ones. The parents have been normal. Parental consanguinity was noted by Halliday (1949). Both males and females have been affected. Autosomal recessive inheritance is likely.

DIAGNOSIS

Craniometaphyseal dysplasia, in both its dominant and recessive forms, exhibits ocular hypertelorism, paranasal bony overgrowth, and impingement of cranial foramina. Both the milder degree of involvement and the metaphyseal flaring of the long bones, especially of the femur, clearly distinguish these two forms of the condition.

2222222222222222

TREATMENT

Therapy is of no avail.

PROGNOSIS

The prognosis is poor. The disorder is relentless in its progress and results in severe mental and somatic retardation, blindness, deafness, and often early death.

SUMMARY

The characteristics of this disorder include: 1) autosomal recessive inheritance, 2) massive enlargement and sclerosis of cranial and facial bones, ribs, and clavicles, 3) cylindrization of long bones and diaphyseal endostosis, 4) bony overgrowth of cranial foramina resulting in blindness and deafness, 5) elevated levels of alkaline phosphatase, and 6) mixed deafness.

REFERENCES

de Souza, O., Leontiasis ossea. *Porto Allegre (Brazil) Faculdade de Med. Rev. Dos. Cursos, 13*:47–54, 1927.

Gemmell, J. H., Leontiasis ossea: a clinical and roentgenographical entity. *Radiology, 25*:723–729, 1935.

Gorlin, R. J., Spranger, J., and Koszalka, M. F., Genetic craniotubular bone dysplasias and hyperostoses: a critical analysis. *Birth Defects, 5*(4):79–95, 1969.

Halliday, J., A rare case of bone dysplasia. *Br. J. Surg., 37*:52–63, 1949.

Joseph, R., Lefebvre, J., Guy, E., and Job, J. C., Dysplasie crânio-diaphysaire progressive. Ses relations avec la dysplasie diaphysaire progressive de Camurati-Engelmann. *Ann. Radiol. (Paris), 1*:477–490, 1958.

Macpherson, R. I., Craniodiaphyseal dysplasia, a disease or group of diseases? *J. Can. Assoc. Radiol., 25*:22–33, 1974.

Stransky, E., Mabilangan, L., and Lara, R. T., On Paget's disease with leontiasis ossea and hypothyreosis, starting in early childhood. *Ann. Paediatr., 199*:393–408, 1962.

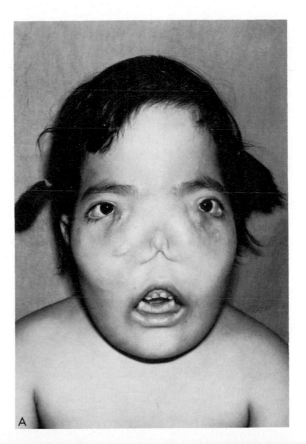

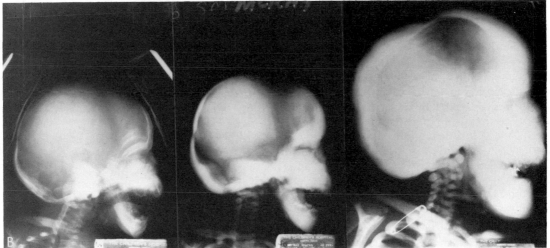

Figure 5-8 *Craniodiaphyseal dysplasia. (A)* Five-year-old patient showing marked enlargement of cranium, facial bones, and mandible. Note severe ocular hypertelorism and dental malocclusion. *(B)* Lateral skull radiographs at 3½ months (left), 18 months (center), and 5 years (right) showing progression of hyperostosis involving cranium, facial bones, mandible, and proximal cervical spine. There is no development of paranasal sinuses and mastoids. *(A* and *B* from R. I. Macpherson, *J. Can. Assoc. Radiol., 25:22,* 1974.)

FRONTOMETAPHYSEAL DYSPLASIA

Gorlin and Cohen (1969) separated frontometaphyseal dysplasia from a number of other craniotubular dysplasias. The condition consists of pronounced bony supraorbital ridge, conduction deafness, and various skeletal alterations. Similar cases were described by Lischi (1967), Walker (1969), Holt *et al.* (1972), Danks *et al.* (1972), Jarvis and Jenkins (1975), and Weiss and Reynolds (1976).

CLINICAL FINDINGS

Physical Findings. The marked supra-orbital ridge, wide nasal bridge, and small pointed chin give the patient a striking appearance (Fig. 5–9*A*). Enlargement of the supraorbital ridge becomes evident before puberty (Danks *et al.*, 1972).

Musculoskeletal System. There is wasting of muscles of the arms and legs, especially the hypothenar and interosseous muscles of the hands. Dorsiflexion of the wrist and extension of the elbows are reduced; pronation and supination are extremely limited. Flexion deformities of the fingers and ulnar deviation of the wrist are progressive (Fig. 5–9*B*). Finger mobility is limited essentially to the metacarpophalangeal joints. Hammer toes have also been noted.

Nervous System. Walker (1969) described headache and reduced sensation of areas supplied by the trigeminal nerve. Jarvis and Jenkins (1975) reported severe mental retardation in their patients.

Other Findings. One patient had a small penis and cryptorchidism (Gorlin and Cohen, 1969). Bundle branch block and right ventricular hypertrophy have been described (Danks *et al.*, 1972).

Missing permanent teeth, retained deciduous teeth, and bifid uvula were noted (Lischi, 1967; Gorlin and Cohen, 1969; Danks *et al.*, 1972).

Auditory System. Gorlin and Cohen (1969) described moderate conductive hearing loss in their 19-year-old patient. Walker (1969) reported a hearing deficit and attacks of tinnitus appearing in his patient at 25 years of age. The deafness was not otherwise characterized. Holt *et al.* (1972)

and Arenberg *et al.* (1974) noted symmetric progressive mixed hearing loss that appeared prior to puberty. A fixed malleus and incus were found on tympanotomy.

Vestibular Findings. No vestibular tests were reported.

LABORATORY FINDINGS

Roentgenograms. Radiographic examination demonstrated a thick toruslike frontal ridge, absence of frontal sinuses, "Hershey kiss" or "top of the mosque" defects of supraorbital rims, arched superior border of maxillary sinuses, and antegonial notching along the lower border of the body of the mandible with marked hypoplasia of the angle and condyloid process (Gorlin and Cohen, 1969; Holt *et al.*, 1972) (Fig. 5–9*C*). The foramen magnum was greatly enlarged and numerous cervical vertebral anomalies have been noted, such as the odontoid process being located too far anteriorly, the atlas having no posterior arch, C2 and C3 being fused, and C3 and C4 being partially dislocated. The long bones manifested an increased density in the diaphyseal region with lack of modeling in the metaphyseal area producing an Erlenmeyer-flask deformity (Fig. 5–9*D*). Marked flaring of the iliac bones, widened elongated middle phalanges, slender ribs, and increased interpediculate distances in the lumbar spine have been observed (Danks *et al.*, 1972). The ribs and vertebrae were irregularly contoured (Holt *et al.*, 1972).

Other Findings. Danks *et al.* (1972) found metachromasia in cultured fibroblasts.

HEREDITY

The disorder may have genetic heterogeneity. Weiss and Reynolds (1976) described the disorder in a mother and son, thereby suggesting autosomal dominant inheritance. Jarvis and Jenkins (1975) reported the disorder in male half sibs who had the same mother, indicating X-linked inheritance. Although the bony abnormalities were similar, the patients exhibited severe mental retardation not found in any of the other cases.

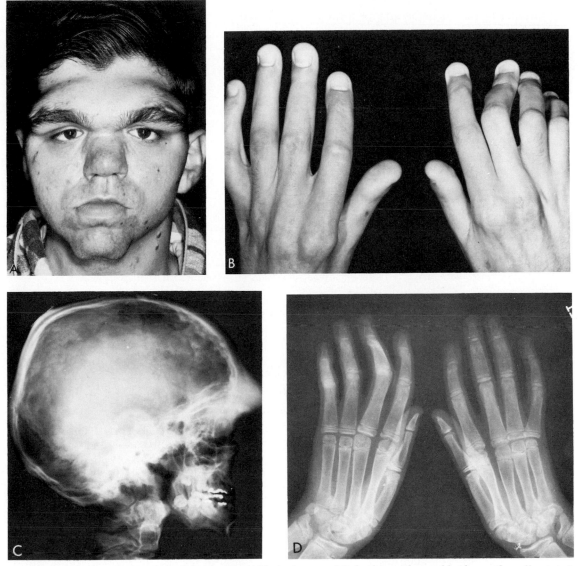

Figure 5-9 *Frontometaphyseal dysplasia.* (A) Marked supraorbital ridge, wide nasal bridge, and small pointed chin give patient a striking appearance. (B) Wasting of interosseous muscles of hands, ulnar deviation of fingers. (C) Radiograph showing supraorbital torus, hypoplasia and dysplasia of mandible, and cervical anomalies. (D) Generalized lack of modeling of long bones. (A–D from R. J. Gorlin and M. M. Cohen, Jr., *Am. J. Dis. Child.*, *118*:487, 1969.)

DIAGNOSIS

Other craniotubular dysplasias, such as *craniometaphyseal dysplasia* and *craniodiaphyseal dysplasia,* should be excluded. These disorders are discussed at length by Gorlin *et al.* (1969).

A thick toruslike frontal ridge has been noted in the end-stage of Jansen's metaphyseal dysostosis, a bone disorder otherwise quite different from frontometaphyseal dysplasia (de Haas *et al.*, 1969).

TREATMENT

A hearing aid may be used to ameliorate the deafness.

SUMMARY

Characteristics of this syndrome incluse: 1) autosomal dominant or X-linked recessive inheritance, 2) characteristic facies marked by pronounced supraorbital ridge and pointed chin, 3) wasting of arm and leg muscles with flexion deformity of joints, 4)

characteristic skeletal changes, and 5) mixed but mostly conductive deafness.

REFERENCES

Arenberg, I. K., Shambaugh, G. E., Jr., and Valvassori, G. E., Otolaryngologic manifestations of frontometaphyseal dysplasia. The Gorlin-Holt syndrome. *Arch. Otolaryngol., 99*:52–58, 1974.
Danks, D. M., Mayne, V., Hall, R. K., and McKinnon, M. C., Fronto-metaphyseal dysplasia. *Am. J. Dis. Child., 123*:254–258, 1972.
de Haas, W. H., de Boer, W., and Griffioen, F., Metaphyseal dysostosis. *J. Bone Joint Surg., 51B*:290–299, 1969.
Gorlin, R. J., and Cohen, M. M., Jr., Frontometaphyseal dysplasia. A new syndrome. *Am. J. Dis. Child., 118*:487–494, 1969.
Gorlin, R. J., Koszalka, M., and Spranger, J. W., Genetic craniotubular bone dysplasia and hyperostoses. A critical analysis. *Birth Defects, 5*(4):79–95, 1969.
Holt, J. F., Thompson, G. R., and Arenberg, I. K., Frontometaphyseal dysplasia. *Radiol. Clin. North Am., 10*:225–243, 1972.
Jarvis, G. A., and Jenkins, E. C., *Syndrome Iden., 3*(1):18–19, 1975.
Lischi, G., Le torus supraorbitalis (variation cranienne rare). *J. Radiol. Electr., 48*:463–466, 1967.
Walker, B. A., A craniodiaphyseal dysplasia or craniometaphyseal dysplasia. ? Type. *Birth Defects, 5*(4):298–300, 1969.
Weiss, L., Reynolds, W. A., and Syzmanowski, R. T., Familial frontometaphyseal dysplasia-evidence for dominant inheritance. *Am. J. Dis. Child. 130*:259–264, 1976.

RECESSIVE OSTEOPETROSIS
(Albers-Schönberg Disease)

Osteopetrosis, sometimes known as "marble bone disease," has been divided by various authors into several different entities. We shall limit our remarks to recessive osteopetrosis, since deafness has been reported only in this form. Autosomal recessive osteopetrosis is characterized by increased density of all bones and by the complications that occur from failure of absorption of the primary spongiosa and its resultant persistence: anemia, hepatosplenomegaly, thrombocytopenia, blindness, deafness, facial paralysis, and osteomyelitis. The disorder may be recognized at birth or even in utero. The infant may be stillborn or may survive only a few months. Death usually results within the first few years of life from anemia or secondary infection.

CLINICAL FINDINGS

Physical Findings. The head may be somewhat enlarged and show frontal and parietal bossing. There may be mild ocular hypertelorism. Growth is retarded in about 35 per cent of the cases.
Skeletal System. There is increased density of all bones. Osteomyelitis of the

jaws, which occurs in about 20 per cent of the cases, is a complication of dental extraction and, presumably, is due to deficient blood supply (Bergman, 1956; Gomez *et al.*, 1966). Fractures have occurred in about 30 per cent of 50 published cases (Johnston *et al.*, 1968).
Ocular System. Visual loss is noted in about 80 per cent of the cases. This loss usually begins in the first year of life, but sometimes it occurs in later childhood and may progress to blindness. Keith (1968) suggested that it resulted from retinal atrophy and not from optic atrophy secondary to pressure on the optic nerve.
Nervous System. Mental retardation has been evident in about 20 per cent of the cases (Johnston *et al.*, 1968). In about 10 per cent, unilateral or bilateral facial palsy occurs in the first few years of life, probably being secondary to pressure of dense bone on the foramen of the seventh cranial nerve.
Hematopoietic System. Although the liver and spleen are normal at birth, in over 50 per cent of the cases they enlarge in childhood because of extramedullary hematopoiesis. Hemolytic anemia and thrombocytopenia are associated with the condition.

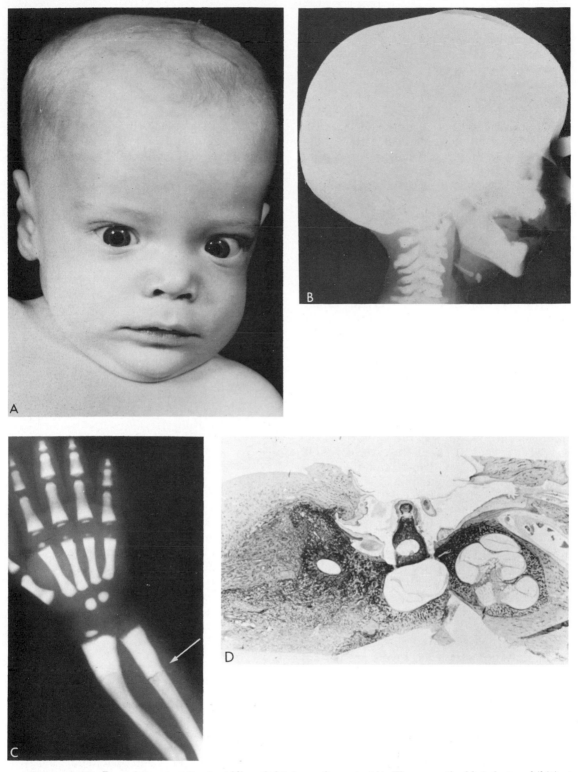

Figure 5–10 *Recessive osteopetrosis (Albers-Schönberg disease). (A)* Three-month-old infant exhibiting "squared" head form, hepatosplenomegaly, blindness, and anemia. (From R. D. Thompson *et al., J. Oral Surg., 27*:63, 1969.) *(B, C)* Marked increased density of all bones. Note fractures of radius and ulna. *(C* from E. N. Myers and S. Stool, *Arch. Otolaryngol., 89*:460, 1969.) *(D)* Section showing striking differences between lighter staining periosteal bone and darker staining osteopetrotic bone in endochondral layer of otic capsule. Abnormal bone obliterates area of mastoid antrum. (Courtesy of E. N. Myers, Pittsburgh, Pa.)

Generalized lymphadenopathy has been noted in about 20 per cent.

Auditory System. Between 25 and 50 per cent of the patients have moderate mixed sensorineural and conductive hearing loss beginning in childhood (Johnston *et al.*, 1968; Myers and Stool, 1969). In general, investigators have not reported detailed audiometric findings. Enell and Pehrson (1958), however, have described the audiogram of their 9-year-old patient as resembling that found in otosclerosis. In about half the cases there is a history of otitis media.

Vestibular System. No vestibular findings have been described.

LABORATORY FINDINGS

Roentgenograms. The radiographic picture is quite characteristic: the entire skeleton shows increased density and thickening; the bones are expanded, splayed, and dense, with the epiphysis, metaphysis, and diaphysis being involved to a similar degree. The cortical and cancellous portions are radiographically indistinguishable.

The skull is thickened and dense (mainly at its base), but the calvaria is involved as well without the recognizable diploë. The mastoid bones and paranasal sinuses are poorly pneumatized, and the facial bones appear denser than normal. Tomograms of the temporal bones have not been described.

Blood. In almost all cases, there is mild to moderate hemolytic anemia, the hemoglobin ranging from about 40 to 80 per cent of normal. Presumably, this condition results from erythrocyte destruction in the spleen (Gamsu *et al.*, 1961). Thrombocytopenia is a frequent finding.

Serum calcium, phosphorus, and acid and alkaline phosphatase levels are normal (Enell and Pehrson, 1958).

PATHOLOGY

Auditory System. Temporal bone changes have been described in a child with moderate hearing loss (Myers and Stool, 1969). The middle ear cavity was smaller than normal; there was marked hypertrophy of the mucosa. A portion of the facial nerve was herniated into the middle ear. There was a small and incomplete fallopian canal. Abnormal otosclerotic bone, evident throughout the temporal bone, covered the periosteal and endosteal layers of the otic capsule. The ossicles, which were composed of otosclerotic bone, lacked medullary cavities. The stapes was thickened, preserving its fetal shape through lack of remodeling. The organ of Corti, vestibular labyrinth, and the spiral ganglion were normal. The round window membrane was markedly thickened. There was no pneumatization of mastoid cells, these areas being filled with chondrocytes and osteoblasts (Fig. 5–10D).

HEREDITY

Since the disorder has occurred frequently in sibs, and increased parental consanguinity has been demonstrated (Enell and Pehrson, 1958; Tips and Lynch, 1962), autosomal recessive inheritance is clearly indicated in the severe form of the syndrome.

DIAGNOSIS

Generalized increased bone density occurs in pyknodysostosis and *sclerosteosis*. Recessive osteopetrosis can be distinguished by mode of transmission from the dominant form, which has later onset, a milder course, and is not associated with anemia, hepatosplenomegaly, or deafness. Fracture (40 per cent), cranial nerve palsies (15 per cent), and osteomyelitis (10 per cent) do occur, however (Johnston *et al.*, 1968).

TREATMENT

Although surgical enlargement of the optic foramina has been carried out, treatment of the facial palsy has not been described. Splenectomy and prednisone have been employed to treat the anemia (Moe and Skjaeveland, 1969). Hearing aids will help those with deafness. The ears should be examined periodically to detect otitis media. Additional temporal bone studies or tympanotomies must be performed to determine whether the stapes always becomes immobilized.

PROGNOSIS

The clinical course is variable. Facial palsy and visual or hearing loss may appear rather rapidly and then may improve slightly.

SUMMARY

The major characteristics of this disease are: 1) autosomal recessive transmission, 2) osteosclerosis with involvement of all bones of the skeleton, 3) facial palsy and visual loss in over half the cases, and 4) mild to moderate conductive hearing loss in about half the cases.

REFERENCES

Bergman, G., Studies on mineralized dental tissues. VII. Dental changes occurring in osteopetrosis. *Acta Odont. Scand., 14*:81–101, 1956.

Enell, H., and Pehrson, M., Studies on osteopetrosis. *Acta Paediatr. (Stockh.), 47*:279–287, 1958.

Gamsu, H., Lorber, J., and Rendle-Short, J., Hemolytic anemia in osteopetrosis. *Arch. Dis. Child., 36*:494–499, 1961.

Gomez, L., Taylor, R., Cohen, M. M., and Shklar, G., The jaws in osteopetrosis. *J. Oral Surg., 25*:67–74, 1966.

Johnston, C. C., Lawy, N., Lord, T., Vellios, F., Merritt, A. D., and Deiss, W. P., Osteopetrosis. A clinical, genetic, metabolic, and morphologic study of the dominantly inherited benign form. *Medicine, 47*:149–167, 1968.

Keith, C. G., Retinal atrophy in osteopetrosis. *Arch. Ophthalmol., 79*:234–241, 1968.

Moe, P. J., and Skjaeveland, A., Therapeutic studies in osteopetrosis. *Acta Paediatr. (Stockh.), 58*:593–600, 1969.

Myers, E. N., and Stool, S., The temporal bone in osteopetrosis. *Arch. Otolaryngol., 89*:460–469, 1969.

Tips, R. L., and Lynch, H. T., Malignant congenital osteopetrosis resulting from a consanguineous marriage. *Acta Paediatr. (Stockh.), 51*:585–588, 1962.

DOMINANT SYMPHALANGISM AND CONDUCTION DEAFNESS

Conduction deafness due to fixation of the footplate of the stapes to the round window in combination with hereditary absence of the proximal interphalangeal joints and carpal and tarsal bone coalition has been described in several kindreds (Vessell, 1960; Strasburger *et al.*, 1965; Gorlin *et al.*, 1970; Maroteaux *et al.*, 1972; Gloede and Stenger, 1974; Spoendlin, 1974; Murakami, 1975). Although the digital anomaly has existed in the Talbot family of England for several centuries ("Talbot fingers"), the contention that John Talbot, the first Earl of Shrewsbury (1388 ?–1453), had the disorder has been discounted after close scrutiny of the evidence. John Talbot was made famous by Shakespeare (Henry VI, Part I, Act IV) (Elkington and Huntsman, 1967).

CLINICAL FINDINGS

Ocular System. The mother and daughter described by Vessel (1960) both had strabismus, as did the sibs described by Gloede and Stenger (1974).

Skeletal System. The fingers are quite striking: little or no movement is possible in the proximal interphalangeal joints, usually from birth. The skin over the affected joint area is shiny and is without hairs or wrinkles. In some cases, the middle phalanges are shorter and wider than normal. If there is multiple finger involvement, all digits ulnar to the most radially affected digit have the same fusion anomaly. Neither the thumb nor the metacarpophalangeal joints are involved, although there are shortening and flattening of the distal head of the first metacarpal in about 25 per cent of the cases. Some degree of clinodactyly of the little finger is not uncommon.

Clinically, the feet often show a prominence on the medial side at the level of the distal end of the navicular bone. Another prominence is usually seen at the base of the fifth metatarsal. Extra bones were noted by Wildervanck *et al.* (1967).

Tarsal coalition results in decreased movement at the subtaloid and metatarsal joints. The feet are usually flat and the ankles broad. The ability to invert and evert the foot is reduced. In some individuals the gait is almost normal, in others the patient walks on the external border of the feet or, occasionally, on his toes. As in the case of the fingers, the toes may be stiff, abbreviated, or even amputated. Occasionally, the elbows may have limited flexion, extension, pronation, and supination (Murakami, 1975).

Auditory System. The mother and daughter described by Vesell had a 10 to 60 dB bilateral conductive hearing loss between the frequencies of 500 and 2000 Hz. Both had hearing loss from childhood; the deafness was probably congenital. Many individuals in the family described by Strasburger *et al.* (1965) were deaf. Conduction hearing loss was noted during the first year of life. Tympanotomy revealed bony fusion between the stapes and the petrous portion of the temporal bone. Gorlin *et al.* (1970) also described total ankylosis of the stapes.

Vestibular System. Vestibular studies have not been described.

LABORATORY FINDINGS

Roentgenograms. By adolescence (in some children much earlier) the hands show complete bony fusion of the proximal interphalangeal joints of the little finger and less complete fusion of this joint in the more radially situated fingers. The middle phalanges may be normal, short and massive, or even hypoplastic. Infrequently, there is distal interphalangeal fusion. In some cases, the fifth fingers appear to consist of a hypoplastic middle phalanx fused with the terminal phalanx. The first metacarpal is shortened, and its proximal end is coniform or fused with the adjacent carpus. The epiphyses of the major metacarpals may be somewhat flattened. The carpal bones may show anomalies, including malsegmentation of the triquetrum and partial fusion to both the lunate and hamate. Talonavicular fusion is a virtually constant finding. Less common fusions—including metatarsal, calcaneocuboid, and talonavicular—have been described. In the toes, the most common abnormality is fusion of the distal interphalangeal joints; a less common abnormality is proximal fusion. In the kindred reported by Spoendlin (1974), carpal and tarsal synostosis was marked, but symphalangism was not present.

HEREDITY

The kindreds described by these authors clearly exhibit autosomal dominant inheritance.

DIAGNOSIS

Proximal symphalangism may occur in diastrophic dwarfism and metatropic dwarfism; these conditions, however, are easily distinguished from the syndrome under discussion here. In distal symphalangism, a dominantly transmitted condition, there is no associated hearing loss (McKusick, 1975).

Dominant symphalangism and conduction deafness must be differentiated from *multiple synostoses and conduction deafness* (symphalangism-brachydactyly syndrome). This disorder also has autosomal dominant inheritance, but it is distinguished by a characteristic facies, it involves other parts of the skeletal system, and it is often associated with aplasia or hypoplasia of the fingers or toes.

There are numerous reports, reviewed by several authors, of the association of symphalangism with fusion of the carpus and tarsus. However, in no cases, other than those cited, has deafness been found (Harle and Stevenson, 1967; Wildervanck *et al.*, 1967; Geelhoed *et al.*, 1969).

TREATMENT

Despite the inability to flex their fingers, the patients do quite well and require no treatment for the symphalangism. The hearing loss can be effectively treated by stapedectomy.

PROGNOSIS

Although the symphalangism is congenital, it generally becomes more marked with age. This progression also applies to the carpal and tarsal coalitions. The hearing loss may be congenital or may appear in childhood. Even though there are no long-term studies to document this, there is no apparent increase in hearing deficit with age.

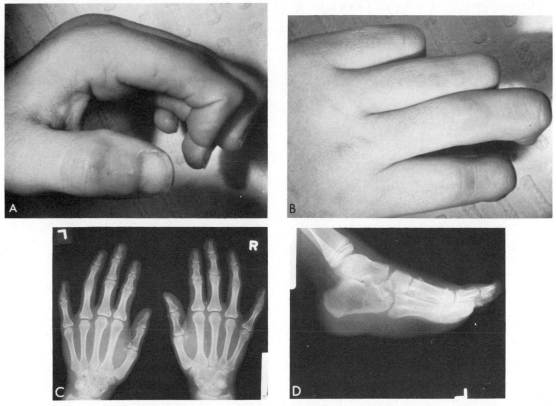

Figure 5–11   *Dominant symphalangism and conduction deafness. (A, B)* Proximal symphalangism prevents normal closure of the hand; fingers not all affected to same degree. Note lack of flexion creases over knuckles. *(C, D)* Radiograph of patient showing mild radial deviation of third through fifth digits; two phalanges in fourth and fifth digits are the result of fusion. Note fusion of lesser multangular with capitate, and triquetral with hamate. In foot, talus is fused with calcaneus. *(A–D from R. J. Gorlin et al., Z. Kinderheilkd., 108:*12, 1970.)

SUMMARY

The characteristics of this syndrome include: 1) autosomal dominant transmission with variable expressivity, 2) symphalangism involving proximal interphalangeal joints, most marked in the ulnar digits, 3) carpal and tarsal coalitions, and 4) mild to severe conductive hearing loss in infancy or early childhood.

REFERENCES

Elkington, S. G., and Huntsman, R. G., The Talbot fingers. A study in symphalangism. *Br. Med. J., 1:*407–411, 1967.

Geelhoed, G. W., Neel, J. V., and Davidson, R. T., Symphalangism and tarsal coalitions. A hereditary syndrome. A report on two families. *J. Bone Joint Surg., 51B:*278–289, 1969.

Gloede, J. F., and Stenger, H. H., Symphalangismus, Strabismus und Mittelohrmissbildungen. *Humangenetik, 22:*23–32, 1974.

Gorlin, R. J., Kietzer, G., and Wolfson, J., Stapes fixation and proximal symphalangism. *Z. Kinderheilk., 108:*12–16, 1970.

Harle, T. S., and Stevenson, J. R., Hereditary symphalangism associated with carpal and tarsal fusions. *Radiology, 89:*91–94, 1967.

McKusick, V. A., *Mendelian Inheritance in Man,* 4th Ed. Baltimore, Johns Hopkins Press, 1975.

Maroteaux, P., Bouvet, J. P., and Briard, M. L., La maladie des synostosis multiples. *Nouv. Presse Méd., 1:*3041–3047, 1972.

Murakami, Y., Nievergelt-Pearlman syndrome with impairment of hearing. *J. Bone Joint Surg. 57B:*367–372, 1975.

Spoendlin, H., Congenital stapesankylosis and fusion of carpal and tarsal bones as a dominant hereditary syndrome. *Arch. Oto-Rhino-Laryngol. 206:*173–179, 1974.

Strasburger, A. K., Hawkins, M. R., Eldridge, R., Hargrave, R. L., and McKusick, V. A., Symphalangism: genetic and clinical aspects. *Bull. Johns Hopkins Hosp., 117:*108–127, 1965.

Vesell, E. S., Symphalangism, strabismus, and hearing loss in mother and daughter. *N. Engl. J. Méd., 263:*839–842, 1960.

Wildervanck, L. S., Goedhard, G., and Meijer, S., Proximal symphalangism of fingers associated with fusion of os naviculare and talus and occurrence of two accessory bones in the feet (os paranaviculare and os tibiale externum) in a European-Indonesian-Chinese family. *Acta Genet. (Basel), 17:*166–177, 1967.

MULTIPLE SYNOSTOSES AND CONDUCTION DEAFNESS
(Symphalangism-Brachydactyly Syndrome)

Maroteaux *et al.* (1972) and Herrmann (1974) reported kindreds with multiple synostoses and conduction deafness. We have seen an isolated case.

CLINICAL FINDINGS

Physical Findings. The nose is long and thin and has minimal alar flare, i.e., it is hemicylindrical (Fig. 5–12*A*). Even though the patient is of normal height, he has abnormal body proportions. The gait is waddling; the patient often walks on the outer border of the feet without resting on the heels.

Musculoskeletal System. The upper arms are short. There is cubitus valgus with dislocation of the head of the radius and limitation of pronation, supination, and extension at the elbow.

The fingers are short. There is absence of creases over all proximal interphalangeal joints of the fingers and over the fifth, or less often the fourth, distal interphalangeal finger joints. One or more fingernails and/or toenails may be hypoplastic. One or more terminal portions of fingers (rarely the third) and/or of toes may be missing (Fig. 5–12*B*). The fifth finger may exhibit clinodactyly. The hallux is often short; there may be an increase in the space between the hallux and the rest of the toes.

Other Findings. Simian creases are a common finding. The absence of some digital triradii and the presence of two palmar axial triradii have been observed (Maroteaux *et al.*, 1972). Strabismus has been noted in several patients (Herrmann, 1974).

Auditory System. Conductive hearing loss appearing during early childhood or adolescence was noted in four of six patients reported by Herrmann (1974) and in four of seven patients examined by Maroteaux *et al.* (1972). The latter authors demonstrated total ankylosis of the stapes. One of their patients had malformed stapes and incus.

Vestibular System. No data have been reported on vestibular function.

LABORATORY FINDINGS

The hands and feet are most severely affected. Starting in childhood, there are progressive coalition of the lesser multangular-capitate-hamate and triquetral bones, short and broad first metacarpal, progressive proximal symphalangism of the second, third, fourth, and fifth digits, and progressive distal symphalangism of the fifth and often the fourth digits. One or more distal phalanges may be hypoplastic and one or more metacarpals and proximal phalanges may be overtubulated.

The forefoot is short and shows coalition of the talus and navicular bone, fusion between the second and third cuneiforms, and coalition between both the first two cuneiforms and the tarsometatarsal joints. There are progressive hallux valgus and proximal symphalangism of the second, third, and fourth digits, and hypoplastic or absent middle and distal phalanges of the fourth and/or fifth digits. The first metatarsal is often short and, like the other metatarsals, may be overtubulated.

The metaphyses of long bones are broad and irregular. The diaphyses may be somewhat bowed. Radiohumeral synostosis, malformed distal humerus and proximal radius, and subluxation of the radial head are common findings.

Spinal anomalies include hypoplastic spinal processes of cervical vertebrae, fused arches, and osteolytic defects in the anterior superior portions of the lower thoracic and upper lumbar vertebrae.

HEREDITY

The syndrome has been clearly shown to have autosomal dominant inheritance.

DIAGNOSIS

Both Lambert (1947) and Pfeiffer (1969) briefly described similarly affected children but neither investigator mentioned deafness. Lacheretz *et al.* (1974) described a boy whose parents were first cousins. He presented obliteration of the coronal and sagittal sutures, a somewhat cylindrical nose, bilateral radiohumeral synostosis, fusion of the trapezius and trapezoid, malformed pinnae, absence of palmar flexion creases, talipes equinovarus, mental retardation, and conduction deafness due to fixation of the footplate of the stapes. Possibly, this unique condition has autosomal

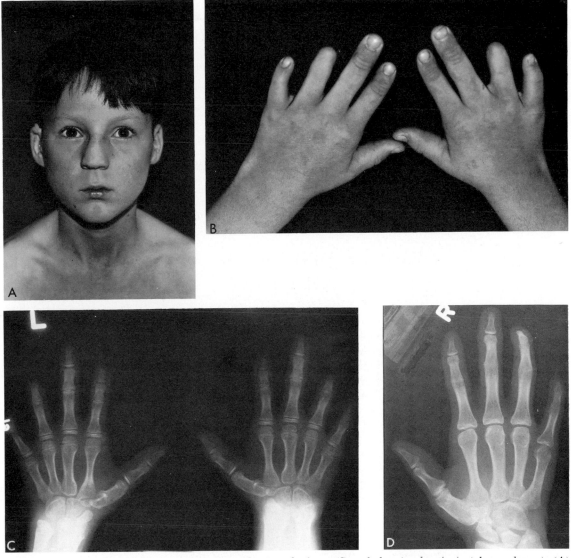

Figure 5-12   Multiple synostoses and conduction deafness (Symphalangism-brachydactyly syndrome). (A) Facies showing somewhat cylindrical nose, lack of alar flare, and hypoplastic septum. *(B)* Failure of development of terminal portions of fourth digits and absence of proximal flexion creases of fingers. *(C, D)* Fusion of carpal bones, proximal symphalangism, amputation of terminal phalanges of fourth fingers, and enlargement of first metacarpal. *(A–D from J. Herrmann, Birth Defects, 10(5):23, 1974.)*

recessive inheritance. *Dominant symphalangism and conduction deafness* can be excluded, since there is no altered facies. The skeletal alterations are limited to the hands and feet. There is no hypoplasia or aplasia of terminal phalanges and/or nails.

PROGNOSIS

The symphalangism and other synostoses as well as the hearing loss are progressive.

TREATMENT

Stapedectomy and insertion of a prosthesis may improve hearing. Orthopedic surgical help should be sought for relief of the skeletal problems.

SUMMARY

The syndrome is characterized by: 1) autosomal dominant inheritance, 2) lack of nasal alar flare, 3) progressive proximal symphalangism of all the fingers and distal symphalangism of the last finger, 4) carpal and tarsal coalition, 5) subluxation of the radial heads, 6) short first metapodial bone, 7) hypoplasia or aplasia of various distal phalanges and corresponding fingernails and toenails, and 8) progressive conduction deafness.

REFERENCES

Herrmann, J., Symphalangism and brachydactyly syndromes. Report of the WL symphalangism–brachydactyly syndrome. *Birth Defects, 10*(5):23–54, 1974.

Lacheretz, M., Walbaum, R., and Tourgis, C., L'acrocéphalo-synankie. A propos d'une observation avec synostoses multiples. *Pédiatrie, 29*:169–177, 1974.

Lambert, L. A., Congenital humeroradial synostotic anomalies. *Pediatrics, 31*:573–577, 1947.

Lenz, W. D., Bone defects of the limbs—an overview. *Birth Defects, 5*(3):1–6, 1969.

Maroteaux, P., Bouvet, J. P., and Briard, M. L., La maladie des synostosis multiples. *Nouv. Presse Méd., 1*:3041–3047, 1972.

Pfeiffer, R. A., Associated deformities of the head and hands. *Birth Defects, 5*(3):18–34, 1969.

PAGET'S DISEASE OF BONE

(Osteitis Deformans)

Paget (1876) described a form of "chronic osteitis" that begins in middle age and is characterized by changes in the shape, size, and direction of involved bones. Usually the disorder symmetrically affects the skull and bones of the lower extremities. The bones enlarge and soften, and those that are weight-bearing yield and become curved and misshapen. With extensive cranial and vertebral changes, neurologic signs or symptoms are not uncommon.

CLINICAL FINDINGS

Physical Findings. Clinical alterations begin in the fifth decade with progressive skull enlargement and frontal bossing. There is tortuosity of the terminal branches of the temporal artery in about 70 per cent of the cases (Fig. 5–13*B*). With time, there are progressive kyphosis and bowing of the legs; most cases, however, are subclinical (Davies, 1968).

Skeletal System. The onset of bony changes is insidious and progresses slowly. When symptoms are a feature, bone pain has been noted in about 50 per cent of the cases. The bones most strikingly involved are the sacrum, pelvis, lumbar vertebrae, femur, and skull. The cranium may gradually enlarge, and the patient may become aware of the disorder when his hat no longer fits. About 15 per cent have involvement of the maxilla or, rarely, the mandible. Kyphosis and bowing of the leg bones result in shortened stature. The involved bones are more susceptible to fracture, but they usually heal well. Sarcomatous changes occur in 1 to 3 per cent.

Nervous System. Neuromuscular disturbances, such as sensory-motor, reflex, gait, or central nervous system changes, are common (Rosenkrantz *et al.*, 1952). About 20 per cent of those with skull involvement experience tinnitus and/or vertigo. In advanced Paget's disease, headache—especially occipital—is an almost constant feature (Davies, 1968). Similar data were presented by Fowler (1937). Occasionally, there is involvement of the optic nerve and, following collapse of an osteoporotic vertebra, there is compression of the spinal cord (Wyllie, 1923). Optic atrophy due to compression of the nerves in the optic foramina is a rare complication (Galbraith, 1954).

Auditory System. Patients may have narrowing and/or tortuosity of the external auditory meatus (Sparrow and Duvall, 1967; Davies, 1968). Marked involvement of the auditory system more often accompanies advanced skull changes. Goldstein *et al.* (1926), in their review of 400 cases, noted hearing impairment in only 5 per cent of the cases. Rosenkrantz *et al.* (1952) noted deafness in 12 per cent. Davies, on the other hand, found hearing loss in 40 per cent. The type of hearing loss varies from conductive to sensorineural and may be unilateral or bilateral (Wyllie, 1923). Barth (1934) described six patients with sensorineural deafness and eight with mixed deafness. Clemis *et al.* (1967), Sparrow and

Duvall (1967), and Calvet *et al.* (1967) found mixed deafness most frequently. Audiometric tests did not suggest evidence of a retrocochlear focus of the disease to account for the sensorineural component. Petasnick (1969), however, found sensorineural deafness more common.

Davies (1968) noted most patients to have conductive deafness in the low frequencies — the air-bone gap being greatest at 500 Hz. SISI scores were low at low frequencies but were high at high frequencies (above 1000 Hz) (Clemis *et al.*, 1967).

We have studied three patients with Paget's disease. In a 79-year-old patient there were bilateral mixed hearing loss at lower frequencies and severe bilateral sensorineural loss at the higher frequencies. The SISI test findings were negative. Another 79-year-old patient had moderate to severe bilateral mixed hearing loss, more marked unilaterally. A third patient, 80 years old, had severe sensorineural hearing loss on one side and moderate sensorineural hearing loss on the other side. Radiographs of all these patients showed extensive skull involvement.

Vestibular System. Among 28 patients complaining of vertigo, Davies (1968) found a diminished caloric reaction in only two individuals. In the three cases we studied, one patient had no response to caloric stimulation, whereas the other two were normal.

LABORATORY FINDINGS

Roentgenograms. The early stage of osteitis deformans is osteoclastic. In later stages, the affected bones assume a "cotton wool" appearance as a result of formation of premature, coarse-fibered bone in discontinuous trabeculae that gradually are replaced by thick trabeculae with a mosaic pattern. Radiographs show increased size of affected bones, coarse trabeculation, and bowing of the extremities. Most frequently involved are the skull, tibias, pelvis, vertebrae, and femurs. Tomography has shown demineralization of the petrous pyramid. About 60 per cent manifest partial or complete demineralization of the cochlea, whereas approximately 50 per cent exhibit changes in the rest of the otic capsule. Thickening of the footplate of the stapes was evident in about 25 per cent. Over 65 per cent of patients with conductive deafness had no radiographic changes in the middle ear (Petasnick, 1969).

Other Findings. Serum alkaline phosphatase levels are greatly elevated. In about 10 per cent of the patients, the urinary calcium level is high. Serum calcium and phosphorus levels are normal.

PATHOLOGY

The skull is enlarged, and the calvaria is markedly thickened and shows narrowing of the diploë. Recently affected long bones may show sharp lines of demarcation between involved areas and the normal cortex, suggesting that Paget's disease begins focally and spreads gradually.

Histologic sections reveal a characteristic mosaic bone pattern. This results from resorption of older, calcified bone and deposition of the new osteoid layers, thereby altering the original body architecture. This alteration is associated with fibrosis and increased vascularity of marrow spaces.

There have been several reports on histopathologic changes in the temporal bones (Anson and Wilson, 1937; Kornfeld, 1967; Davies, 1968; Lindsay and Lehman, 1969; Gussen, 1970; Nager, 1975). The earliest changes include increased remodeling of bone surrounding vascular channels near the labyrinthine capsule and finally encroaching upon the endosteum of the membranous labyrinth (Gussen, 1970). There is a variable degree of degeneration of sensory cells of the saccular and utricular maculae and cristae of the semicircular canals (Lindsay and Lehman, 1969). In the organ of Corti there is degeneration of the stria vascularis and hair cells, edema of the tectorial membrane, and dilatation of the cochlear duct. Kornfeld (1967), studying seven temporal bones affected with osteitis deformans, showed that when the innermost portion of the capsule was affected, there was thickening of the stria vascularis, atrophy of portions of the stria adjacent to the thickenings, and formation of intravascular concrements. There were also occasional findings of microaneurysms. None of the authors found compression of the auditory nerve in the internal auditory meatus. Thus, the pathologic changes appear to originate from encroachment on the labyrinthine capsule by the altered bone and possibly by the attendant vascular changes.

HEREDITY

The disorder occurs much more frequently than is supposed. Autopsy evidence suggests that Paget's disease is present in about 3 per cent of those over 40 years of age and occurs possibly in as many as 10 per cent in their ninth decade.

Most data support the view that Paget's disease has autosomal dominant inheritance with incomplete penetrance and variable expressivity (Galbraith, 1954; Evens and Bartter, 1968; McKusick, 1972).

DIAGNOSIS

The clinical appearance and radiographic alterations of affected bones are characteristic.

TREATMENT

A hearing aid is currently the best treatment for the hearing loss. Attempts to mobilize the stapes have met with generally poor results (Davis, 1968). Therapy for the generalized disease includes a high-protein diet with adequate vitamin C, a high intake of calcium unless the patient is immobilized, and anabolic steroids for increasing bone repair. Corticosteroid treatment relieves pain but aggravates the osteoporosis. Calcitonin, mithramycin, and diphosphonates have been employed in treatment (Ryan et al., 1969; Haddad et al., 1970; Smith et al., 1971; Woodhouse et al., 1971).

PROGNOSIS

The disease is slowly progressive but does not appear to shorten life. Fractures are frequent, but there is minimal trauma. Only a small proportion of patients develop severe neurologic or renal complications, or sarcomatous degeneration of bone. Increased vascularity may induce high-output cardiac failure.

SUMMARY

Major features of this syndrome include: 1) autosomal dominant transmission with incomplete penetrance and variable expressivity, 2) onset in middle age, 3) involvement of the sacrum, pelvis, vertebrae, long bones of the legs, and skull, 4) neurologic deficits and spinal cord compression in a small percentage of patients, and 5) mixed hearing loss.

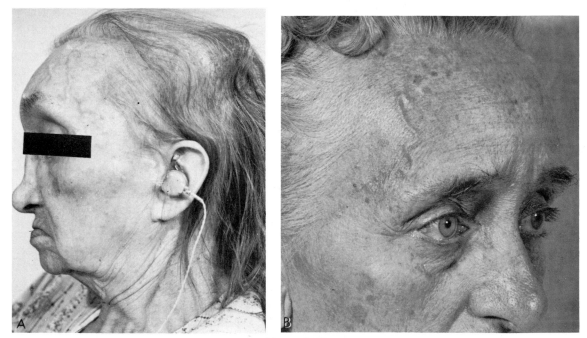

Figure 5–13

See legend on the opposite page.

Figure 5-13 *Paget's disease (osteitis deformans).* *(A)* Seventy-seven-year-old woman with long-standing history of head enlargement and deformity as well as diminished hearing. *(B)* Increased tortuosity and enlargement of anterior branch of superficial temporal artery. (From D. G. Davies, *Acta Otolaryngol., Suppl. 242*:1, 1968.) *(C)* "Cotton-wool" appearance of skull. (*A* and *C* from S. M. Gage *et al., Oral Surg., 20*:616, 1965.) *(D)* Photomicrograph of cochlear duct of patient with Paget's disease. Labyrinthine capsule is extensively replaced by Paget bone. Note dilated duct, absorption of walls of posterior canal, fibrosis in middle ear, scala tympani, and posterior canal. Also note fracture from posterior canal ampulla to scala tympani and round window niche *(A)*. (Courtesy of J. R. Lindsay and R. H. Lehman, *Laryngoscope, 79*:213, 1969.) *(E)* Temporal bone section showing Pagetic projections (s) arising from epitympanic wall and lying in close proximity to head of malleus (m) and incus (i). (From D. G. Davies, *Acta Otolaryngol., Suppl. 242*:1, 1968.)

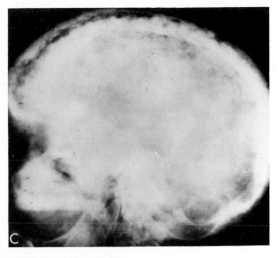

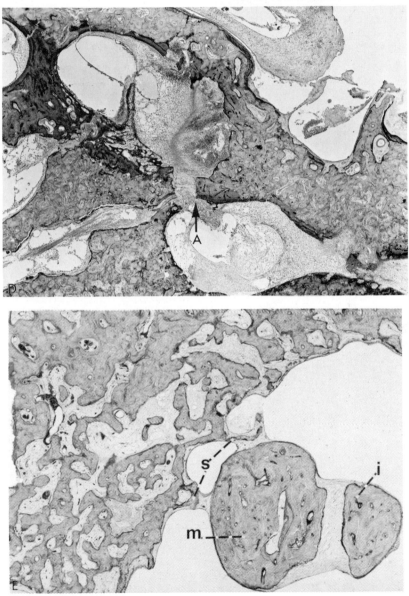

REFERENCES

Anson, B. J., and Wilson, J. G., Structural alterations in the petrous portion of the temporal bone in osteitis deformans. *Arch. Otolaryngol., 25*:560–580, 1937.

Barth, H., Klinische Befunde am Hör-und Gleichgewichtsapparat bei den metapoetischen Knochenerkrankungen. *Z. Hals- Nasen- Ohrenheilkd, 35*:305–324, 1934.

Calvet, J., Coll, J., Dussert, J., and Pelletier, L., Les surdités dans la maladie de Paget. *Int. Audiol., 6*:68–71, 1967.

Clemis, J. D., Boyles, J., Harford, E. R., and Petasnick, J. P., The clinical diagnosis of Paget's disease of the temporal bone. *Ann. Otol., 76*:611–623, 1967.

Davies, D. G., Paget's disease of the temporal bone. A clinical and histopathological survey. *Acta Otolaryngol. (Stockh.), Suppl. 242*:1–47, 1968.

Evens, R. G., and Bartter, F. C., The hereditary aspects of Paget's disease: (Osteitis deformans). *J.A.M.A., 205*:900–902, 1968.

Fowler, E. P., Jr., Nerve deafness from noninflammatory lesions. *Trans. Am. Otol. Soc., 27*:381–392, 1937.

Galbraith, H. J. B., Familial Paget's disease of bone. *Br. Med. J., 2*:29, 1954.

Goldstein, H., Goldstein, L., and Goldstein, H. Z., Paget's disease of the bones (osteitis deformans), with report of seven additional cases. *Med. Times, 54*:194–200, 1926.

Goodhill, V., *Stapes Surgery for Otosclerosis.* New York, P. B. Hoeber, 1961, p. 37.

Gussen, R., Early Paget's disease of the labyrinthine capsule. *Arch. Otolaryngol., 91*:341–345, 1970.

Haddad, J. G., Jr., Birge, S. J., and Avioli, L. V., Effects of prolonged thyrocalcitonin administration on Paget's disease of bone. *N. Engl. J. Med., 283*:549–556, 1970.

Kornfeld, M., Pathological changes in the stria vascularis in Paget's disease. *Pract. Oto-rhino-laryngol., 29*:406–432, 1967.

Lindsay, J. R., and Lehman, R. H., Histopathology of the temporal bone in advanced Paget's disease. *Laryngoscope, 79*:213–227, 1969.

McKusick, V. A., *Heritable Disorders of Connective Tissue,* 4th Ed. St. Louis, C. V. Mosby Company, 1972.

Nager, G. T., Paget's disease of the temporal bone. *Ann. Otol., Suppl. 22*:1–32, 1975.

Paget, J., On a form of chronic inflammation of bones (osteitis deformans). *Proc. R. Med. Chir. Soc. (Lond.), 8*:127–128, 1876.

Petasnick, J. P., Tomography of the temporal bone in Paget's disease. *Am. J. Roentgenol., 105*:838–843, 1969.

Rosenkrantz, J. A., Wolf, J., and Kaicher, J. J., Paget's disease (osteitis deformans). Review of one hundred eleven cases. *Arch. Intern. Med., 90*:610–633, 1952.

Ryan, W. G., Schwartz, T. B., and Perlea, C. P., Effects of mithramycin on Paget's disease of bone. *Ann. Intern. Med., 70*:549–557, 1969.

Smith, R., Russell, R. G., and Bishop, M., Diphosphonates and Paget's disease of bone. *Lancet, 1*:945–947, 1971.

Sparrow, N. L., and Duvall, A. J., Hearing loss and Paget's disease. *J. Laryngol., 81*:601–611, 1967.

Tamari, M., Histopathologic changes of the temporal bone in Paget's disease. *Ann. Otol., 51*:170–208, 1942.

Woodhouse, N. J., Reiner, M., Bordier, P., Kalu, D., *et al.,* Human calcitonin in the treatment of Paget's bone disease. *Lancet, 1*:1139–1143, 1971.

Wyllie, W. G., The occurrence in osteitis deformans of lesions of the central nervous system, with a report of four cases. *Brain, 46*:336–351, 1923.

HYPEROSTOSIS CORTICALIS GENERALISATA
(van Buchem's Disease)

A syndrome characterized by osteosclerosis of the skull, mandible, clavicles, and ribs and by hyperplasia of the diaphyseal cortex of the long and short bones was reported in seven cases by van Buchem *et al.* in 1962. An earlier example is that of Garland (1946). An isolated case was described by Fosmoe *et al.* (1968). Van Buchem (1971) documented another eight patients.

The disorder begins during puberty and results in narrowing of cranial nerve foramina, in some individuals producing facial paralysis and visual or hearing loss.

CLINICAL FINDINGS

Physical Findings. The facial changes develop slowly but usually become apparent before the second decade. A most striking finding is a wide and thickened mandible, suggesting acromegaly. Rarely is skull circumference enlarged. Occasionally, there is mild exophthalmos. The extremities appear grossly normal.

Skeletal System. Enlargement of the mandible and skull generally is noted when the patient is about 10 years old. The calvaria is thickened and the skull base becomes dense. In adult patients, the thickened clavicles become palpable. This thickening progresses slowly, and there are no other signs until facial paralysis, hearing loss, or visual loss develops. The long tubular bones become thickened. There is no increased tendency to fracture.

Ocular System. Three of seven patients described by van Buchem *et al.* (1962) had visual loss, beginning with papilledema at 30 years of age and progressing to optic atrophy and blindness.

Nervous System. Headache is a common complaint. Facial palsy, which is not uncommon, is transient, appearing during the early years of life. Two of fifteen patients had unilateral and one had bilateral facial paralysis (van Buchem *et al.*, 1962). Of eight patients, all had facial palsy: bilateral in the five adults and unilateral in the three children (van Buchem, 1971).

Auditory System. Of fifteen patients described, thirteen had hearing loss (van Buchem *et al.*, 1962). Gradual impairment of hearing began at about 15 years of age. One patient was severely deaf by the age of 38 years. Of seven patients described by van der Wouden (1968), all had bilateral symmetric hearing loss. Some cases showed sensorineural hearing loss whereas others manifested mixed deafness. Speech audiometry often demonstrated loss of discrimination. Tone-decay and SISI tests were positive in some cases.

LABORATORY FINDINGS

Roentgenograms. The skeletal changes include marked thickening of the skull and enlargement of the mandible. The clavicles, ribs, and diaphyses of long bones show a marked increase in density and are rough-textured. The medullary cavity is often occluded. The diameter of the ribs and clavicles is increased throughout.

Other Findings. Serum calcium and inorganic phosphate levels are normal, but alkaline phosphatase levels are usually increased from 50 to 250 per cent above normal.

PATHOLOGY

Autopsy findings have been described in only one case (van Buchem *et al.*, 1962). The skull was greatly enlarged and thickened with compact bone, lacked the diploe, and showed numerous bony excrescences on the surface. All foramina were narrowed (van Buchem, 1971). Long bones exhibited a thickened diaphysis.

Histologic sections showed mature lamellar bone that had narrow haversian canals and rare osteoblastic activity. Histologic sections of the temporal bone were not described.

HEREDITY

The disorder exhibits autosomal recessive inheritance. Parents have been normal and affected sibs have been described. Consanguinity has been demonstrated (van Buchem *et al.*, 1962; van Buchem, 1971).

DIAGNOSIS

In *osteopetrosis*, all the bones are increased in density. Marked thickening of the skull and mandible does not occur. In pachydermoperiostosis, irregular subperiosteal bone is formed as in van Buchem's disease, but it is more pronounced at the distal ends of long bones and at insertions of tendons and ligaments. Massive endostosis is not present. There may be two or more genetic forms of the disorder. The patient described by Dyson (1972) may have had *sclerosteosis*.

TREATMENT

A hearing aid may lessen the effects of the hearing loss. Possible decompression of the optic or facial nerves should be considered when there are signs of involvement.

PROGNOSIS

The disorder becomes manifest when affected persons are about 10 years old and progresses slowly thereafter. One patient died when she was 52 years old (van Buchem *et al.*, 1962). All other patients, ranging in age from 23 to 48 years, were normal except for evidence of the disease and associated cranial nerve palsies.

SUMMARY

Characteristics of this disorder include: 1) autosomal recessive transmission, 2) generalized osteosclerotic overgrowth of the skeleton (including mandible, skull, ribs, long and short bones), 3) markedly increased levels of serum alkaline phosphatase in most patients, and 4) narrowing of skull foramina, causing cranial nerve palsies with visual and mixed hearing loss.

REFERENCES

Dyson, D. P., Van Buchem's disease (hyperostosis corticalis generalisata familiaris). *Br. J. Oral Surg., 9*:237–245, 1972.

Fosmoe, R. J., Holm, R. S., and Hildreth, R. C., Van Buchem's disease (hyperostosis corticalis generalisata familiaris). *Radiology, 90*:771–774, 1968.

Garland, L. H., Generalized leontiasis ossea. *Am. J. Roentgenol., 55*:37–43, 1946.

van Buchem, F. S., Hadders, H. N., Hansen, J. F., and Woldring, M. G., Hyperostosis corticalis generalisata. *Am. J. Med., 33*:387–397, 1962.

van Buchem, F. S., Hyperostosis corticalis generalisata. Eight new cases. *Acta Med. Scand., 189*:257–267, 1971.

van der Wouden, A., Deafness caused by hyperostosis corticalis generalisata. *Pract. Otorhinolaryngol., 30*:91–92, 1968.

Figure 5-14 *Hyperostosis corticalis generalisata (van Buchem's disease). (A)* Broad chin, thick clavicles. *(B)* Thickening of skull and mandible. *(C)* Base of skull formed of thickened sclerotic bone without diploë. Note multiple excrescences. *(D)* Thickening of diaphysis of tibia. *(A–D* from F. S. van Buchem *et al., Am. J. Med., 33*: 387, 1962.)

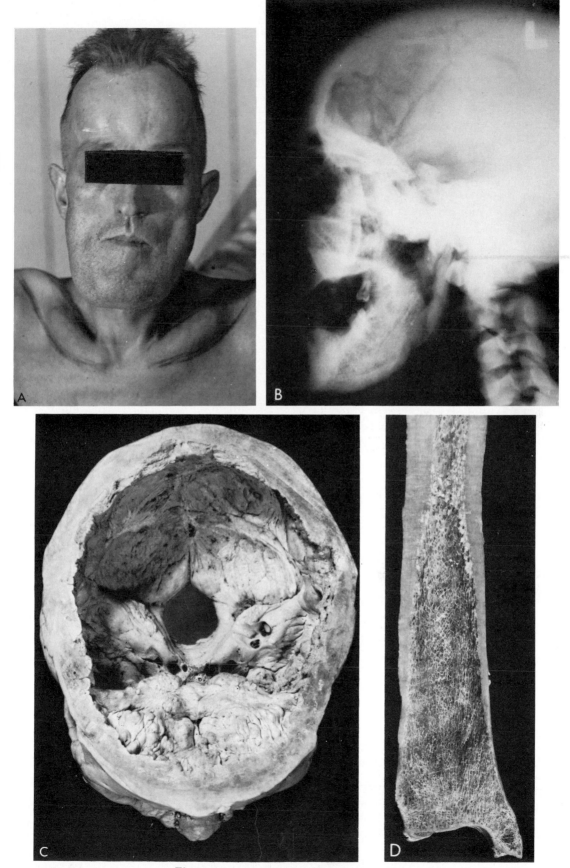

Figure 5-14   *See legend on the opposite page*

SCLEROSTEOSIS

Sclerosteosis is characterized by generalized osteosclerosis and hyperostosis of the calvaria, mandible, clavicles, and pelvis. Frequently, it is combined with syndactyly and other abnormalities of digits. Hirsch (1929) probably described the first cases. Additional examples are those of Kretzmar and Roberts (1936), Falconer and Ryrie (1937), Higinbotham and Alexander (1941), Kelley and Lawlah (1946), Pietruschka (1958), Truswell (1958), Klintworth (1963) and Sugiura (1975). Witkop (1958) described other members of the same kindred noted earlier by Kelley and Lawlah. Beighton et al. (1976) reported 25 affected individuals from 15 kindreds in South Africa.

CLINICAL FINDINGS

Physical Findings. The typical facies is evident in early childhood but becomes progressively marked with age. It is characterized by steep high forehead, ocular hypertelorism, broad flat nasal root, midfacial hypoplasia, and a prognathic, broadened, squared mandible. Frequently, there is exophthalmos. Head circumference is enlarged. Body height is increased—affected males not uncommonly exceed 198 cm. and affected females, 183 cm.

Skeletal System. About 90 per cent of patients exhibit asymmetric cutaneous syndactyly of the index and middle fingers. This condition often extends only to the proximal interphalangeal joint; there is radial deviation of the distal phalanx of the index fingers. Occasionally, syndactyly of a milder degree involves the third and fourth fingers. The nails of the involved fingers commonly are dysplastic. There is no increased tendency to fracture.

Nervous System. Facial nerve paralysis may be congenital; more frequently, it appears in infancy or childhood. Characteristically, it is unilateral for many years but becomes bilateral in late adolescence. Chronic headache and decreased sensory function of the first and second divisions of the trigeminal nerve are common findings. Increased intracranial pressure has been documented and may have been responsible for several unexplained early adult deaths. Anosmia has also been described (Pietruschka, 1958; Klintworth, 1963; Beighton

et al., 1976). Cervical plexus compression has been reported (Beighton et al., 1976).

Ocular System. In early adult life there may be unilateral or bilateral compression of optic nerves, papilledema, optic atrophy, and reduced visual fields. Convergent strabismus, nystagmus, and exophthalmos are common.

Auditory System. Bilateral sensorineural, mixed, or conductive deafness—a constant feature of the disorder—may appear early in infancy, during childhood, or late in adolescence. Beighton et al. (1976) described fixed ossicles.

Vestibular System. Pietruschka (1958) found negative reaction to caloric stimulation.

LABORATORY FINDINGS

Roentgenograms. Radiologic changes first become evident in early childhood and progress through the end of the third decade. The calvaria is greatly thickened and dense, the inner and outer tables not being recognizable. Especially thickened is the skull base. The inner acoustic meatus and the optic canal are narrowed; the orbits are usually flattened. The body of the mandible is greatly thickened and prognathic, and the angle is opened. There is only minimal involvement of the mandibular rami.

The clavicles and ribs are broadened as a result of cortical thickening. The scapulae, pelvis, and vertebral bodies are uniformly sclerotic. The tubular bones, in addition to showing increased density, exhibit a lack of diaphyseal modeling. The index finger may have no middle phalanx or only a small triangular bone; in some cases, however, it is normal.

Other Findings. Serum alkaline phosphatase levels are markedly elevated in nearly all patients (Beighton et al., 1976).

PATHOLOGY

No histopathologic studies have been reported.

HEREDITY

The syndrome is inherited as an autosomal recessive trait. Affected sibs have been described by Hirsch (1929), Falconer

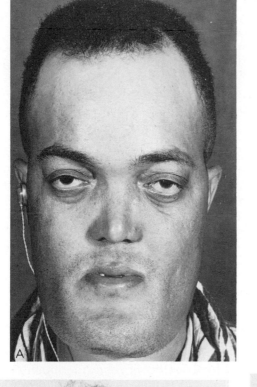
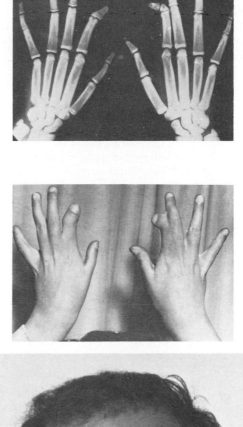
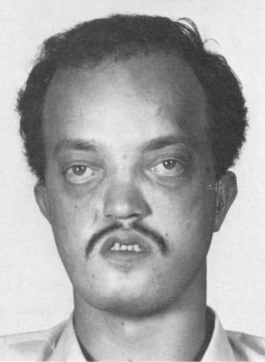
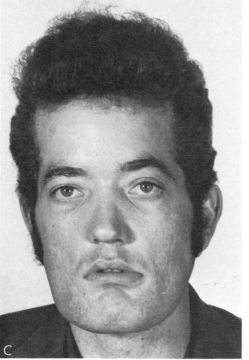

Figure 5–15 *Sclerosteosis.* (A) Marked mandibular growth following puberty; mandible assumes square form. Mixed deafness, facial palsy, headache, exophthalmos, and blindness are common complications. (Courtesy of C. J. Witkop, Jr., Minneapolis, Minnesota.) (B) Soft tissue syndactyly of second and third fingers was present bilaterally. Third and fourth fingers were partly fused unilaterally. Radiograph shows hypoplasia or absence of middle phalanx of second digit together with radial deviation of terminal phalanx. (Courtesy of A. S. Truswell, *J. Bone Joint Surg., 40B*:208, 1958.) (C) Grossly enlarged cranial vault and mandible. Expressionless facies is due to seventh nerve involvement. (D) Exophthalmos and facial palsy. Lips cannot close over teeth. (C and D from H. Hamersma, *Laryngoscope, 80*:1518, 1970.)

and Ryrie (1937), Higinbotham and Alexander (1941), Kelley and Lawlah (1946), Truswell (1958), Klintworth (1963) and Beighton *et al.* (1976). Parental consanguinity was noted in the cases of Falconer and Ryrie (1937), Truswell (1958), and Beighton *et al.* (1976).

DIAGNOSIS

While the typical facial palsy, deafness, visual disturbances, and syndactyly should readily distinguish sclerosteosis, one should exclude *benign dominant osteopetrosis* and *van Buchem disease.* Facial and radiographic features virtually identical to those found in sclerosteosis were illustrated by Montgomery and Standard (1960). Although parental consanguinity was present, the father of eight affected children was reported to have mild but definite sclerosis of the skull base and diffuse sclerosis throughout the pelvis and femora. Serum alkaline phosphatase levels were elevated in seven of the eight affected children.

TREATMENT

Surgical intervention may be indicated for relief of cranial nerve compression and raised intracranial pressure. Tarsorraphy or orbital decompression may be indicated for the proptosis. The syndactyly and mandibular prognathism can be surgically corrected. A hearing aid may provide relief for the conductive component of the hearing loss.

PROGNOSIS

The facial palsy, at first transient and unilateral, usually becomes bilateral. It often appears within the first few years of life. The deafness is progressive, but its onset is variable—almost without exception appearing before the end of the second decade. In sibs described by Beighton *et al.* (1976) death resulted from compression of the medulla.

SUMMARY

Characteristics include: 1) autosomal recessive inheritance, 2) square appearance of mandible, 3) generalized osteosclerosis and hyperostosis of calvaria, mandible, clavicles, and pelvis, 4) frequent asymmetric cutaneous syndactyly of index and middle fingers, 5) bony impingement on cranial foramina producing mixed deafness, facial palsy, or optic atrophy.

REFERENCES

Beighton, P., Hamersma, H., and Durr, L., The clinical features of sclerosteosis—a review of the manifestations in 25 affected individuals. *Ann. Intern. Med., 84*:393–397, 1976.

Falconer, A. W., and Ryrie, B. J., Report on a familial type of generalized osteosclerosis. *Med. Press, 195*:12–24, 1937.

Higinbotham, N. L., and Alexander, S. F., Osteopetrosis. Four cases in one family. *Am. J. Surg., 53*:444–454, 1941.

Hirsch, I. S., Generalized osteitis fibrosa. *Radiology, 13*:44–84, 1929 (see Fig. 36).

Kelley, C. H., and Lawlah, J. W., Albers-Schönberg disease—a family survey. *Radiology, 47*:507–513, 1946.

Klintworth, G. K., The neurologic manifestations of osteopetrosis (Albers-Schönberg's disease). *Neurology (Minneap.), 13*:512–519, 1963.

Kretzmar, J. H., and Roberts, R. A., Case of Albers-Schönberg's disease. *Br. Med. J., 1*:837–838, 1936.

Montgomery, R. D., and Standard, K. L., Albers-Schönberg's disease. A changing concept. *J. Bone Joint Surg., 42B*:303–312, 1960.

Pietruschka, G., Weitere Mitteilungen über die Marmorknochenkrankheit. (Albers-Schönbergsche Krankheit) nebst Bemerkungen zur Differentialdiagnose. *Klin. Monatsbl. Augenheilkd., 132*:509–525, 1958.

Sugiura, Y., and Yasuhara, T., Sclerosteosis—a case report. *J. Bone Joint Surg., 57A*:273–276, 1975.

Truswell, A. S., Osteopetrosis with syndactyly. A morphologic variant of Albers-Schönberg's disease. *J. Bone Joint Surg., 40B*:208–218, 1958.

Witkop, C. J., Genetic disease of the oral cavity. In Tiecke, R. W., *Oral Pathology.* New York, McGraw-Hill Book Company, 1965.

ECTRODACTYLY, ECTODERMAL DYSPLASIA, CLEFTING, AND MIXED HEARING LOSS

(EEC Syndrome)

The syndrome of lobster-claw deformity of the hands and feet, nasolacrimal duct obstruction, and cleft lip–palate was possibly first described by Eckoldt and Martens (1804).

CLINICAL FINDINGS

Physical Findings. The combination of ectrodactyly and cleft lip and/or cleft palate is striking.

Cleft lip–palate, more often bilateral, has been described in about 60 per cent of the cases. Oligodontia or even anodontia has been frequently observed. Not uncommonly, teeth with conical crown form have been noted (Rüdiger *et al.*, 1970; Beckerman, 1973; Gorlin *et al.*, 1976).

The mucous membranes are dry and subject to candidal infection (Pashayan *et al.*, 1974).

Musculoskeletal System. The lobster-claw deformity (ectrodactyly) usually involves all four extremities but is remarkable in its variability of expression, even among members of the same family. Occasionally, there has been some degree of soft tissue syndactyly, especially of the toes.

Ocular System. Absent lacrimal puncta have been noted in most cases. This defect is associated with tearing, blepharitis, dacrocystitis, keratoconjunctivitis, and photophobia (Cockayne, 1936; Bixler *et al.*, 1971; Kaiser-Kupfer, 1973; Beckerman, 1973; Ernest and Pullon, 1974). The eyebrows and lashes may be sparse.

Integumentary System. An albinoid alteration in the skin and hair has been noted in several cases; the scalp hair, eyebrows, and lashes have been sparse (Ahrens, 1967; Rüdiger *et al.*, 1970; Bixler *et al.*, 1971; Pashayan *et al.*, 1974). The sebaceous and meibomian glands are reduced in number (Pashayan *et al.*, 1974). The nails may be hypoplastic (Bixler *et al.*, 1971; Beckerman, 1973).

Nervous System. Microcephaly and/or mental retardation have been described in about 20 per cent of the cases (Ahrens, 1967; Berndorfer, 1970; Rüdiger *et al.*, 1970; Bixler *et al.*, 1971; Brill *et al.*, 1972).

Genitourinary System. Renal and ureteral malformations (absent kidney, hydronephrosis, hydroureter) have been noted in about 20 per cent of the cases (Walker and Clodius, 1963; Maisels, 1970; Brill *et al.*, 1972; Kaiser-Kupfer, 1973; Preus and Fraser, 1973; Ernest and Pullon, 1974).

Auditory System. Deafness has been a relatively uncommon component of this syndrome. Wildervanck (1963) described 40 to 100 dB sensorineural hearing loss in brothers with the syndrome. Meller (1893) and Birch-Jensen (1949) described patients who were deaf-mutes without otherwise categorizing the deafness. Kellner (1934) and others (Hillman and Fraser, 1969; Bixler *et al.*, 1971) also noted decreased hearing.

Conductive deafness of an unspecified degree was noted by Patterson and Stevenson (1964), Robinson *et al.* (1973), Beckerman (1973) and Pashayan *et al.* (1974). Ernest and Pullon (1974) described a mild to moderate conductive hearing loss in two of three affected siblings and Bystrom *et al.* (1974) described moderate conductive hearing loss. We have also seen a patient with moderate conductive deafness. After performing tympanotomy, Robinson *et al.* (1973) found absence of the stapes and part of the incus in one patient. Bystrom *et al.* (1974) noted absence of the incus. Robinson *et al.* (1973) described abnormal modeling of the pinna; Berndorfer (1970) noted absence of pinnae and lack of inner ears. Swallow *et al.* (1973) described moderate low-frequency conductive deafness.

Vestibular System. A caloric vestibular test on one patient showed marked depression of the vestibular response and minimal nystagmus produced by cold water (Wildervanck, 1963).

LABORATORY FINDINGS

Roentgenograms. Radiographs of the hands and feet show variable absent axial or paraxial phalanges and metapodial bones. No other bony abnormalities have been noted.

HEREDITY

Although most cases have been isolated examples, there have been affected sibs with normal parents (Walker and Clodius, 1963; Ahrens, 1967) and several cases in which the disorder has been transmitted from a parent to one or more children (Cockayne, 1936; Walker and Clodius, 1963; Brill *et al.*, 1972; Pfeiffer and Verbeck, 1973; Preus and Fraser, 1973; Robinson *et al.*, 1973). The syndrome appears to have autosomal dominant inheritance with poor penetrance and very variable expressivity. There is no sex predilection.

DIAGNOSIS

Lobster-claw deformity usually occurs as an isolated autosomal dominant trait. Although lacrimal duct obstruction occurs in 1 to 6 per cent of the general childhood population, it has been found in about 10 per cent of the cleft lip–palate population.

Reed *et al.* (1974) described a mother and daughter with ectrodactyly, lacrimal duct obstruction, early graying of the hair with pili torti and subtotal alopecia, and atrophic pigmented macules on the exterior surfaces of the body.

TREATMENT

Hearing aids may be of help to those with residual hearing. The cleft lip and/or palate should be corrected by plastic surgery. In cases of obstruction of the inferior lacrimal puncta, a plastic tube should be inserted to carry away the tears (Beckerman, 1973). The ectrodactyly is remarkably variable in form and degree; the hands and feet usually are quite functional. In some cases, correction by plastic surgery is indicated for cosmetic improvement.

PROGNOSIS

There appears to be progression in the degree of hearing loss. Apparently, patients adapt well to the deformity of their extremities.

SUMMARY

Characteristics of this syndrome include: 1) autosomal dominant inheritance with incomplete penetrance and variable expressivity, 2) hand and foot deformities, including absent phalanges and metapodial bones and syndactyly of some remaining digits, 3) absence of lacrimal puncta, 4) occasional cleft lip–palate, 5) occasional albinoid changes in the skin and hair, 6) mixed hearing loss (mostly conductive), and 7) depressed vestibular function.

REFERENCES

Ahrens, K., Chromosomale Untersuchungen bei craniofacialen Missbildungen. *HNO, 15*:106–109, 1967 (cases 3A, B).

Beckerman, B. L., Lacrimal anomalies in anhidrotic ectodermal dysplasia. *Am. J. Ophthalmol., 75*:728–730, 1973.

Berndorfer, A., Gesichtsspalten gemeinsam mit Hand-und Fussspalten. *Z. Orthop., 107*:344–354, 1970.

Birch-Jensen, A., *Congenital Deformities of the Upper Extremities.* Copenhagen, Denmark, E. Munksgaard, 1949, pp. 181–182.

Bixler, D., Spivack, J., Bennett, J., and Christian, J. C., The ectrodactyly-ectodermal dysplasia-clefting (EEC) syndrome. *Clin. Genet., 3*:43–51, 1971.

Brill, C. B., Hsu, L., and Hirschhorn, K., The syndrome of ectrodactyly, ectodermal dysplasia, and cleft lip and palate: report of a family demonstrating a dominant inheritance pattern. *Clin. Genet., 3*:295–302, 1972.

Bystrom, E., Sanger, R., and Stewart, R., EEC: heterogeneity in a syndrome of meso-ectodermal dysmorphia. *J. Dent. Res. (IADR Abst. #534), 53*:188, 1974.

Cockayne, E. A., Cleft palate, hare lip, dacrocystitis, and cleft hand and feet. *Biometrika, 28*:60–63, 1936.

Eckoldt, J. G., and Martens, F. H., *Über eine sehr komplicierte Hasenscharte.* Leipzig, Steinacker, 1804.

Ernest, M. A., and Pullon, P. A., A cleft lip–palate, ectodermal dysplasia, syndactyly, and genitourinary syndrome of autosomal recessive inheritance. *J. Dent. Res. (IADR Abstract, #535), 53*:188, 1974.

Gorlin, R. J., Pindborg, J. J., and Cohen, M. M., Jr., *Syndromes of the Head and Neck,* 2nd Ed. New York, McGraw-Hill Book Company, 1976.

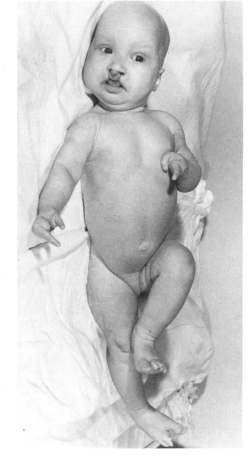

Figure 5-16 *Ectrodactyly, ectodermal dysplasia, clefting, and mixed hearing loss (EEC syndrome).* Female infant with ectrodactyly and bilateral cleft-lip and palate. A deficiency of hair and sebaceous glands has been found in many patients. In most the lacrimal puncta are absent. (From R. A. Rüdiger *et al., Am. J. Dis. Child., 120*:160, 1970.)

Hillman, D. A., and Fraser, F. C., Artificial sweeteners and fetal malformations: a rumored relationship. *Pediatrics, 44*:299–300, 1969.

Kaiser-Kupfer, M., Ectrodactyly, ectodermal dysplasia and clefting syndrome. *Am. J. Ophthalmol., 76*:992–998, 1973.

Kellner, A. W., Über Spalthand und fuss mit Oligodaktylie. *Klin. Wochenschr., 13*:1507–1509, 1934.

Maisels, D. O., Lobster-claw deformity of the hands and feet. *Br. J. Plast. Surg., 23*:269–282, 1970 (case 1).

Meller, J., Ein Fall von angeborener Spaltbildung der Hände und Füsse. *Berl. Klin. Wschr., 30*:232–233, 1893.

Pashayan, H. M., Pruzansky, S., and Solomon, L., The EEC syndrome. *Birth Defects, 10*(7):105–127, 1974.

Patterson, T. J. S., and Stevenson, A. C., Craniofacial dysostosis and malformations of feet. *J. Med. Genet., 1*:112–114, 1964.

Pfeiffer, R. A., and Verbeck, C., Spalthand und Spaltfuss, ektodermal Dysplasie und Lippen-Kiefer-Gaumen-Spalte: ein autosomal-dominant vererbtes Syndrom. *Z. Kinderheilkd., 115*:235–244, 1973.

Preus, M., and Fraser, F. C., The lobster-claw defect with ectodermal defects, cleft lip–palate, tear duct anomaly, and renal anomalies. *Clin. Genet., 4*:369–375, 1973.

Reed, W. B., Brown, A. C., Sugarman, G. I., and Schlesinger, L., The REEDS syndrome. *Birth Defects, 10*(5):61–73, 1974.

Robinson, G. C., Wildervanck, L. S., and Chiang, T. P., Ectrodactyly, ectodermal dysplasia and cleft lip–palate. Its association with conductive hearing loss. *J. Pediatr., 82*:107–109, 1973.

Rüdiger, R. A., Haase, W., and Passarge, E., Association of ectrodactyly, ectodermal dysplasia, and cleft lip–palate. The EEC syndrome. *Am. J. Dis. Child., 120*:160–163, 1970.

Swallow, J. N., Gray, O. P., and Harper, P. S., Ectrodactyly, ectodermal dysplasia, and cleft lip and palate (EEC syndrome). *Br. J. Derm., Suppl. 9*:54–56, 1973.

Walker, J. C., and Clodius, L., The syndromes of cleft lip, cleft palate, and lobster-claw deformities of hands and feet. *Plast. Reconstr. Surg., 32*:627–636, 1963.

Wildervanck, L. S., Perceptive deafness associated with split-hand and -foot—a new syndrome? *Acta Genet. (Basel), 13*:161–169, 1963.

UNNAMED BONE DYSPLASIA(S) AND SENSORINEURAL DEAFNESS

Insley and Astley (1974) described a syndrome of bone dysplasia, sunken nasal bridge, and sensorineural deafness in two sisters. Nance and Sweeney (1970) reported what might be the same disorder in an adult male, his deceased sibs, and female cousins.

CLINICAL FINDINGS

Physical Findings. The facies is characterized by a severely depressed nasal bridge and small mandible. One sib described by Insley and Astley had cleft palate; the patient reported by Nance and Sweeney also had this defect. The latter patient had calcified pinnae as well.

Skeletal System. Height was at the tenth to twenty-fifth percentile. The adult height of the patient of Nance and Sweeney was 51 inches.

Patients exhibited intermittent joint pains and limitation of movement after the fourth year of life. Kyphosis and/or scoliosis developed after 10 years of age, and there was limitation of movement at the metacarpophalangeal joints.

Auditory System. Both sibs described by Insley and Astley exhibited sensorineural deafness; one had a conductive component thought to be due to otitis media. The patient studied by Nance and Sweeney had slowly progressive mixed hearing loss that was more severe at high frequencies.

Vestibular System. No vestibular studies were reported.

LABORATORY FINDINGS

Radiographic examination showed marked hypoplasia of nasal bones. The long bones were shortened and the epiphyses and metaphyses were enlarged. After the age of 3 years, progressive platyspondylia was noted. The vertebral bodies had irregular surfaces. The interpediculate distances did not increase in the lumbar spine. Progressive fusion of carpal bones was also noted (capitate-hamate-trapezoid, scaphoid-trapezium). Bowing of the tibias was noted by Nance and Sweeney.

HEREDITY

In the kindred of Insley and Astley (1974), the parents and the other sib of the proband were normal, suggesting that the disorder has autosomal recessive inheritance. Several affected sibs and parental consanguinity noted by Nance and Sweeney (1970) confirm that impression.

DIAGNOSIS

The syndrome must be distinguished from *Marshall syndrome* and *Stickler syndrome* (if the latter two disorders are not, in fact, identical). In this disorder, the fusion of carpal bones, the absence of myopia, and the recessive inheritance pattern appear to be distinguishing factors.

TREATMENT

The depressed nasal bridge can be corrected by plastic surgery.

PROGNOSIS

Insufficient information is available to determine the prognosis in this disorder.

SUMMARY

The characteristics of this syndrome include: 1) autosomal recessive inheritance, 2) severely depressed nasal bridge, 3) skeletal alterations, including platyspondylia and carpal fusion, and 4) sensorineural or mixed deafness.

REFERENCES

Insley, J., and Astley, R., A bone dysplasia with deafness. *Br. J. Radiol.,* 47:241–251, 1974.
Nance, W. E., and Sweeney, A., A recessively inherited chondrodystrophy. *Birth Defects,* 6(4): 25–27, 1970.

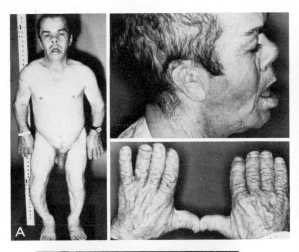

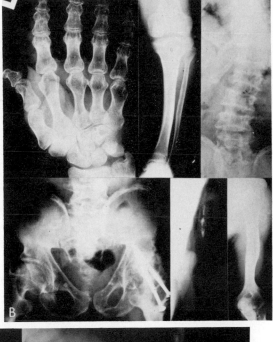

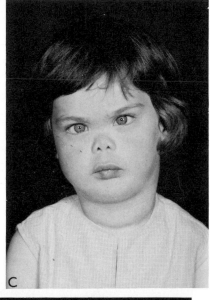

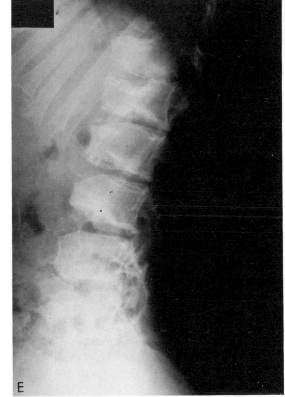

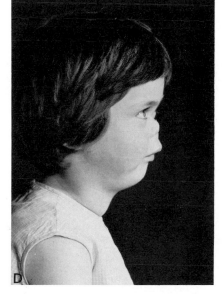

Figure 5–17   *Unnamed bone dysplasia(s) and sensorineural deafness. (A)* Adult male showing short stature, large head, saddle nose, deformed pinnae, limitation of elbow extension, stubby fingers, and thick leathery skin. Patient also had cleft palate. *(B)* Radiographs of same patient, showing short tubular bones, curvature of tibias, scoliosis, abnormal pelvis, calcified pinnae, and deformed humerus. *(A* and *B* from W. E. Nance and A. Sweeney, *Birth Defects,* 6(4):25, 1970.) *(C, D)* Younger of two affected sibs showing hypoplastic nasal bones. *(E)* Spine of sib at 12 years of age showing osteochondrosislike defects of upper and lower anterior angles of vertebral bodies. With time, these defects became more extensive, resulting in a generalized platyspondyly.

Illustration continued on the following page

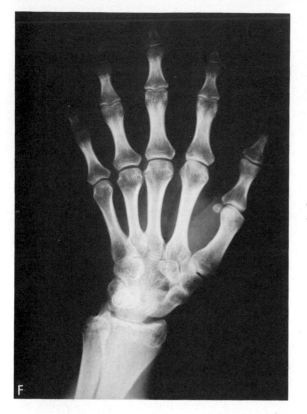

Figure 5–17 Continued (*F*) General fusion of carpal bones. (*C, D, E,* and *F* from J. Insley and R. Astley, *Br. J. Radiol.,* 47:241, 1974.)

METAPHYSEAL DYSOSTOSIS, MENTAL RETARDATION, AND CONDUCTION DEAFNESS

Rimoin and McAlister (1971) reported three male sibs with short-limbed dwarfism, metaphyseal dysostosis, mild mental retardation, and conductive deafness.

CLINICAL FINDINGS

Physical Findings. The short stature, due to abbreviated limbs, was striking in all three sibs. Height was below the third percentile. Birth weight and length were normal. Head circumference was large.

Musculoskeletal System. Short stature in one sib was first noted by school authorities at registration for primary school. At that time, his 3-year-old and 1-year-old brothers were also noted to be short. Pains in the knees and genua vara were noted in late childhood in two of the children. Another child had unilateral genu valgum. The feet and hands were short and broad, and the fingers were loose-jointed. Scoliosis and/or lumbar lordosis were noted in two of the three sibs.

Nervous System. I.Q. was estimated in the three children at about 70 to 80.

Ocular System. Two of three sibs wore glasses. Two had hyperopia and alternating esotropia; the other had strabismus. Anterior polar cataract was found in one sib.

Auditory System. Hearing difficulties were first noted at adolescence, bilateral moderate conductive deafness being found in the three sibs. Recurrent ear infections were observed in all the sibs.

Vestibular System. No vestibular tests were described.

LABORATORY FINDINGS

Radiographically, the major changes were limited essentially to the metaphyses of the long bones, including those of the hands and feet. Relative to body height the skull was large. The vertebrae appeared proportionally small in all dimensions but

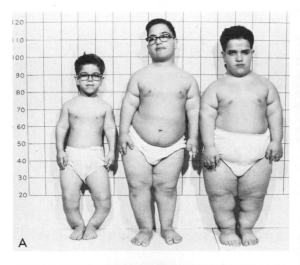

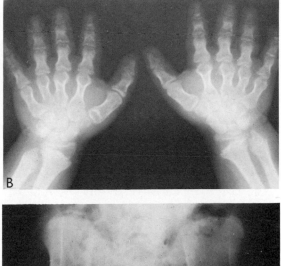

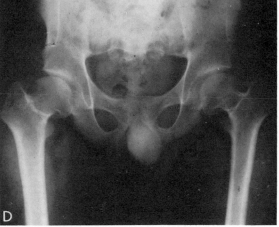

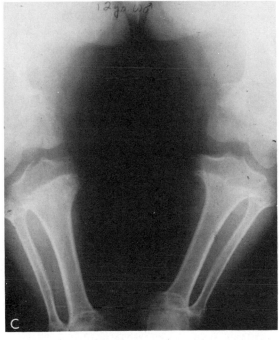

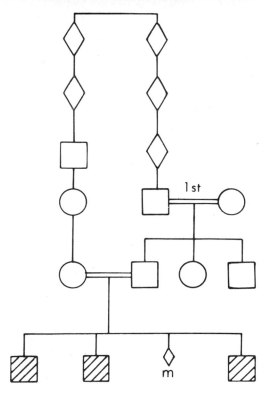

Figure 5–18 Metaphyseal dysostosis, mental retardation, and conductive deafness. *(A)* Three brothers with short-limbed dwarfism. Note genua vara and genu valgum in two of the sibs. *(B)* Radiograph of hands showing shortened tubular bones with widened metaphyses and cone-shaped epiphyses. Note metaphyseal flaring and irregularity of radius and ulna. *(C)* Fibulas are relatively long distally with genu varum. Note shortening and minimal eiphyseal deformity. Metaphyses are irregular and flared. *(D)* Iliac wings are narrow, pelvic inlet is flattened; note coxa vara. *(E)* Pedigree of kindred. Parents are fourth cousins. Sex of common ancestors is unknown, hence diamond-shaped symbols. (*A* and *E* from D. L. Rimoin and W. H. McAlister, *Birth Defects*, 7(4):116, 1971; *B, C,* and *D* courtesy of D. L. Rimoin, Torrance, Calif.)

were not deformed. Increased lumbar lordosis was evident in the two older brothers, one of whom had rotary scoliosis. The ribs were short and widened anteriorly and showed cupping and irregularity of the costochondral margins. Premature sternal fusion was noted. The vertical and transverse diameters of the iliac bones were decreased; the iliac wings were narrowed and their lateral margins were angulated. All the long tubular bones were markedly shortened. The femoral neck was remarkably short, resulting in severe coxa vara. The greater trochanters appeared relatively prominent. The lower limbs were bowed, and the fibula was longer than the tibia, especially distally.

The most severe changes were seen in the metaphyses, which were widened and irregular and had broad zones of irregular dense calcification and focal radiolucent areas. The epiphyses tended to fuse early, but they fused asymmetrically. The glenoid fossas were flattened and there was loss of the normal humeral neck angle. The distal ulnas were shortened and deformed relative to the radius. The hands and feet were short and broad. The short tubular bones of the hands were also severely abbreviated and showed marked epiphyseal-metaphyseal flaring. The phalanges were wide, and with the exception of the second and fifth distal phalanges, showed early epiphyseal fusion.

Polytomography of the mastoid areas revealed bilateral low placement of the ossicles as well as striking upward angulation of the internal auditory canals.

HEREDITY

The syndrome occurred in three brothers. The parents were fourth cousins, suggesting autosomal recessive inheritance.

DIAGNOSIS

There are several types of metaphyseal dysostosis that differ in several respects from the syndrome under discussion. The most common (Schmid type) is milder and does not involve the hands and feet; there is coxa vara, however. Associated anomalies are not found. Inheritance is autosomal dominant. Although the Spahr type is similar to the Schmid type, inheritance is autosomal recessive. Cartilage-hair hypoplasia is characterized by sparse hair, malabsorption, congenital megacolon, and autosomal recessive inheritance. The Maroteaux type, also autosomal recessive, is spotty in its involvement, sparing the proximal femoral metaphyses. Metaphyseal dysostosis may also occur with thymic aplasia and lymphopenic agammaglobulinemia (Rimoin and McAlister, 1971).

TREATMENT

A hearing aid may lessen the effects of the deafness. Orthopedic therapy may be used to correct the genua vara or valga.

PROGNOSIS

The deafness and mental retardation are not thought to be progressive.

SUMMARY

Characteristics of this syndrome include: 1) autosomal recessive inheritance, 2) short stature due to metaphyseal dysostosis, 3) mild mental retardation, and 4) bilateral moderate conduction deafness that appears around adolescence.

REFERENCE

Rimoin, D. L., and McAlister, W. H., Metaphyseal dysostosis, conductive hearing loss, and mental retardation: a recessively inherited syndrome. *Birth Defects,* 7(4):116–122, 1971.

KNIEST SYNDROME

Kniest (1952) described a rare form of disproportionate dwarfism, characterized by depressed nasal bridge, cleft palate, and prominent knees.

CLINICAL FINDINGS

Physical Findings. The face is round and the nasal bridge is depressed. The neck is short and the head appears to sit upon the thorax. At birth, the patient is frequently noted to have cleft palate, shortened extremities, club feet, and prominent knees.

Musculoskeletal System. Lumbar lordosis with dorsal kyphosis usually develops within the first few years of life, together with platyspondylia; the combination of these conditions reduces the height of the trunk. The child may not sit until the age of 2 years, and not begin to walk until 3 years of age. By the fourth year, most joints become progressively enlarged, stiff, and painful. The knees, elbows, and wrists become especially enlarged, and flexion and extension of most joints become progressively reduced. The feet and legs are externally rotated. Gait shows marked waddling. Thoracic scoliosis may develop later in the course of the disorder. Adult height is rarely greater than 140 cm.

Ocular System. Myopia of greater than 10 diopters and lattice degeneration with or without retinal detachment and/or cataract formation have been present in about 40 per cent of published cases (Roaf *et al.*, 1967).

Other System. Cleft palate has been noted in about 50 per cent of reported cases (Larose and Gay, 1969; Maroteaux and Spranger, 1973).

Auditory System. Conductive deafness has been described by a number of authors (Roaf *et al.*, 1967; Maroteaux and Spranger, 1973; Siggers *et al.*, 1974).

Vestibular System. No studies have been reported.

LABORATORY FINDINGS

Radiographically, in the infant the long bones are squat and have enlarged meta-physes. The skull often shows basilar impression. The bones of the upper limbs are short. The metaphyses of long bones flare, and the epiphyses around the knee are large, irregular, and transparent.

In childhood, the distal ends of the proximal phalanges of the fingers have pseudoepiphyses. Even though the proximal row of carpal bones is small, bone age is normal or advanced. The iliac wings are broad and reduced in height, especially in relation to the large capital femoral epiphysis and proximal femoral metaphysis. The capital femoral epiphysis may form as late as adolescence; the neck is wide and short with a poorly ossified central area. Usually there is coxa vara. The trochanter is prominent. The vertebral height is reduced, and there is anterior wedging of the vertebral bodies.

PATHOLOGY

Rimoin *et al.* (1974) reported a "Swiss cheese" appearance to the cartilage. Ultrastructural studies have shown chondrocytes filled with dilated cisternae of endoplasmic reticulum and abnormalities in collagen (Silberberg, 1974).

HEREDITY

Since Maroteaux and Spranger (1973) described Kniest syndrome in a mother and her child, autosomal dominance is likely.

DIAGNOSIS

This disorder during infancy must be distinguished from metatropic dwarfism and *spondyloepiphyseal dysplasia congenita.* In the former, the thorax is narrow in contrast to the thorax being broad in Kniest syndrome. The flaring of the distal femur and the proximal tibia is far more marked in metatropic dwarfism.

In spondyloepiphyseal dysplasia congenita, ossification of the pubic bones, the talus, and the calcaneus is very delayed. The tubular bones exhibit more metaphyseal widening, especially in the proximal femora, in Kniest syndrome.

TREATMENT

Referral for periodic ophthalmologic examination is mandatory. The talipes equinovarus and cleft palate can be corrected.

PROGNOSIS

As indicated above, the patients become progressively deformed. Gait is difficult. Retinal detachment is a distinct hazard in this disorder.

SUMMARY

Characteristics of this syndrome are: 1) autosomal dominant inheritance, 2) short extremities, club feet, and large knees, all noted at birth, 3) late development of walking, 4) stiff joints and waddling gait, 5) severe myopia and often retinal detachment, 6) cleft palate, 7) characteristic radiographic alterations, and 8) conduction deafness.

REFERENCES

Hobaek, A., *Problems of Hereditary Chondrodysplasia.* Oslo, Oslo University Press, 1961, (Family XVIII).

Kim, H. J., Beratis, N. G., Brill, P., Raab, E., Hirschhorn, K., and Matalon, R., Kniest syndrome with dominant inheritance and mucopolysacchariduria. *Am. J. Hum. Genet.,* 27(6):755, 1975.

Kniest, W., Zur Abgrenzung der Dysostosis enchondralis von der Chondrodystrophie. *Z. Kinderheilkd.,* 70:663–640, 1952.

Larose, J. H., and Gay, B. B., Metatropic dwarfism. *Am. J. Roentgenol., 106*:156–161, 1969 (Case 1).

Maroteaux, P., and Spranger, J., La maladie de Kniest. *Arch. Franç Pédiatr., 30*:735–750, 1973.

Rimon, D. L., Hollister, D. W., Lachman, R. S., Kaufman, R. L., McAlister, W. H., Rosenthal, R. E., and Hughes, G. N. F., Histologic studies in the chondrodystrophies. *Birth Defects, 10*(12): 274–294, 1974.

Roaf, R., Longmore, J. B., and Forrester, R. M., A childhood syndrome of bone dysplasia, retinal detachment, and deafness. *Dev. Med. Child. Neurol.,* 9:464–472, 1967 (Case 2).

Siggers, D. C., Kniest disease. *Birth Defects, 10*(12):432–442, 1974.

Siggers, D. C., Rimoin, D. L., Dorst, J. P., *et al.,* The Kniest disease. *Birth Defects, 10*(9):193–208, 1974.

Silberberg, R., Ultrastructure of cartilage in chondrodystrophies. *Birth Defects, 10*(12):306–313, 1974.

Silverman, F. N., Discussion. *Birth Defects, 5*(4):45–47, 1969.

Spranger, J., and Maroteaux, P., Kniest disease. *Birth Defects 10*(12):50–56, 1974.

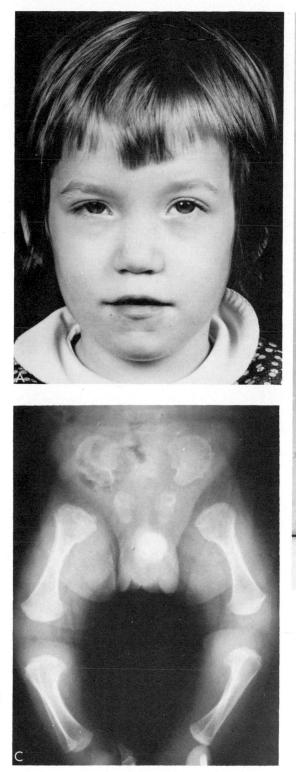

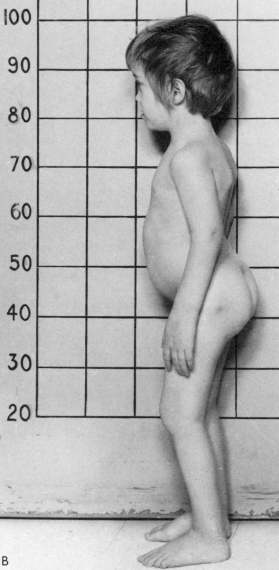

Figure 5–19 Kniest syndrome. (A) The nasal bridge is depressed. *(B)* Lumbar lordosis with dorsal kyphosis develops within first few years of life. Joints become enlarged and stiff and result in waddling gait. *(A* and *B* from D. C. Siggers *et al., Birth Defects, 10*(9): 193, 1974.) *(C)* Radiograph showing shortened long bones with enlarged metaphyses. The iliac wings are broad and reduced in height, especially in relation to the large capital femoral epiphysis and proximal femoral metaphysis. Note delayed appearance of epiphyses. *(C* from F. N. Silverman, *Birth Defects, 5*(4): 45, 1969.)

ARTHROGRYPOTIC HAND ANOMALY AND SENSORINEURAL DEAFNESS

Stewart and Bergstrom (1971) reported a combination of an arthrogrypotic hand anomaly and sensorineural deafness in 12 individuals in 5 generations.

CLINICAL FINDINGS

Physical Findings. Clinical alterations are limited to deafness and to changes in the hands and arms.

Musculoskeletal System. Height and weight of the affected persons were usually below the tenth percentile. Flexion creases over both proximal and distal interphalangeal finger joints were absent; there was limitation of both passive flexion and extension. The thenar, hypothenar, and interosseous muscle masses were decreased. Ulnar deviation of the wrists and of the fingers at the proximal interphalangeal joints was noted as well as difficulty in dorsiflexion at the wrist. Muscle weakness was most marked on the ulnar side of the arm. Limitation of elbow extension and flexion of the toes was observed in some individuals. Other patients exhibited some limitation of pronation and supination of the hands.

Auditory System. Seven of 12 affected persons manifested sensorineural deafness. In some, it was unilateral, in others bilateral. It varied from moderate to profound and apparently was congenital.

Vestibular System. No studies were reported.

LABORATORY FINDINGS

Radiographs of the hands and feet showed osteoporotic changes and poor bone modeling.

Dermatoglyphic analysis revealed striking vertical orientation of the palmar digital lines with variable missing digital triradii.

HEREDITY

The syndrome was inherited as an autosomal dominant trait with complete penetrance and variable expressivity.

DIAGNOSIS

Arthrogryposis multiplex congenita, which may be seen as an isolated phenomenon or in association with several syndromes (Drachman and Banker, 1961), must be excluded. Of interest is the similarity between dermatoglyphic findings in the syndrome described here and those in arthrogryposis (Brehme and Baitsch, 1966).

TREATMENT

In most cases, a hearing aid benefitted the patients.

PROGNOSIS

The deafness and hand anomalies were nonprogressive.

SUMMARY

Characteristics of this syndrome include: 1) autosomal dominant inheritance with variable expressivity, 2) growth retardation, 3) arthrogrypotic alterations of the hands, 4) some limitation of joint mobility, and 5) congenital sensorineural deafness of moderate to profound degree, which may be unilateral or bilateral.

REFERENCES

Brehme, H., and Baitsch, H., Hautleistenbefunde bei 15 Patienten mit Arthrogryposis multiplex congenita. *Humangenetik,* 2:344–354, 1966.

Drachman, D. B., and Banker, B. Q., Arthrogryposis multiplex congenita. *Arch. Neurol.,* 5:77–93, 1961.

Stewart, J. M., and Bergstrom, L., Familial hand abnormality and sensorineural deafness: a new syndrome. *J. Pediatr.,* 78:102–110, 1971.

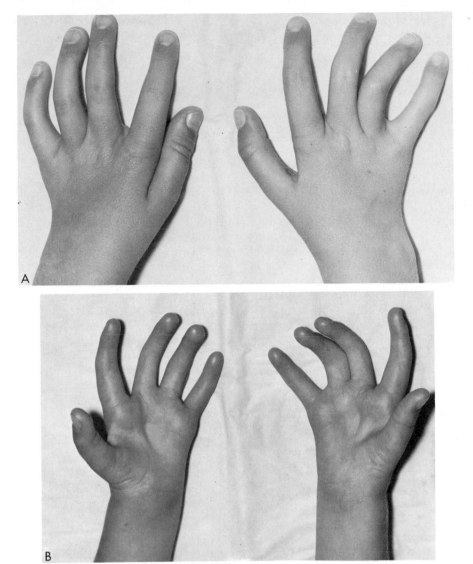

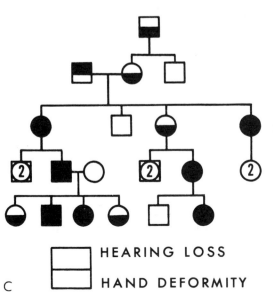

Figure 5–20 *Arthrogrypotic hand anomaly and sensorineural deafness.* *(A, B)* Dorsal and palmar views of hands showing absence of flexion creases and diminished muscle mass. *(C)* Pedigree of kindred. *(A, B,* and *C* from J. M. Stewart and L. Bergstrom, *J. Pediatr.,* 78:102, 1971.)

HEARING LOSS

HAND DEFORMITY

KLIPPEL-FEIL ANOMALAD AND ABDUCENS PARALYSIS WITH RETRACTED BULB AND SENSORINEURAL OR CONDUCTION DEAFNESS

(Wildervanck Syndrome, Cervico-oculoacoustic Dysplasia)

Although Wildervanck and colleagues (1952, 1960, 1966) brought attention to the syndrome of Klippel-Feil anomalad, abducens palsy with retracted bulb (Duane syndrome), and severe congenital sensorineural deafness, earlier cases were buried in the literature. For example, Jalladeau (1936) described 20 cases of Klippel-Feil anomalad. Six were noted to be deaf-mutes. Mein (1968), in analysis of 77 cases of Duane syndrome, found three with the Klippel-Feil anomalad and two with deafness. Kirkham (1969b), in an analysis of 112 patients with Duane syndrome, reported that while 12 were deaf and 5 had the Klippel-Feil anomalad, only two had the complete triad. These cases were described more fully by Kirkham (1970a), who also noted cleft palate.

CLINICAL FINDINGS

Physical Findings. The appearance is striking. The head seems to sit directly upon the trunk; lateral mobility and flexion and extension of the neck are greatly reduced. Not uncommonly, there is facial asymmetry and/or torticollis of variable degree. The posterior hairline is low.

Skeletal System. There is variable fusion of one or more cervical vertebrae.

Nervous System. Mental retardation has been noted in several cases (Wildervanck, 1963; Everberg *et al.,* 1963; Bintliff, 1965; Fraser and MacGillivray, 1968; McLay and Maran, 1969). Kirkham (1969b) noted arrested hydrocephalus. We have also seen such a case.

Ocular System. Abducens paralysis prevents the external rotation of the eyeballs. On lateral gaze, the abducted eye becomes retracted as the eye slit narrows (convergent squint). This phenomenon, known as Duane syndrome, may be unilateral or bilateral (around 15 to 20 per cent). When the condition is unilateral, it is more often left-sided. Occasionally, it is absent (Wildervanck, 1966). Kirkham (1969b) described associated pseudopapilledema.

Unilateral epibulbar dermoids have been reported by Franceschetti and Klein (1954), Wildervanck *et al.* (1966), Kirkham (1969b), Cross and Pfaffenbach (1972), and others cited by the latter authors.

Oral Findings. Several authors have noted cleft palate (Witzel, 1959; Bintliff, 1965; Fraser and MacGillivray, 1968; Kirkham, 1970a).

Auditory System. Of 112 patients with the Duane syndrome, Kirkham (1970b) found 11 per cent to have unilateral or bilateral moderate to severe sensorineural deafness, whereas less than 5 per cent had the Klippel-Feil anomalad. However, Fraser and MacGillivray (1968) found a much higher correlation. Various ear anomalies have been described: preauricular tags, malformation, atresia or absence of external auditory canal, abnormal ossicles, stenosis or bony septum within the internal auditory meatus, absence of oval window, abnormal semicircular canals, and underdevelopment of the bony labyrinth (Everberg *et al.,* 1962; Fraser and MacGillivray, 1968; Cross and Pfaffenbach, 1972; Baumeister and Terrahe, 1974).

Vestibular System. Vestibular response has usually been abnormal (Everberg *et al.,* 1963; Wildervanck *et al.,* 1966).

LABORATORY FINDINGS

Klippel-Feil anomalad is a feature of the disorder. Radiographically, there is fusion of several cervical vertebrae. Spina bifida and elevation of one or both scapulae (Sprengel's deformity) as well as kyphoscoliosis have been noted. Hemivertebrae have also been observed (Witzel, 1959; Cross and Pfaffenbach, 1972; Stark and Borton, 1973).

HEREDITY

An overwhelming preponderance of patients with the Wildervanck syndrome are female. This has led to the conjecture that the disorder is X-linked dominant with lethality in the male. We find no evidence to support this contention. Franceschetti *et al.* (1965) and Kirkham (1970b) suggested that the syndrome is inherited as a dominant trait with poor penetrance and variable expressivity. Other authors have suggested autosomal recessive inheritance. We find little to support the belief that single-gene transmission is responsible. At this writing, multifactorial inheritance would appear most likely, in our opinion.

DIAGNOSIS

Incomplete forms abound; in some cases, the stigmata overlap with those of oculoauriculovertebral syndrome (Goldenhar syndrome), causing us to wonder whether we are dealing with a teratogenic spectrum of multifactorial nature. Kirkham (1969a) reported five generations of patients with sensorineural deafness that appeared at puberty. Among these patients, the proposita and her maternal aunt exhibited the Duane syndrome. Cohney (1963) described six patients with cleft palate and Klippel-Feil anomalad, two of whom were deaf; Cohney did not mention lateral rectus palsy or squint. Magnus (1944) noted a patient with kyphoscoliosis, torticollis, abducens paralysis, and winged scapulae; he did not mention deafness. Fickentscher (1954) described deafness in a male patient with Klippel-Feil anomalad, but he did not mention eye problems. Everberg (1968) reported a boy with Klippel-Feil anomalad, deafness due to absence of the oval window, and various skeletal anomalies (missing ribs, absent right radius, left thumb, first metacarpal, and some carpal bones) but there was no abducens palsy. Stark and Borton (1973) described four patients with cervical fusion of varying degrees. They documented conductive, sensorineural, and mixed hearing loss but did not mention eye problems. Douglas (1964) described Duane syndrome, limbal dermoids, and ear tags in two patients, but he did not report Klippel-Feil anomalad or deafness. Bauman (1932) noted a female child with Klippel-Feil anomalad, torticollis, mental retardation, and deafness (type not specified) but did not mention abducens paralysis. Ffooks (1963) described a male child with Klippel-Feil anomalad, abducens paralysis, coloboma of the outer canthus, and ear tags, but he did not observe deafness. Dem-

jen and Marcinková (1965) described a girl with Klippel-Feil anomalad, torticollis, deaf-mutism, and cleft palate, but they did not report eye problems.

Pintucci and De Tizio (1961) described a male patient with minimal Klippel-Feil anomalad, abducens paralysis, but no deafness. The girl reported by Sherk and Nicholson (1972) had Klippel-Feil anomalad, abducens paralysis, bilateral radial hemimelia, and ear tags, but normal hearing. Jaffee (1968) and Singh *et al.* (1969) noted Klippel-Feil anomalad and mixed hearing loss.

Troy (1968) described a girl with Klippel-Feil anomalad, sensorineural deafness, mental retardation, and torticollis but not abducens palsy. Martin and Trabue (1952) reported Klippel-Feil anomalad in combination with cleft palate and congenital deafness in three children. Graf (1968) documented a girl with Klippel-Feil anomalad, severe congenital sensorineural deafness, unilateral facial palsy, no abducens palsy, normal vestibular function, and some malformation of the labyrinth. Jarvis and Sellars (1974) reported congenital conductive deafness in Klippel-Feil anomalad due to fixation of the footplate of the stapes. Hensinger *et al.* (1974) noted "hearing impairment" in 15 of 50 patients with Klippel-Feil anomalad. They did not otherwise define the hearing loss.

TREATMENT

The restriction of abduction of the eye can be partly or completely corrected by temporal transplantation of the superior and inferior recti combined with resection of the internal rectus (Gobin, 1971).

PROGNOSIS

The disorder is congenital and is not progressive.

SUMMARY

Characteristics of this syndrome include: 1) multifactorial inheritance, 2) fusion of cervical vertebrae, 3) abducens palsy with retracted bulb (Duane syndrome), 4) occasional cleft palate and/or torticollis, and 5) severe congenital sensorineural or conductive hearing loss.

REFERENCES

Bauman, G. I., Absence of the cervical spine. *J.A.M.A.*, *98*:129–132, 1932.

Baumeister, S., and Terrahe, K., Innenohrmissbildungen beim Klippel-Feil-Syndrom. *Laryngol. Rhinol. Otol.*, *53*:120–130, 1974.

Bauman, G. I., Absence of the cervical spine. *J.A.M.A.*, *98*:129–132, 1932.

Bintliff, S. J., Klippel-Feil syndrome. *J. Am. Med. Women's Assoc.*, *20*:547–550, 1965.

Cohney, B. C., The association of cleft palate with the Klippel-Feil syndrome. *Plast. Reconstr. Surg.*, *31*:179–187, 1963 (cases 5, 6).

Cross, H. E., and Pfaffenbach, D. D., Duane's retraction syndrome and associated congenital malformations. *Am. J. Ophthalmol.*, *73*:442–449, 1972.

Demjen, S., and Marcinková, V., Klippel-Feil syndrome and cleft palate. *Acta Chir. Plast.*, *7*:297–300, 1965.

Douglas, A. A., Nature and cause of squint of early onset. *Br. Orthopt. J.*, *21*:29–33, 1964.

Edwards, W. G., Congenital middle-ear deafness with anomalies of the face. *J. Laryngol.*, *78*:152–171, 1964.

Everberg, G., Congenital absence of the oval window. *Acta Otolaryngol. (Stockh.)*, *66*:320–332, 1968.

Everberg, G., Ratjen, E., and Sørensen, H., Wildervanck's syndrome. Klippel-Feil's syndrome associated with deafness and retraction of the eyeball. *Br. J. Radiol.*, *36*:562–567, 1963.

Ffooks, O. O., Encanthoschisis. *Br. J. Ophthalmol.*, *47*:500–503, 1963.

Fickentscher, H., Klippel-Feil Syndrom und Schwerhörigkeit. *Arch Klin. Exp. Ohren Nasen Kehlkopfheilkd.*, *164*:297–307, 1954.

Franceschetti, A., and Klein, D., Dysmorphie cervico-oculo-faciale avec surdité familiale. *J. Génét. Hum.*, *3*:176–183, 1954.

Franceschetti, A., Klein, D., Brocher, J. E. W., and Ammann, F., An extensive form of cervico-oculo-facial dysmorphia (Wildervanck-Franceschetti-Klein). *Acta Fac. Med. Univ. Brun.*, *25*:53–61, 1965.

Fraser, G. R., Profound childhood deafness. *J. Med. Genet.*, *1*:118–161, 1964.

Fraser, W. I., and MacGillivray, R. C., Cervico-oculo-acoustic-dysplasia. *J. Ment. Defic. Res.*, *12*:322–329, 1968.

Gobin, M. H., The surgical treatment of Duane's retraction syndrome. *Ophthalmologica, 162*:284, 1971.

Graf, K., Angeborene Taubstummheit und okzipito-zervikale Skelettmissbildung (Wildervanck-Syndrom). *Prac. Otorhinolaryngol.*, *30*:82–89, 1968.

Hensinger, R. N., Lang, J. E., and MacEwen, G. D., Klippel-Feil Syndrome. *J. Bone Joint Surg.*, *56A*:1246–1253, 1974.

Jaffee, I. S., Congenital shoulder-neck-auditory anomalies. *Laryngoscope, 78*:2119–2139, 1968 (case 2).

Jalladeau, J., *Malformations congénitales associées au syndrome de Klippel-Feil*. Paris, Thesis, 1936.

Jarvis, J. F., and Sellars, S. L., Klippel-Feil deformity associated with congenital conductive deafness. *J. Laryngol. Otol.*, *88*:285–289, 1974.

Kirkham, T. H., Duane's syndrome and familial perceptive deafness. *Br. J. Ophthalmol.*, *53*:335–339, 1969a.

Kirkham, T. H., Cervico-oculo-acusticus syndrome with pseudopapilloedema. *Arch. Dis. Child.*, *44*:504–508, 1969b.

Kirkham, T. H., Duane's retraction syndrome and cleft palate. *Am. J. Ophthalmol.*, *70*:209–212, 1970a.

Kirkham, T. H., Inheritance of Duane's syndrome. *Br. J. Ophthalmol.*, *54*:323–329, 1970b.

Livingstone, G., and Delahunty, J. E., Malformation of the ear associated with congenital ophthalmic and other conditions. *J. Laryngol.*, *82*:495–504, 1968.

McLay, K., and Maran, A. G., Deafness and the Klippel-Feil syndrome. *J. Laryngol.*, *83*:175–184, 1969.

Magnus, J. A., Congenital paralysis of both external recti treated by transplantation of eye muscles. *Br. J. Ophthalmol.*, *28*:241–245, 1949.

Martin, B. C., and Trabue, J. C., Klippel-Feil syndrome with associated deformities. *Plast. Recontr. Surg.*, *9*:59–62, 1952.

Mein, J., Clinical features of the retraction syndrome. In *Transactions of the First International Congress of Orthoptics*. London, Kingston, 1968, p. 165.

Pintucci, F., and di Tizio, A., Dysmorphie cervico-oculo-faciale. *J. Génét. Hum.*, *10*:156–171, 1961.

Sherk, H. H., and Nicholson, J. T., Cervico-oculo-acusticus syndrome. *J. Bone Joint Surg.*, *54A*:1776–1778, 1972.

Singh, S. P., Rock, E. H., and Shulman, A., Klippel-Feil syndrome with unexplained conductive hearing loss. *Laryngoscope, 79*:113–117, 1969.

Stark, E. W., and Borton, T. E., Klippel-Feil syndrome and associated hearing loss. *Arch. Otolaryngol.*, *97*:415–419, 1973.

Troy, J. J., A case of Klippel-Feil syndrome. *Ir. J. Med. Sci.*, *1*:15–18, 1968.

Whetnall, E., and Fry, D. B., *The Deaf Child*. London, William Heinemann, Ltd. 1964, p. 103.

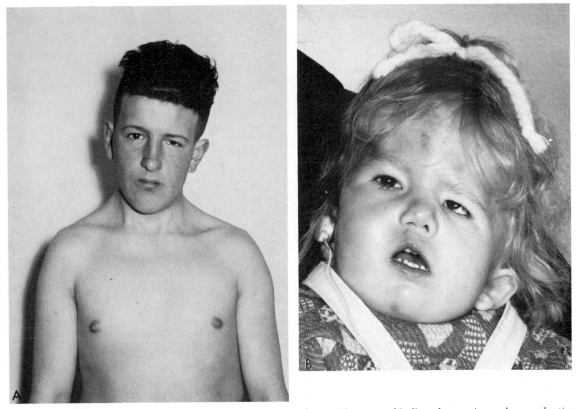

Figure 5-21 *Klippel-Feil anomalad and abducens paralysis with retracted bulb and sensorineural or conductive deafness (Wildervanck syndrome; cervico-oculoacoustic dysplasia). (A)* Twenty-two-year-old male with facial asymmetry and torticollis. Left eye exhibits strabismus, narrowed palpebral fissure, and retracted globe. Patient had unilateral sensorineural deafness and epibulbar dermoid. (From A. Franceschetti and D. Klein, *J. Génét. Hum., 3*:176, 1954.) *(B)* Two-year-old girl with asymmetry of head, severe Klippel-Feil anomalad, strabismus, arrested hydrocephalus, and sensorineural deafness.

Wildervanck, L. S., En geval van aandoening van Klippel-Feil gecominieerd met abducens paralyse, retractio bulbi en doofstomheid. *Ned. Tijdschr. Geneeskd., 104*:2600–2605, 1960.

Wildervanck, L. S., A cervico-oculo-acusticus syndrome belonging to the status dysraphicus. *Proc. 2nd Int. Cong. Hum. Genet. (Rome), 1961, 3*:1409–1412, 1963.

Wildervanck, L. S., Hoeksema, P. E., and Penning, L., Radiological examination of the inner ear of deaf-mutes presenting the cervico-oculo-acusticus syndrome. *Acta Otolaryngol. (Stockh.), 61*:445–453, 1966.

Witzel, S. H., Congenital paralysis of lateral conjugate gaze. Occurrence in a case of Klippel-Feil syndrome. *Arch. Ophthalmol., 59*:463–464, 1959.

CRANIOFACIAL DYSOSTOSIS

(Crouzon Syndrome)

Craniofacial dysostosis is characterized by premature craniosynostosis, midface hypoplasia with relative mandibular prognathism, ocular proptosis, and hypertelorism.

CLINICAL FINDINGS

Physical Findings. Clinical changes are limited to the cranium and face. The nose may be somewhat unusual in shape as a result of vertical hypoplasia of the middle-third of the face. Relative mandibular prognathism, drooping lower lip, short upper lip, and protruding tongue are frequent findings. Dental malocclusion is a constant feature.

Skeletal System. The shape of the cranium depends upon which sutures are involved. Brachycephaly, scaphocephaly, trigonocephaly, and, rarely, the Kleeblattschädel anomalad have been observed. Palpable ridging is usually evident. A prominent bulge may be present at the bregma (Bertelsen, 1958). Premature craniosynostosis is variable in onset but frequently commences during the first year of life and is usually complete by 2 to 3 years of age. In some cases, synostosis may not be evident until 10 years of age.

Ocular System. Proptosis is secondary to shallow orbits. Divergent strabismus and nystagmus may be observed. Hypertelorism is a constant feature. Bertelsen (1958) noted that 80 per cent of patients with craniofacial dysostosis had optic nerve involvement. Spontaneous luxation of the globes, megalocornea, ectopia lentis, iris coloboma, and corectopia have been noted occasionally.

Auditory System. Boedts (1967) estimated that one third of the patients with the Crouzon syndrome have hearing loss, mostly conductive. In surgical exploration and postmortem studies he found deformity of the ossicles or fixation of the stapes to the oval window. Aubrey (1935), Nager, and de Reynier (1948), Wiegand (1954), and Baldwin (1968) noted bilateral atresia of the external auditory canal and mixed or conductive deafness. Schurmans and Hariga (1963) found diminished bone conduction, absence of recruitment and, by means of tomography, deformity of the acoustic meatus.

Vestibular System. Aubrey (1935) described normal vestibular function.

LABORATORY FINDINGS

Roentgenograms. The coronal, sagittal, and lambdoidal sutures are most frequently involved in premature fusion. Other findings may include digital impressions, shallow orbits, basilar kyphosis, widening of the hypophyseal fossa, and small paranasal sinuses (Bertelsen, 1958).

As noted above, Schurmans and Hariga (1963), in tomographic study, observed deformity of the acoustic meatus. Radiographs have shown well-developed labyrinths (Wiegand, 1954). The elegant tomographic studies by Terrahe (1968) of the temporal bones showed outward rotation of the petrous pyramids secondary to cranial base dysplasia resulting in obliquity of the ear canals, atypical course of the facial nerve, and hyperostosis. Terrahe emphasized that the primary changes were ossicular fixation with intratympanic bony masses, ossicular anomalies, and closure of the oval window.

PATHOLOGY

Temporal bone study has shown stenosis or atresia of the external auditory canal as well as absence of the drum, deformity of the stapes and bony fusion to the promontory, ankylosis of the malleus to the outer wall of the epitympanum, distortion, and narrowing of the middle ear and mastoid air spaces (Nager and de Reynier, 1948). Baldwin (1968) also found the periosteal portion of the labyrinth to be underdeveloped. The malleus and incus were ankylosed to the lateral wall of the epitympanic recess and the crura of the stapes were oblique to the footplate with the incudostapedial joint in contact with the promontory. Either the round window or the oval window or both were narrower than normal. The tympanic membrane was missing.

HEREDITY

Inheritance is autosomal dominant with full penetrance (Schiller, 1959; Vulliamy and Normandale, 1966). Almost one third of the cases are new mutations.

DIAGNOSIS

Craniofacial dysostosis should be distinguished from isolated craniosynostosis, *Apert syndrome, Pfeiffer syndrome,* and the *Saethre-Chotzen syndrome* (Gorlin *et al.*, 1976).

TREATMENT

Cosmetic and functional correction has been carried out by morcellation of prematurely fused sutures and by surgically produced blepharophimosis to prevent luxation of the eyeballs. Tessier (1971) described an excellent radical surgical approach for correction of the facial deformities.

PROGNOSIS

With age, binocular vision often becomes impossible and there is divergent, alternating and concomitant strabismus. Frequently, optic atrophy and loss of vision occur. Occasionally, due to the shallow orbits there is complete proptosis of one or both eyeballs. Premature fusion of sutures produces a bregmatic bump. The normal growth of the

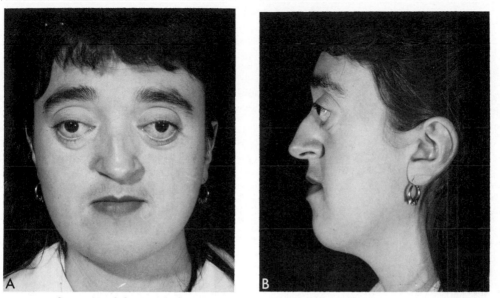

Figure 5-22 *Craniofacial dysostosis (Crouzon syndrome). (A, B)* Note mild ocular hypertelorism, proptosis of globes, and midfacial hypoplasia with relative mandibular prognathism. (Courtesy of P. Tessier, Paris, France.)

mandible and the hypoplastic midface become more accentuated with age.

SUMMARY

Characteristics of Crouzon syndrome include: 1) autosomal dominant inheritance, 2) premature variable craniosynostosis, 3) ocular hypertelorism, shallow orbits and exophthalmos, 4) beaked nose, 5) maxillary hypoplasia with relative mandibular prognathism, and 6) occasional bilateral atresia of the external auditory canals, ossicular anomalies and mixed hearing loss.

REFERENCES

Aubrey, M., Examen otologique de 10 cas de dysostose cranio-faciale de Crouzon. *Rev. Neurol.,* 63:302–305, 1935.
Baldwin, J. L., Dysostosis craniofacialis of Crouzon. *Laryngoscope, 78:*1660–1676, 1968.
Bertelsen, T. I., *The Premature Synostosis of the Cranial Sutures.* Copenhagen, Munksgaard International Booksellers & Publishers, Ltd., 1958.
Boedts, D., La surdité dans la dysostose crâniofaciale ou maladie de Crouzon. *Acta Otorhinolaryngol. Belg., 21:*143–155, 1967.
Gorlin, R. J., Pindborg, J. J., and Cohen, M. M., Jr., *Syndromes of the Head and Neck,* 2nd Ed. New York, McGraw-Hill Book Company, 1976.
Kittel, G., and Fleischer-Peters, A., Das Ohr bei Dysostosesyndromen des Schädels. *Z. Laryngol. Rhinol., 42:*384–397, 1963.
Nager, F. R., and de Reynier, J., Das Gehörorgan bei den angeborenen Kopfmissbildungen. *Pract. Otorhinolaryngol., 10(Suppl. 2):*1–128, 1948.
Schiller, J. G., Craniofacial dysostosis of Crouzon: a case report and pedigree with emphasis on heredity. *Pediatrics, 23:*107–112, 1959.
Schurmans, P., and Hariga, J., Dysostose crâniofaciale familiale et malformations nerveuses associeés. *Acta Neurol. Belg., 63:*794–820, 1963.
Terrahe, K., Das Gehörorgan bie den kraniofazialen Missbildungssyndromen nach Crouzon und Apert. *Z. Laryngol. Rhinol., 50:*794–802, 1971.
Tessier, P., Relationship of craniostenoses to craniofacial dysostoses and to faciostenoses. A study with therapeutic implications. *Plast. Reconstr. Surg., 48:*224–237, 1971.
Tessier, P., The definitive plastic surgical treatment of the severe facial deformities of craniofacial dysostosis. Crouzon's and Apert's diseases. *Plast. Reconstr. Surg., 48:*419–442, 1971.
Vulliamy, D. G., and Normandale, P. A., Craniofacial dysostosis in a Dorset family. *Arch. Dis. Child., 41:*375–382, 1966.
Wiegand, R., Dysostosis craniofacialis (Morbus Crouzon 1912) mit beidseitiger (häutiger) Gehörgangsatresie. *Arch. Ohr.-Nas. Kehlk.-heilk., 166:*128–139, 1954.

APERT SYNDROME

(Acrocephalosyndactyly, Type I)

Apert type acrocephalosyndactyly is a rare developmental deformity syndrome characterized by craniosynostosis leading to turribrachycephaly and syndactyly of hands and feet. Other features include various ankyloses and progressive synostoses of the hands, feet, and cervical spine. Apert (1906) was credited with the discovery of the disorder, although the condition had been reported earlier. Over 200 cases have been reported to date. Although the frequency of the syndrome is about 1 in 160,000 births, because of the high neonatal mortality rate, the disorder is seen in about 1 in 2,000,000 in the general population.

In the Anglo-American literature prior to 1960, all acrocephalosyndactylies were thought to constitute a single syndrome. Blank (1960) divided acrocephalosyndactyly into typical and atypical forms. Typical (Apert type) acrocephalosyndactyly included only those patients who had a mid-digital hand mass consisting of osseous and soft tissue syndactyly of digits 2 through 4.

CLINICAL FINDINGS

Facies. The forehead is high and steep, and during infancy a horizontal groove may be present above the supraorbital ridges. The occiput is flattened. Hypertelorism is commonly observed. Proptosis and antimongoloid obliquity of the palpebral fissures vary in the degree of expression. Strabismus is present in some cases. Nasal morphology is quite variable. The middle third of the face is underdeveloped, lending prominence to the mandible and causing the often unusual nasal form.

Musculoskeletal System. The skull is turribrachycephalic. The frontal and occipital bones are flattened, and the apex of the cranium is located near or anterior to the bregma. The maxilla is underdeveloped.

Deformities of the hands and feet are symmetric. A mid-digital hand mass with soft tissue syndactyly of the second, third, and fourth fingers is always found. The first and fifth digits may be joined to the second and fourth or may be separate. In the feet, the second, third, and fourth are joined by soft tissue syndactyly. The first and fifth are at times free and at times joined by soft tissue to the second and fourth toes, respectively. The interphalangeal joints of the fingers are stiff. Fingernails of the mid-digital hand mass may be completely or partially continuous; toenails may be partially united or show some segmentation. The thumb usually deviates radially at the metacarpophalangeal joint.

The upper extremities are shortened. Aplasia or ankylosis of several joints, especially the elbow, shoulder, and hip, is commonly observed.

Nervous System. Some degree of mental retardation is found in most patients, although normal intelligence has been observed in some cases.

Oral Findings. The palate is high-arched, constricted, and may have a marked median furrow. Cleft soft palate is observed in approximately 30 per cent of the cases.

Auditory System. Perhaps because of the frequent mental retardation, the relatively mild congenital conductive deafness associated with the syndrome has been largely ignored. Data concerning the frequency of hearing loss in the syndrome are nonexistent; the only information available is case reports. Cooper (1953) reported bilateral conduction deafness in his patient, and Grebe (1944) noted that one of eight patients was "completely deaf." Bergstrom *et al.* (1972), in their excellent survey, described conduction deafness in four patients, two of whom were mother and daughter. The daughter had noted progressive hearing loss since puberty. Tympanotomy showed congenital fixation of the footplate of the stapes. The stapes was removed and a perilymphatic gusher ensued—possibly as a result of a widened cochlear aqueduct. Later, some sensorineural loss was noted. Petrous pyramid polytomography performed on another patient showed no internal auditory meatus. Acoustic bridge studies on still another patient indicated increased impedance and absence of the stapedius reflex, a finding consistent with ossicular fixation. Lindsay *et al.* (1975) reported cartilaginous fixation of the stapes footplate, an incompletely developed annular ligament, and an enlarged subarcuate fossa.

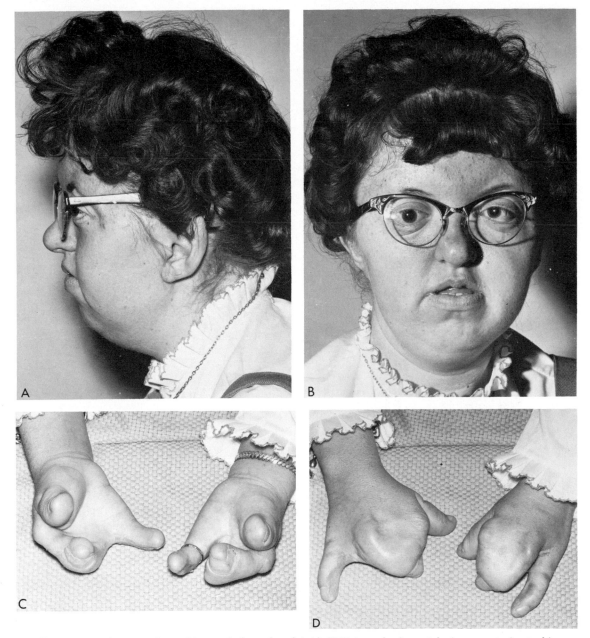

Figure 5-23 *Apert syndrome (Acrocephalosyndactyly). (A, B)* Note ocular hypertelorism, proptosis, strabismus, and hypoplasia of maxilla. Patient's mother was similarly affected. *(C, D)* Syndactyly of hands showing mid-digital hand mass with common nail. *(A–D* from L. Bergstrom *et al., Arch. Otolaryngol.,* 96:117, 1972.)

Vestibular System. No studies have been reported.

LABORATORY FINDINGS

Radiologically, there is irregular, early obliteration of cranial sutures, especially the coronal, but frequently other sutures as well. Digital markings are usually accentuated. The anterior fontanel may remain open longer than normal. The orbits are hyperteloric and the maxilla is hypoplastic. Progressive synostosis of the bones of the hands, feet, and cervical spine has been reported. In several cases, six metatarsals have been observed (Gorlin *et al.,* 1976).

HEREDITY

Most cases are sporadic. On a few occasions, a female with Apert syndrome has given birth to an affected child (Weech, 1972; Hoover et al., 1970; Roberts and Hall, 1971; Bergstrom et al., 1972). Increased paternal age at the time of conception was found by Blank (1960). The few familial cases, the lack of sex predilection, the increased paternal age at conception, and the large number of sporadic cases suggest autosomal dominant transmission.

DIAGNOSIS

One should exclude *Pfeiffer syndrome, Crouzon syndrome,* Carpenter syndrome, Summitt syndrome, and various other craniostenotic syndromes. Marked syndactyly resembling that in Apert syndrome may be seen in *cryptophthalmos syndrome* (Gorlin et al., 1976).

TREATMENT

The hands should be corrected by plastic surgery. Tessier (1971) has devised a major surgical procedure for correction of the maxillofacial anomalies.

PROGNOSIS

The disorder is congenital and, in general, does not progress with age.

SUMMARY

Characteristics of the disorder are: 1) autosomal dominant inheritance (although nearly all cases are sporadic, representing new mutations), 2) craniostenosis, eventuating in turribrachycephaly, 3) soft tissue syndactyly and progressive synostoses of hands and feet, 4) mental retardation, and 5) conduction deafness (occasionally).

REFERENCES

Apert, E., De l'acrocephalosyndactylie. *Bull. Soc. Med. (Paris), 23*:1310–1330, 1906.

Bergstrom, L. V., Neblett, L. M., and Hemenway, W. G., Otologic manifestations of acrocephalosyndactyly. *Arch. Otolaryngol., 96*:117–123, 1972.

Blank, C. E., Apert's syndrome (a type of acrocephalosyndactyly): observations on a British series of thirty-nine cases. *Ann. Hum. Genet., 24*:151–164, 1960.

Cooper, R., Acrocephalosyndactyly. *Br. J. Radiol., 26*:533–538, 1953.

Gorlin, R. J., Pindborg, J. J., and Cohen, M. M., Jr., *Syndromes of the Head and Neck,* 2nd Ed. New York, McGraw-Hill Book Company, 1976.

Grebe, H., Die Akrocephalosyndaktylie: eine klinisch-ätiologische Studie. *Z. Menschl. Vererb. Konstit.-lehre., 28*:211–261, 1944.

Hoover, G. H., Flatt, A. E., and Weiss, M. W., The hand in Apert's syndrome. *J. Bone Joint Surg., 52A*:878–895, 1970.

Lindsay, J. R., Black, F. O., and Donnelly, W. N., Jr., Acrocephalosyndactyly (Apert's syndrome). Temporal bone findings. *Ann. Otol., 84*:174–178, 1975.

Roberts, K. B., and Hall, J. B., Apert's acrocephalosyndactyly in mother and daughter. Cleft palate in the mother. *Birth Defects, 7*(7):262–263, 1971.

Tessier, P., The definitive plastic surgical treatment of the severe facial deformities of craniofacial dysostosis, Crouzon's and Apert's diseases. *Plast. Recontr. Surg., 48*:419–442, 1971.

Weech, A. A., Combined acrocephaly and syndactylism occurring in mother and daughter. *Bull. Johns Hopkins Hosp., 40*:73–76, 1927.

HEREDITARY HYPERPHOSPHATASIA

(Juvenile Paget's Disease; Hyperostosis Corticalis Juvenilis Deformans)

Hereditary hyperphosphatasia is characterized by progressive skeletal deformities that become apparent during the second or third year of life and result in sporadic cranial nerve involvement. Consistently elevated levels of serum alkaline and acid phosphatase are also associated with this disorder. It was possibly first described by Sorrell and LeGrand-Lambling (1938).

CLINICAL FINDINGS

Musculoskeletal System. Swelling of the extremities occurs during the first year of life and may be accompanied by pain (Eyring and Eisenberg, 1968). Soon thereafter, the circumference of the calvaria enlarges—up to 65 cm. or more. Bending and thickening of the bones of the extremities occur; in particular, there is anterior bowing of the legs and a general broadening of the diaphyseal areas of the tubular bones with loss of normal cortical outline from epiphysis to epiphysis. Cysts have been described in the metaphyses of the long bones (Fanconi *et al.*, 1964). The spine and ribs may be osteoporotic; dorsal kyphoscoliosis is common. The chest is barrel-shaped, and usually there is coxa vara (Mitsudo, 1971).

Chondral ossification is not markedly disturbed, i.e., the epiphyses are normally formed and the joints are not involved. Since muscle weakness is frequent, walking, running, and jumping are retarded. Because of the severe bending of the legs, some patients are confined to a wheelchair. Flexion deformities have been noted in several cases.

Ocular System. Visual acuity may be diminished because of optic atrophy. Angioid streaks and/or macular hemorrhage have been noted (Thompson *et al.*, 1969, Mitsudo, 1971).

Nervous System. Intelligence is normal. Headache is common. Motor sensory and cerebellar functions as well as deep tendon reflexes are normal.

Cardiovascular System. Hypertension has been reported in several cases (Marshall, 1962; Thompson *et al.*, 1969; Mitsudo, 1971; Caffey, 1972).

Auditory System. Progressive mixed 60 to 80 dB hearing loss has been evident from the fourth to the fourteenth year of life (Thompson *et al.*, 1969). The ear canals are narrowed. Eyring and Eisenberg (1968) described high-frequency sensorineural hearing loss. Mitsudo (1971) noted "diminished hearing" bilaterally.

Vestibular System. Studies have not been reported.

LABORATORY FINDINGS

Roentgenograms. Radiographic examination of the skull reveals changes remarkably like those seen in Paget's disease. Long bones exhibit bending, overcylindrization, and general diaphyseal cortical widening. The bone structure is coarse. Short bones are involved to a lesser degree, almost entirely on the endosteal side. The facial bones, except in the patient reported by Marshall (1962) and Rubin (1964), have not been involved.

Other Findings. Both serum acid and alkaline phosphatase levels are elevated, but calcium and phosphorus levels are normal. The alkaline phosphatase may range from 100 to 500 King-Armstrong units. Urinary hydroxyproline and proline-containing peptides are increased (Seakins, 1963; Thompson *et al.*, 1969). Mild microcytic hypochromic anemia has been noted in several cases (Swoboda, 1958; Thompson *et al.*, 1969). Eyring and Eisenberg (1968) described elevated leucine aminopeptidase.

PATHOLOGY

There is intensive metaplastic fibrous bone formation as well as markedly increased osteoblastic and osteoclastic activity that is very similar to that seen in Paget's disease but is without typical mosaic or regression lines (Choremis *et al.*, 1958; Fanconi *et al.*, 1964; Thompson *et al.*, 1969). Thus, there is a marked rapid turnover of lamellar bone and a failure to lay down compact cortical bone. This deviation from the normal pattern of bone formation is reflected not only by the histopathologic picture but also by the elevated levels of hydroxyproline, proline-containing peptides, and acid and alkaline phosphatases determined by tetracycline labelling studies (Stemmermann, 1966; Eyring and Eisenberg, 1968).

HEREDITY

The disorder has been described in sibs with normal parents (Swoboda, 1958; Stemmermann, 1966; Eyring and Eisenberg, 1968; Thompson *et al.*, 1969) and parental consanguinity has been noted (Swoboda, 1958). Thus, inheritance appears to be autosomal recessive.

DIAGNOSIS

Although the sibs described by Bakwin and coworkers (1956, 1964) had similar clinical and radiologic appearance, they also exhibited multiple fractures and intermittent elevated serum alkaline phosphatase only following fractures. Bowing of the extremities and enlargement of the head occurred about the age of 2 to 3 years. Macular degeneration, grossly constricted visual fields, and angioid streaks were noted. Audiometry revealed mild to moderate mixed hearing loss. Whether these children had hereditary hyperphosphatasia is not known.

Clinically or radiologically, hereditary hyperphosphatasia may be distinguished from such disorders as polyostotic fibrous dysplasia, *van Buchem's disease, Paget's disease,* and *osteogenesis imperfecta.*

TREATMENT

Sodium fluoride, at a dose of 1 mg./kg./day, was given by Eyring and Eisenberg (1968) with mildly encouraging results.

SUMMARY

Characteristics of hereditary hyperphosphatasia include: 1) autosomal recessive inheritance, 2) progressive enlargement of the head and bending and thickening of long bones of the extremities, 3) elevated alkaline and acid phosphatase levels, and 4) occasionally mixed hearing loss.

REFERENCES

Bakwin, H., and Eiger, M. S., Fragile bones and macrocranium. *J. Pediatr., 49*:558–564, 1956.

Bakwin, H., Golden, A., and Fox, S., Familial osteoectasia with macrocranium. *Am. J. Roentgenol., 91*:609–617, 1964.

Caffey, J., *Pediatric X-ray Diagnosis,* 6th Ed. Chicago, Year Book Medical Publishers, 1972, pp. 1231–1237.

Choremis, C., Yannakos, D., Papadatos, C., and Baroutsou, E., Osteitis deformans (Paget's disease) in an 11-year-old boy. *Helv. Paediatr. Acta, 13*:185–188, 1958.

Eyring, E. J., and Eisenberg, E., Congenital hyperphosphatasia: a clinical, pathological, and biochemical study of two cases. *J. Bone Joint Surg., 50A*:1099–1117, 1968.

Fanconi, G., Moreira, G., Uehlinger, E., and Giedion, A., Osteochalasia desmalis familiaris. *Helv. Paediatr. Acta, 19*:279–295, 1964.

Koenen, H. P. J., Ostitis deformans fibrosa (Paget) bij een zuigeling. *Maandschr. Kindergeneeskd., 1*:533–536, 1932.

Marshall, W. C., A chronic progressive osteopathy with hyperphosphatasia. *Proc. R. Soc. Med., 55*:238–239, 1962.

Mitsudo, S. M., Chronic idiopathic hyperphosphatasia associated with pseudoxanthoma elasticum. *J. Bone Joint Surg., 53A*:303–314, 1971.

Rubin, P., *Dynamic Classification of Bone Dysplasia.* Chicago, Year Book Medical Publishers, Inc., 1964, pp. 340–344.

Seakins, J. W., Peptiduria in an unusual bone disorder. *Arch. Dis. Child., 38*:215–219, 1963 (same case as Marshall).

Sorrell, E., and LeGrand-Lambling, Dystrophie osseuse generalisée. *Bull. Soc. Pédiatr. (Paris), 36*:86–92, 1938.

Stemmermann, G. N., A histologic and histochemical study of familial osteoectasia. *Am. J. Pathol., 48*:641–651, 1966.

Swoboda, J. W., Hyperostosis corticalis deformans juvenilis: Ungewöhnliche generalisierte Osteopathie bei zwei Geschwistern. *Helv. Paediatr. Acta, 13*:292–312, 1958.

Thompson, R. C., Jr., Gaull, G. E., Horwitz, S.. J., and Schenk, R. K., Hereditary hyperphosphatasia. Studies of three siblings. *Am. J. Med., 47*:209–219, 1969.

Wagner, J. M., and Solomon, A., Hyperostosis corticalis infantilis (Caffey's disease). *S. Afr. Med. J., 43*:754–755, 1969.

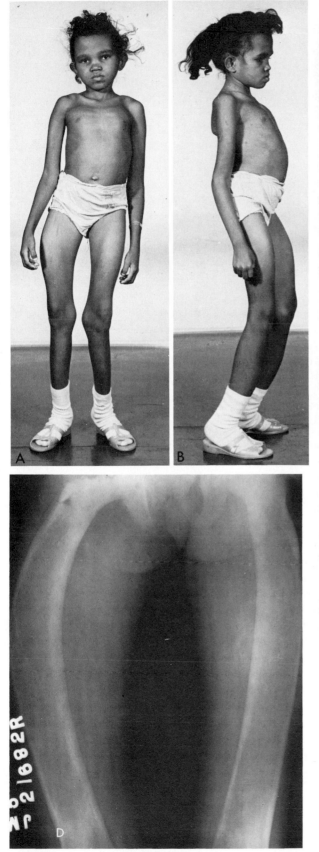

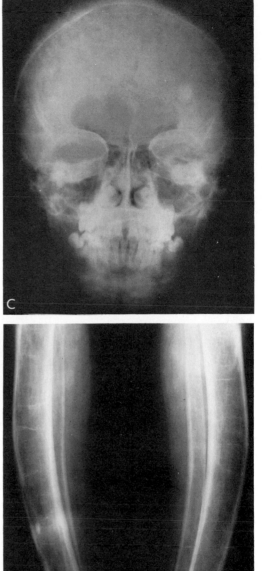

Figure 5-24 Hereditary hyperphosphatasia (Juvenile Paget's disease). (A, B) Eleven-year-old child with enlargement of skull, high forehead, wide face, and bowing of lower extremities. (C, D, and E) Calvaria greatly thickened and exhibiting patches of increased density. Long bones of lower extremities are expanded and bowed. (A-E from H. Bakwin *et al., Am. J. Roentgenol., 91*:609, 1964.)

HEREDITARY ARTHRO-OPHTHALMOPATHY

(Stickler Syndrome)

First defined by Stickler and coworkers (1965, 1967), the condition consists of progressive multiple dysplasia of the epiphyses and of other skeletal changes, joint hypermobility, myopia, retinal detachment, cleft palate, and hearing loss. An earlier example was described by David (1953).

CLINICAL FINDINGS

Facies. About 50 per cent of the patients that we have seen have exhibited midfacial flattening. The nose is often saddle-shaped (David, 1954; Spranger, 1968; Falger *et al.,* 1970). Cleft palate was noted by Stickler and Pugh (1967), Spranger (1968), Falger *et al.* (1970), and by many others (see Diagnosis)—perhaps in 50 per cent of the cases.

Musculoskeletal System. There is bony enlargement of the ankles, knees, and wrists within the first few years of life. The joints are sometimes painful with use and become stiff at rest. Rarely, they are reddened and warm. The patient may experience difficulty in walking and may tire easily. Thoracic kyphosis, noted in about 30 per cent of the cases, makes the arms appear long (David, 1954; Stickler *et al.*, 1965). Other skeletal anomalies, including pectus carinatum, genua valga, hypermobility of joints, talipes equinovarus, and pes planus, occur in over 60 per cent.

Ocular System. Congenital progressive myopia as great as 18 diopters has been noted in about 70 per cent of the cases. Before the tenth year of life, broad zones of retinal detachment are experienced in about 20 per cent. Secondary cataract, keratopathy and/or glaucoma occur in 10 per cent.

Auditory System. Stickler and Pugh (1967) described sensorineural hearing loss of about 25 to 30 dB. Spranger (1968) reported conductive hearing loss. David (1958) did not further characterize the deafness noted in his patients. Our personal experience would suggest that about 15 per cent experience sensorineural or mixed deafness. A similar figure has been estimated by J. Herrmann (personal communication, 1974). Popkin and Polomeno (1974) reported two large kindreds in which sensorineural deafness was found in about 10 per cent.

Vestibular System. No studies have been reported.

LABORATORY FINDINGS

Radiographically, in about one third of the patients, there are multiple epiphyseal ossification disturbances and diminution of the width of the shaft of tubular bones. The overly thin diaphyses contrast with the normally broad metaphyses. The pelvic bones are hypoplastic, and the femoral neck is poorly modeled, plump, and in coxa valga position. The vertebral bodies are flattened and irregular with a tendency to anterior wedging. Thoracic kyphosis is common.

HEREDITY

There are numerous pedigrees exhibiting autosomal dominant inheritance.

DIAGNOSIS

Cohen *et al.* (1971) described the problems in separation of the Stickler syndrome from what they have called the Cervenka syndrome (midfacial flattening, cleft palate, myopia, retinal detachment, autosomal dominant inheritance) (Frandsen, 1966; Smith, 1969; van Balen and Falger, 1970; Hirose *et al.*, 1973). Hall (1974) demonstrated convincingly that Cervenka syndrome is only a mild expression of hereditary arthro-ophthalmopathy. The kindred described by Schreiner *et al.* (1973) demonstrated the markedly variable expressivity of the Stickler syndrome.

The findings on the patient of Kozlowski *et al.* (1972) were not sufficiently well documented for us to discern whether he had the Stickler syndrome or another skeletal-deafness syndrome.

TREATMENT

Early referral to an ophthalmologist is mandatory.

PROGNOSIS

The arthropathy becomes progressively worse. The retinal detachment usually recurs in spite of surgery.

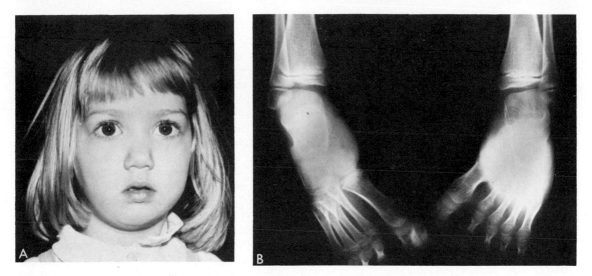

Figure 5-25 Hereditary arthro-ophthalmopathy (Stickler syndrome). (A) Note round face with midfacial hypoplasia. *(B)* Radiograph showing irregularity and underdevelopment laterally of distal tibial epiphysis. (*A* and *B* from J. Hall, *Birth Defects, 10*(8):157, 1974.)

SUMMARY

Characteristics of this syndrome are: 1) autosomal dominant inheritance, 2) numerous but often subtle ossification disturbances, including epiphyseal abnormalities, diaphyseal narrowing and platyspondylia, 3) joint hypermobility, 4) hypoplasia of the midface, 5) severe myopia and, often, retinal detachment, 6) occasionally, cleft palate, submucous cleft palate, or bifid uvula, and 7) mixed deafness.

REFERENCES

Cohen, M. M., Jr., Knobloch, W. H., and Gorlin, R. J., A dominantly inherited syndrome of hyaloideoretinal degeneration, cleft palate and maxillary hypoplasia (Cervenka syndrome). *Birth Defects, 7*(7):83–86, 1971.

David, B., Über einen dominanten Erbgang bei einer polytopen enchondralen Dysostose Typ Pfaundler-Hurler. *Z. Orthopäd., 84*:657–660, 1954.

Falger, E. L., Van Balen, A. T., Binkhorst, P. G., *et al.,* Hereditary hyaloideo-retinal degeneration and palatoschisis. *Ophthalmologie (Basel), 160*:384, 1970.

Frandsen, E., Hereditary hyaloideoretinal degeneration (Wagner) in a Danish family. *Acta Ophthalmol. (Kbh.), 44*:223–232, 1966.

Hall, J., Stickler syndrome: presenting as a syndrome of cleft palate, myopia, and blindness inherited as a dominant trait. *Birth Defects, 10*(8):157–171, 1974.

Hirose, T., Lee, K. V., and Schapens, C. L., Wagner's hereditary vitreoretinal degeneration and retinal detachment. *Arch. Ophthalmol., 89*:176–185, 1973.

Kozlowski, K., Barylak, A., and Niedzwiedzki, T., Spondylo-epiphyseal dysplasia with unusual skull changes. *Acta Radiol. [Diagn.] (Stockh.), 12*:141–144, 1972.

Popkin, J. S., and Polomeno, R. C., Stickler's syndrome (hereditary progressive arthro-ophthalmopathy. *Can. Med. Assoc. J., 111*:1071–1076, 1974.

Schreiner, R. L., McAlister, W. H., Marshall, R. E., and Shearer, W. T., Stickler syndrome in a pedigree of Pierre Robin syndrome. *Am. J. Dis. Child., 126*:86–90, 1973.

Smith, W. K., Pierre Robin syndrome in brothers. *Birth Defects, 5*(2):220–221, 1969.

Spranger, J., Arthro-ophthalmopathia hereditaria. *Ann. Radiol. (Paris), 11*:359–364, 1968.

Stickler, G. B., Belau, P. G., Farrell, F. J., Jones, J. D., Pugh, D. G., Steinberg, A. G., and Ward, L. E., Hereditary progressive arthro-ophthalmopathy. *Mayo Clin. Proc., 40*:433–455, 1965.

Stickler, G. B., and Pugh, D. G., Hereditary progressive arthro-ophthalmopathy. II. Additional observation on vertebral anomalies, a hearing defect, and a report of a similar case. *Mayo Clin. Proc., 42*:495–500, 1967.

van Balen, A. T., and Falger, E. L., Hereditary hyaloideoretinal degeneration and palatoschisis. *Arch. Ophthalmol., 83*:152–162, 1970.

OSTEOGENESIS IMPERFECTA

The syndrome consists of fragile bones, clear or blue sclerae, conductive deafness, loose ligaments, and, frequently, changes in the teeth resembling those seen in dentinogenesis imperfecta. Credit is usually given to Ekman (1788) for performing the first comprehensive study of this syndrome and for discussing its inheritance. Lobstein (1833) and Vrolik (1849) first described the adult and infantile forms, respectively. Van der Hoeve and de Kleijn (1918) first mentioned deafness as part of the syndrome. The incidence varies from about 2 to 5 per 100,000 births in different populations (Seedorff, 1949; Schröder, 1964; McKusick, 1972).

CLINICAL FINDINGS

Physical Findings. Most reported cases (about 90 per cent) represent a type that has been referred to as the "tarda form" of osteogenesis imperfecta. Findings include blue sclerae (90 per cent), brittle bones (60 per cent), impaired hearing (60 per cent), dentin defects (50 per cent), and hyperelasticity of joints and ligaments (30 per cent). The age of onset of clinical symptoms varies, but usually multiple fractures occur in the tarda type. Since there may also be individuals in the same family with the "congenital" type, classification according to age of onset and clinical severity seems inappropriate. Furthermore, there is evidence that the massive bones noted at birth become gracile with age.

Facies. The facies is similar to that seen in cleidocranial dysplasia. The skull appears disproportionally large, and there is temporal bulging that causes the pinnae to extend outward and forward.

Musculoskeletal System. In the congenital type, intrauterine fractures may be so numerous that the child may be born dead or may survive for only a short time. Micromelia is often quite striking (Remigio and Grinvalsky, 1970; McKusick, 1972).

The skull is large, the forehead being especially broad and bossed and showing temporal bulging, an overhanging occiput, decreased vertical dimension, and platybasia, which gives the skull a "mushroom" or "soldier's helmet" appearance.

The long bones, especially those of the lower extremities, are bowed or unevenly shortened. Subperiosteal fractures of the shaft and multiple microfractures at the epiphyses due to minor trauma or sudden muscle pulls are frequently observed.

The tendency to fracture decreases with age; however, pregnancy, lactation, or senile involution may enhance the likelihood. Laxity of ligaments or rupture of tendons, resulting in habitual dislocation of joints, flatfoot, and distortions is not uncommon; it is seen in at least 25 per cent. Hernia occurs with high frequency.

Spinal cord compression resulting from abnormally shaped vertebrae, kyphoscoliosis, pectus carinatum and excavatum, and pseudoarthroses are frequently encountered.

Ocular System. The presence of clear (blue) sclerae is one of the most constant features of the syndrome. It may be the only expression but may be more common in mild cases. The intensity of the blueness varies from family to family and from case to case. There is no direct correlation between intensity of blueness and severity of bone involvement. The blue color may be due in part to thinning of the sclera, to allowing the color of the choroid to be transmitted, to increased translucency related to deficiency of collagen fibers, or to an increase in mucopolysaccharide content.

Dental Changes. Chiefly the dentin is affected. Although the enamel frequently cracks off, it is not considered to be involved. In the tarda type, the deciduous teeth are affected in about 80 per cent of the patients—the permanent teeth in only 35 per cent. Upon eruption, the teeth are translucent or opalescent, and the color darkens with age.

Auditory System. Severely impaired hearing is found in 30 to 60 per cent of patients with the tarda type (Dessoff, 1934; Seedorff, 1949). Complete deafness is rarely observed; hearing appears to be more severely impaired in patients with marked bone involvement (Caniggia et al., 1958). Deafness usually begins in the third decade and increases progressively with time, becoming profound in some individuals (Robertson and Gregory, 1962). The deafness, usually conductive and symmetric, can be mixed or purely sensorineural (Robertson and Gregory, 1962; Kosoy and Maddox,

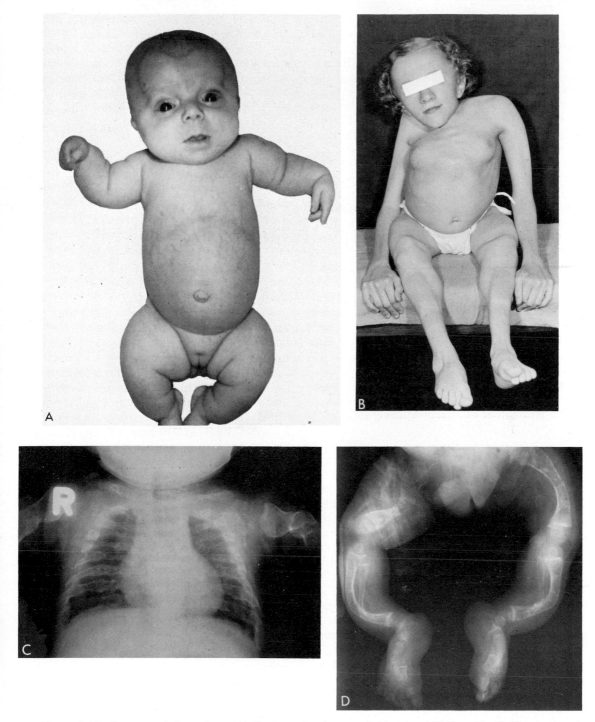

Figure 5–26 *Osteogenesis imperfecta.* (A) Newborn showing rounded head and "doll-position" of bent extremities. (B) Fourteen-year-old female with rounded calvaria, severe scoliosis, and bent extremities. She had suffered numerous fractures. (C) Radiograph of newborn showing evidence of numerous intrauterine fractures. (D) Radiograph showing severely bent, osteoporotic bones of lower extremities.

1971). In some patients the typanic membrane has been found to be thinned and bluish in color.

Although there has been much discussion about the possible relationship between otosclerosis and osteogenesis imperfecta, it is clear that the hearing loss in osteogenesis imperfecta is not due to otosclerosis. Kosoy and Maddox (1971), performing stapedectomies on five patients, found that in each case the body of the stapes footplate had a heavy growth of white, chalky, soft, mounded bone, but the footplate margins were discrete and showed only slight fixation, in contrast to the firm fixation found in otosclerosis. Hall and Røhrt (1968) found a normal footplate. Opheim (1968), Hall and Røhrt (1968), Bretlau et al. (1971), and Müller (1974) noted degeneration of the stapes crura with replacement by fibrous threads. The stapes footplate and adjacent oval window showed no evidence of otosclerosis. However, the otosclerotic change may involve the labyrinthine capsule and may possibly be responsible for the sensorineural hearing loss found in some cases (Bretlau and Jørgensen, 1969; Bretlau et al., 1970; Müller, 1974).

LABORATORY FINDINGS

Radiographic examination reveals remarkably thin calvaria (caput membranaceum) and numerous Wormian bones in the occipital area, giving rise to a mosaic picture (Maroteaux and Gilles, 1965). Hypercallosity at the site of healing fractures may be erroneously interpreted as osteogenic sarcoma.

On radiologic examination, the changes in the teeth are quite striking. The roots are thin and disproportionately shortened. The pulp chamber and canal are greatly diminished in size or totally obliterated by formation of irregular dentin.

PATHOLOGY

Histologic section shows that instead of compact cortical bone there is a thin, loose, and poorly formed and arranged spongy layer. The bony spicules are small, irregular, and nonanastomosing. They are poorly endowed with osteoblasts and osteoid matrix. The mucoid component of the connective tissue seems to be increased.

The basic defect probably is a generalized mesenchymal change in maturation of collagen beyond the reticulum fiber stage. Bone formation rates have been found to be at least three times the normal rate.

HEREDITY

The syndrome is transmitted as an autosomal dominant trait with a wide range in expressivity and incomplete penetrance.

DIAGNOSIS

Wormian bones are also seen in cleidocranial dysplasia and in pyknodysostosis. Brittle bones unassociated with other stigmata may be inherited as a dominant trait (McKusick, 1972). In osteopetrosis, the bones are brittle, but radiographic examination shows that bone density is increased.

Blue sclerae may be seen in normal infants, may be inherited as an isolated autosomal dominant trait, may be observed in other connective tissue disorders such as Ehlers-Danlos syndromes and Marfan syndrome, or may be seen with hydrocephalus and mental retardation as an autosomal recessive trait (Gorlin et al., 1976).

Similar dental changes may be seen in hereditary opalescent dentin, a dominantly inherited disorder. This condition involves all teeth of both dentitions in contrast to osteogenesis imperfecta, which shows marked variation.

TREATMENT

Stapedectomy is the treatment of choice. Special care should be taken in curetting the soft, brittle bone in the external canal. If the tympanic ring is fractured, the chorda tympani and/or seventh nerve may be injured (Kosoy and Maddox, 1971).

SUMMARY

Characteristics of the syndrome include: 1) autosomal dominant transmission, 2) osteogenesis imperfecta with frequent fractures, 3) blue sclerae, and 4) mild to moderate conductive hearing loss.

REFERENCES

Bretlau, P., and Jørgensen, M. B., Otosclerosis and osteogenesis imperfecta. *Acta Otolaryngol. (Stockh.), 67*:269–276, 1969.

Bretlau, P., Jørgensen, M. B., and Johansen, H., Osteogenesis imperfecta. Light and electron-microscopic studies of the stapes. *Acta Otolaryngol. (Stockh.), 69*:172–184, 1970.

Caniggia, A., Stuart, C., and Guideri, R., Fragilitas ossium hereditaria tarda (Ekman-Lobstein disease). *Acta Med. Scand., Suppl.340*:1–172, 1958.

Dessoff, J., Blue sclerotics, fragile bones, and deafness. *Arch. Ophthalmol., 12*:60–71, 1934.

Ekman, O. J., *Dissertatio Medica Descriptionem et Casus Aliquot Osteomaliaciae Sistens,* 1788.

Gorlin, R. J., Pindborg, J. J., and Cohen, M. M., Jr., *Syndromes of the Head and Neck.* 2nd Ed. New York, McGraw-Hill Book Company, 1976.

Hall, J. G., and Røhrt, T., The stapes in osteogenesis imperfecta. *Acta Otolaryngol. (Stockh.), 65*:345–348, 1968.

Ibsen, K. H., Distinct varieties of osteogenesis imperfecta. *Clin. Orthop., 50*:279–290, 1967.

Kosoy, J., and Maddox, H. E., Surgical findings in van der Hoeve's syndrome. *Arch. Otolaryngol., 93*:115–122, 1971.

Lobstein, J. B., *Traite de l'Anatomie Pathologique.* Vol. 2. Paris, F. G. Lerrault, 1883, p. 204.

Maroteaux, P., and Gilles, M., Etude radiologique de l'osteogenesis imperfecta. *Ann. Radiol., 8*:571–583, 1965.

McKusick, V. A., *Heritable Disorders of Connective Tissue,* 1972, 4th Ed., St. Louis, C. V. Mosby Company, 1972, pp. 390–454.

Müller, E., Die Schwerhörigkeit bei Osteogenesis imperfecta. *Laryngol. Rhinol. Otol., 53*:805–808, 1974.

Opheim, O., Loss of hearing following the syndrome of van der Hoeve-de Kleijn. *Acta Otolaryngol. (Stockh.), 65*:337–344, 1968.

Remigio, P. A., and Grinvalsky, H. T., Osteogenesis imperfecta congenita. *Am. J. Dis. Child., 119*:524–528, 1970.

Robertson, M. S., and Gregory, J., Deafness, blue sclerotics, and fragilitas ossium. *J. Laryngol., 76*:655–660, 1962.

Schröder, G., Osteogenesis imperfecta. *Z. Menschl. Vererb. Konstit-Lehre, 37*:632–676, 1964.

Seedorff, K. S., *Osteogenesis Imperfecta: A Study of Clinical Features and Heredity Based on 55 Danish Families Comprising 180 Affected Persons,* Thesis. Copenhagen, Munksgaard Press, 1949, pp. 1–229.

Van der Hoeve, J., and de Kleijn, A., Blaue Sclerae, Knochenbrüchigkeit und Schwerhörigkeit. *Arch. Ophthalmol., 95*:81–93, 1918.

Vrolik, W., *Tabulae ad Illustrandum Embryogenesis Hominis et Mammalium tam Naturalem quam Abnormen,* 1849, Amsterdam.

SPONDYLOEPIPHYSEAL DYSPLASIA CONGENITA AND SENSORINEURAL DEAFNESS

Spondyloepiphyseal dysplasia congenita, first defined by Spranger and Wiedemann (1966), is a skeletal dysplasia recognizable at birth. It is characterized by short trunk and proximal extremities as well as delayed ossification and distinctive skeletal changes. Other frequent findings are severe myopia and retinal detachment, cleft palate, and sensorineural deafness. Earlier probable cases were reported by Uhlig (1954) and Braun and Meythaler (1962). The disorder constituted as much as 10 per cent of cases of dwarfism (excluding rickets, osteogenesis imperfecta, and arthrogryposis) admitted to one pediatric orthopedic hospital (Bailey, 1973).

CLINICAL FINDINGS

Birth length has ranged from 16 to 19 inches (40–48 cm.). Commonly, one notes frontal bossing, mild ocular hypertelorism, mild mongoloid obliquity of the palpebral fissures, saddle nose, and short neck (Fig. 5–27A). Adult height ranges from 37 to 52 in. (85 to 125 cm.) (Spranger and Langer, 1970). Neonatal death may result from respiratory failure (Holthusen, 1972).

Musculoskeletal System. The mildly shortened extremities are evident at birth. There is diminished muscle tone and delayed motor development, which together with severe coxa vara lead to a waddling gait. Walking may not occur until 30 months of age or later. In infancy difficulty is experienced in swallowing fluids (Michaelis *et al.,* 1973). Marked lumbar lordosis develops early. The chest is barrel-shaped with pectus carinatum. Genua vara, genua valga, and flexion contractures of the elbow, hips, and knees are common (Bailey, 1973; Michaelis *et al.,* 1973). Talipes equinovarus, metatarsus adductus, and dislocation of the hips and knees as well as genu recurvatum and laterally dislocated patellae are occasionally noted. Some patients exhibit hyperextensibility of finger joints. Kyphoscoliosis may develop during childhood or adolescence. Hernia has also been described (Bach *et al.*, 1967).

Ocular System. During adolescence visual problems become manifest in about 60 per cent of the cases. These problems include myopia of 10 to 20 diopters, strabismus, primary and/or secondary cataracts, buphthalmos, and secondary glaucoma (Kozlowski *et al.*, 1968; Fraser *et al.*, 1969; Rupprecht, 1969; Spranger and Langer, 1970).

Oral Findings. Cleft palate has been noted in about 40 per cent of the cases (Spranger and Wiedemann, 1966; Fraser *et al.*, 1969; Bach *et al.*, 1969; Spranger and Langer, 1970; Holthusen, 1972; Michaelis *et al.*, 1973).

Nervous System. Mental retardation has been described in about 10 per cent (Fraser *et al.*, 1969; Bach *et al.*, 1969; Michaelis *et al.*, 1973).

Auditory System. Moderately severe (30 to 60 dB) sensorineural deafness, especially marked in the high tones, was described by a number of authors (Fraser *et al.*, 1969; Michaelis *et al.*, 1973). Deafness is not a constant feature. Our impression is that it occurs in about 30 per cent.

Vestibular System. No studies have been reported.

LABORATORY FINDINGS

The radiographic findings are distinctive at birth. The principal alterations occur in the pelvis and vertebrae. There is markedly delayed ossification of the pubic bones, the epiphyses of the knee, the talus, and the calcaneus. The iliac wings are short with flattened lateral margins and rather horizontal acetabular roofs. The sacrosciatic notch is not narrowed. The odontoid process is hypoplastic. The bodies of the thoracic vertebrae are flattened posteriorly, giving

them a pear-shape (Spranger and Langer, 1970).

In the older infant, there is delayed ossification of the femoral heads and severe coxa vara. The humerus is mildly shortened (Fig. 5–27*B–D*).

HEREDITY

Inheritance is clearly autosomal dominant; new mutations account for most cases. A paternal age effect has been demonstrated (Spranger and Wiedemann, 1966; Fraser *et al.*, 1969; Michaelis *et al.*, 1973).

DIAGNOSIS

One must exclude Morquio syndrome, which is characterized by growth retardation and skeletal deformity which become evident during the second year of life, corneal clouding, keratosulfaturia, and autosomal recessive inheritance.

TREATMENT

Therapy consists of early correction of the talipes equinovarus and surgical closure of the cleft palate. Referral to an ophthalmologist for evaluation and/or correction of the myopia and retinal detachment is extremely important.

PROGNOSIS

While life expectancy is not shortened, gait becomes progressively more difficult and scoliosis becomes more severe with age. Many affected persons have severe myopia and/or retinal detachment.

SUMMARY

Characteristics of this disorder include: 1) autosomal dominant inheritance, 2) short trunk and proximal extremities, 3) distinctive skeletal changes, 4) severe myopia and, at times, retinal detachment, 5) cleft palate in about 40 per cent, and 6) sensorineural deafness in about 30 per cent.

REFERENCES

Bach, C., Maroteaux, P., Schaeffer, P., Bitan, A., and Crumiere, C., Dysplasie spondyloepiphysaire congénitale avec anomalies multiples. *Arch. Franç. Pédiatr.,* 24:24–33, 1967.
Bailey, J. A., *Disproportionate Short Stature.* Philadelphia, W. B. Saunders Company, 1973, pp. 439–456.
Braun, O. H., and Meythaler, H., Dysostosis enchondralis (typus Bartenwerfer). *Arch. Kinderheilkd.,* 168:89–96, 1962.

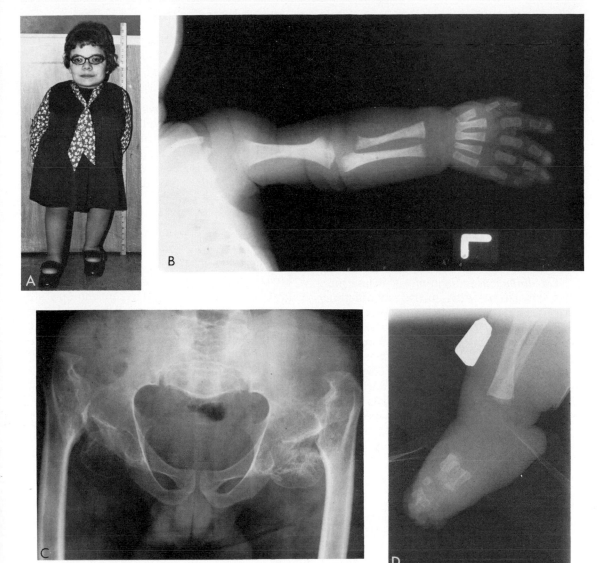

Figure 5-27 Spondyloepiphyseal dysplasia congenita and sensorineural deafness. (A) Adult with short stature, severe myopia, retinal detachment, scoliosis, and sensorineural hearing loss. Patient had severe coxa vara, which produced a waddling gait. *(B)* Radiograph of newborn, showing abbreviation of humerus. *(C)* Note femoral heads in acetabular area, unassociated with displaced femoral necks. *(D)* Absent talus and calcaneus in newborn.

Fraser, G. R., Friedmann, A. I., Maroteaux, P., Glen-Bott, A. M., and Mittwoch, U., Dysplasia spondyloepiphysaria congenita and related generalized skeletal dysplasias among children with severe visual handicaps. *Arch. Dis. Child., 44*:490–498, 1969.

Holthusen, W., The Pierre Robin syndrome: unusual associated developmental defects. *Ann. Radiol. (Paris), 15*:253–262, 1972 (Cases 3, 4).

Kozlowski, K., Bittel-Dobrzynska, N., and Budzynska, A., Spondylo-epiphyseal dysplasia congenita. *Ann. Radiol. (Paris), 11*:367–375, 1968.

Michaelis, E., Kemperdick, H., and Spranger, J., Dysplasia spondyloepiphysaria congenita. *Fortschr. Roentgenstr., 119*:429–438, 1973.

Roaf, R., Longmore, J. B., and Forrester, R., A childhood syndrome of bone dysplasia, retinal detachment, and deafness. *Dev. Med. Child. Neurol., 9*:464–473, 1967 (Case 1 same as Fraser *et al.*; Case 2).

Rupprecht, E., Dysplasia spondyloepiphysaria congenita. *Kinderärztl. Prax., 37*:161–166, 1969.

Spranger, J. W., and Langer, L. O., Spondyloepiphyseal dysplasia congenita. *Radiology, 94*:313–322, 1970.

Spranger, J. W., and Wiedemann, H. R., Dysplasia spondyloepiphysaria congenita. *Helv. Paediatr. Acta, 21*:598–611, 1966.

Uhlig, H., Dysostosis enchondralis—Typ Bartenwerfer. *Arch. Kinderheilkd., 148*:22–31, 1954.

JOINT FUSIONS, MITRAL INSUFFICIENCY, AND CONDUCTION HEARING LOSS

A mother and two daughters having conductive hearing loss, fusion in the carpus, tarsus, and cervical vertebrae, and mitral insufficiency were described by Forney, Robinson, and Pascoe (1966).

CLINICAL FINDINGS

Physical Findings. All affected were short in stature, both children being below the third percentile in height.

Integumentary System. Large numbers of freckles were noted on the face, particularly on the cheeks, and shoulders.

Cardiovascular System. Cardiac murmurs consistent with mitral insufficiency were heard in all affected individuals.

Auditory System. A moderate hearing loss was present in childhood and may have been congenital. Puretone audiograms on each patient showed a 30 to 70 dB conductive hearing loss. Surgical exploration of one ear in each of the two children showed fixation of the footplate of the stapes.

Vestibular System. No vestibular findings were described.

LABORATORY FINDINGS

Roentgenograms. From two to five vertebrae were fused in each patient. In one, the capitate and hamate as well as the lunate and navicular were fused bilaterally. In another patient, the lunate and triquetrum were fused. The phalanges were shortened. The navicular, first cuneiform, and cuboidal bones were fused in both feet in one patient. In another patient, the tarsal bones were normal.

Other Findings. Routine blood and urine studies showed no abnormalities.

An electrocardiogram showed incomplete bundle branch block in each patient. Cardiac catheterization in two cases revealed moderate mitral insufficiency.

PATHOLOGY

No histopathologic findings were described.

HEREDITY

The pedigree shows a mother and two of her four daughters affected. The mother's father was short in stature; her grandfather had had a chronic nonprogressive hearing loss and had also been short. Thus, autosomal dominant transmission of this syndrome appears likely.

DIAGNOSIS

Patients with the *"leopard"* syndrome have multiple lentigines, heart block, hypertrophic cardiomyopathy, pulmonary stenosis, short stature, and sensorineural hearing loss and thus should be readily distinguished from persons having the syndrome discussed here.

TREATMENT

The mitral insufficiency is of only moderate degree and does not warrant surgical correction. The hearing loss may be minimized by use of a hearing aid and by insertion of a prosthesis.

PROGNOSIS

The hearing loss, joint fusions, and mitral insufficiency are apparently nonprogressive. Although mitral insufficiency may result in cardiac failure later in life, there was no indication that this was true in the cases reported.

SUMMARY

The syndrome is characterized by: 1) autosomal dominant transmission with variable expressivity, 2) skeletal abnormalities, including fusion of the cervical vertebrae and carpal and tarsal bones, 3) mild to moderate mitral insufficiency, and 4) moderate, probably congenital, conductive hearing loss.

REFERENCE

Forney, W. R., Robinson, S. J., and Pascoe, D. J., Congenital heart disease, deafness, and skeletal malformations: a new syndrome? *J. Pediatr., 68*:14–26, 1966.

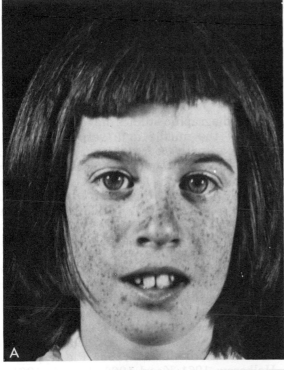
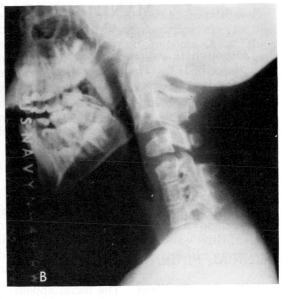
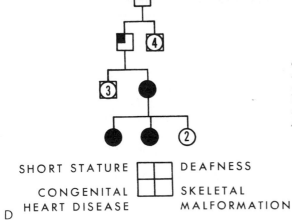
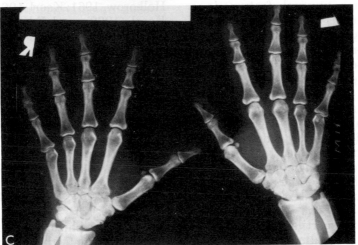

Figure 5-28 Mitral insufficiency, joint fusion, and conductive hearing loss. (A) Numerous freckles on face and shoulders were present in all affected members. (B) Fusion of cervical vertebrae. (C) Fusion of carpal bones. Tarsal bones similarly affected. (D) Pedigree of affected kindred. (A–D from W. R. Forney et al., J. Pediatr. 68:14, 1966.)

SHORT STATURE ☐ DEAFNESS
CONGENITAL ☐ SKELETAL
HEART DISEASE MALFORMATION

Partsch, C. J., and Hülse, M., Verschiedene Schwerhörigkeitsformen innerhalb einer Franceschetti-Familie. *Laryngol. Rhinol., 54*:385–388, 1975.

Pavsek, E. J., Mandibulo-facial dysostosis (Treacher Collins syndrome). *Radiology, 79*:598–602, 1958.

Plester, D., Missbildung des Stapes bei der Dysostosis mandibulo-facialis. *Acta Otolaryngol. (Stockh.), 53*:55–60, 1961.

Rogers, B. O., Berry–Treacher Collins syndrome. A review of 200 cases. *Br. J. Plast. Surg., 17*:109–137, 1964.

Sando, I., Hemenway, W. G., and Morgan, W. R., Histopathology of the temporal bones in mandibulofacial dysostosis. *Trans. Am. Acad. Ophthalmol. Otol., 72*:913–924, 1968.

Snyder, C. C., Bilateral facial agenesia. *Am. J. Surg., 92*:81–87, 1956.

Stovin, J. J., Lyon, J. A., and Clemens, R. L., Mandibulofacial dysostosis. *Radiology, 74*:225–231, 1960.

Terrahe, K., Das Gehörorgan bei der Dysostosis mandibulofacialis. *Z. Laryngol. Rhin. Otol., 47*:591–600, 1968.

Thomson, A., Notice of several cases of malformation of the external ear, together with experiments on the state of hearing in such persons. *Month. J. Med. Sci., 7*:420, 1846–7.

Treacher Collins E., Cases with symmetrical congenital notches in the outer part of each lid and defective development of the malar bones. *Trans. Ophthalmol. Soc. U.K., 20*:190–192, 1900.

Figure 5–29. *Mandibulofacial dysostosis.* (*A, B*) Patient exhibiting typical facies showing antimongoloid obliquity of palpebral fissures, hypoplasia of zygomatic bones, straight nasofrontal angle, and micrognathia. The pinnae in the patient are essentially normal. (*C*) Deformed pinna lacking external auditory canal. (*D*) Schematic diagram of dwarfing of stapes deformity. The stapes, columnar in form, has its footplate ankylosed in the oval window. (*A, B, D* from G. Keerl, *Ophthalmologica, 143*:5, 1962.) (*E*) Stapes showing crurae fused into monopodal structure onto neck of which stapedius tendon was inserted. (From W. G. Edwards, *J. Laryngol. Otol., 78*:152, 1964.) (*F*) The tensor tympani muscle (tt) of the right ear is attached to a bony ossicular mass (bm) in the mesotympanum. These structures are covered laterally only by soft tissue and not by bone. The facial nerve (fn) exits almost directly laterally from its position in the internal auditory meatus. It curves in the middle ear around the bony ossicular mass (bm) before leaving the temporal bone. The bone between the cochlea (c) and tensor tympani (tt) is markedly thickened. (From I. Sando *et al.*, *Trans. Am. Acad. Ophthalmol. Otolaryngol., 72*:913, 1968.)

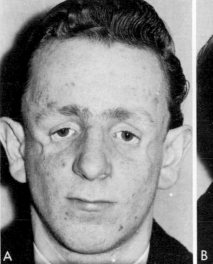

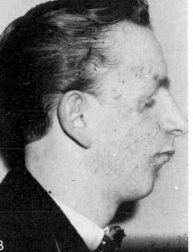

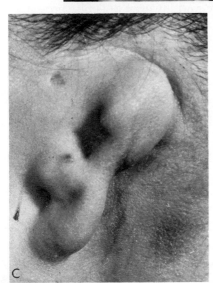

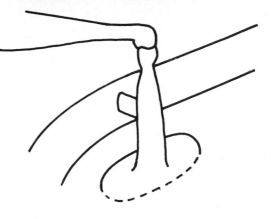

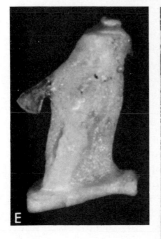

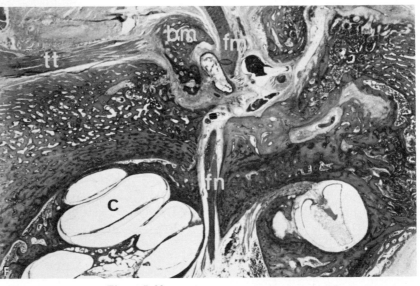

Figure 5–29

See legend on the opposite page

CALCIFICATION OF CARTILAGES, BRACHYTELEPHALANGY, MULTIPLE PERIPHERAL PULMONARY STENOSES, AND MIXED DEAFNESS

Keutel, Jörgenson, and Gabriel (1971, 1972) reported a syndrome of multiple peripheral pulmonary stenoses, brachytelephalangy, calcification and/or ossification of cartilages, and mixed deafness in two sibs.

CLINICAL FINDINGS

Physical Findings. Both sibs had a history of recurrent bronchitis and otitis media.

Musculoskeletal System. The female sib had short, plump thumbs and halluces. The terminal phalanges of the first and third digits were bilaterally abbreviated. Her brother exhibited shortening of the first through fourth terminal phalanges on the right hand and first, third, and fourth on the left hand.

Cardiovascular System. A grade 2/4 systolic murmur, first noted at 8 or 9 years of age, was also heard over the carotid area. Electrocardiographic tracing showed an incomplete right bundle branch block in one child. P_2 was greater than A_2 (see Laboratory Findings).

Auditory System. The pinnae were somewhat too large and prominent. They were pale, stiff, and hard in consistency. The ear drums were perforated bilaterally.

Deafness was noted prior to admission to school. Mixed hearing loss of 40 to 75 dB, being greater at higher frequencies, was found in both children. The conductive component was thought to be related to recurrent middle-ear infections experienced by both sibs.

Vestibular System. Normal caloric response was noted.

LABORATORY FINDINGS

Roentgenograms. Radiographic studies performed at 8 to 9 years of age showed calcification of the cartilaginous portions of the ribs and of the tracheal, bronchial, and nasal cartilages. The mastoid processes were abnormally dense.

In the girl there was shortening of the terminal phalanges of the first and third digits and premature fusion of the epiphyses of these phalanges. In the brother there were corresponding alterations in the terminal phalanges of the first through fourth digits on the right hand and first, third, and fourth digits on the left. In the halluces of both children the terminal phalanges were short and showed premature epiphyseal fusion.

Other Findings. Angiocardiography revealed systolic pressure elevation in the right ventricle and in the main pulmonary artery and lowered diastolic pressure in the pulmonary vein together with a systolic pressure gradient — a picture compatible with multiple peripheral pulmonary stenoses.

HEREDITY

The parents were first cousins once removed. They and their three other children were normal. Inheritance appears to be autosomal recessive.

DIAGNOSIS

Multiple pulmonary stenosis and sensorineural deafness are seen in rubella embryopathy (Arvidsson *et al.*, 1961). Familial multiple pulmonary stenoses have been reported by Gyllenswärd *et al.* (1957) in mother and son, and by van Epps (1957), Arvidsson *et al.* (1961), and McCue *et al.* (1965) in sibs, suggesting two modes of inheritance. One patient (case 10) had associated deafness (Arvidsson *et al.*, 1961). Gyllenswärd *et al.* (1957) noted "malformation of the external ears" in two of their patients with multiple peripheral pulmonary stenoses, but they did not further define the abnormality. Multiple peripheral pulmonary stenoses can be seen in combination with supravalvular aortic stenosis.

Calcification and/or ossification of the auricular cartilage can occur following frostbite, physical trauma, perichondritis, and in the autosomal recessively inherited

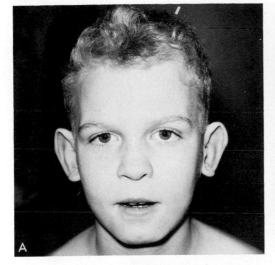
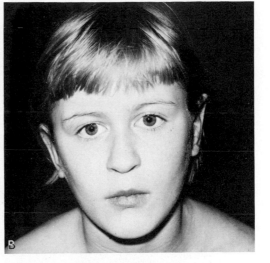

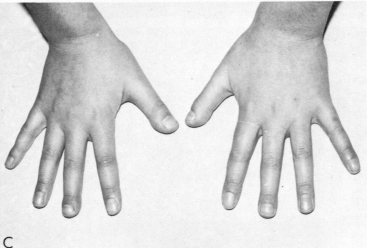

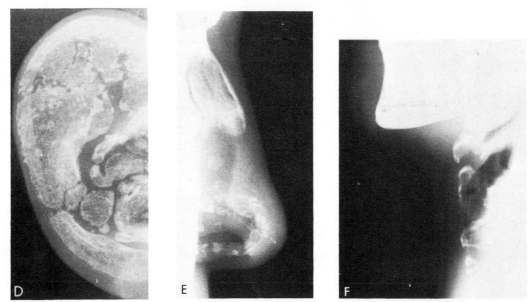

Figure 5-30 *Calcification of cartilages, brachytelephalangy, multiple peripheral pulmonary stenoses, and sensorineural deafness. (A, B) Sibs with syndrome. Facies is essentially normal except for calcified pinnae. (C) Note abbreviated terminal phalanges of middle fingers. (D, E, and F) Calcification of cartilages of ear, nose, and trachea.*

Illustration continued on the following page

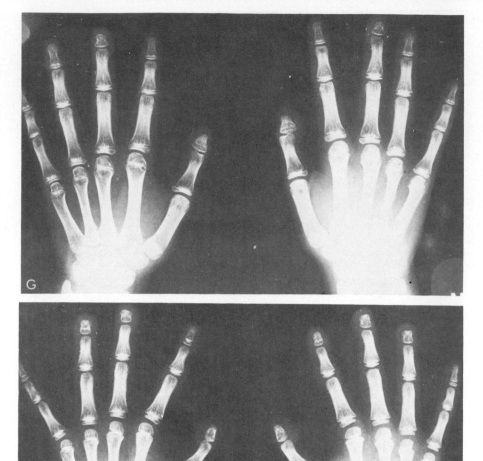

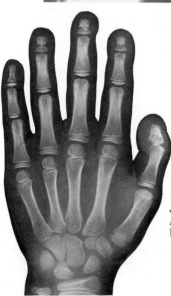

Figure 5-30   Continued (G, H, and I) Radiographs showing abbreviation of terminal phalanges of several fingers. (*A, B, G,* and *H* courtesy of G. Jörgensen, Göttingen, West Germany; *D, E,* and *F* from G. Jörgensen, *Arch. Klin. Exp. Ohren. Nasen. Kehlkopfheilkd, 202*:1, 1972; *I* courtesy of R. Walbaum, Roubaix, France.)

disorder, diastrophic dwarfism. Auricular ossification has also been reported as a dominant trait (Kirsch, 1953).

Walbaum (1974) reported a Moroccan boy with brachytelephalangism, extensive calcifications of the trachea, bronchi, and ribs. The boy had bronchial dilatation and saddle nose but no cardiovascular lesions or auricular calcification.

Say *et al.* (1973) reported a girl with severe growth retardation, frontal bossing, hypoplastic midface with saddle nose, calcification of pinnae and tracheal and costal cartilages, premature fusion of the epiphyses of the terminal phalanges of the fingers and a 55 to 60 dB conductive hearing loss.

We have recently examined a 22-year-old male who has extensive ossification of his pinnae, marked mental retardation, and sensorineural deafness.

TREATMENT

No treatment is required for the pulmonary stenoses. The deafness may be ameliorated with a hearing aid.

PROGNOSIS

Prognosis for an essentially normal life is good.

SUMMARY

Characteristics of this syndrome include: 1) autosomal recessive inheritance, 2) brachytelephalangy, 3) calcification and/or ossification of cartilages of nose, auricles, trachea, bronchi, and ribs, 4) multiple peripheral pulmonary stenoses, 5) recurrent otitis media and bronchitis, and 6) mixed deafness.

REFERENCES

Arvidsson, H., Carlsson, E., Hartmann, A., Tsifutis, A., and Crawford, C., Supravalvular stenoses of the pulmonary arteries: report of eleven cases. *Acta Radiol. (Stockh.), 56*:466–480, 1961.

Gyllenswärd, A., Lodin, H., Lundberg, A., and Möller, T., Congenital multiple peripheral stenoses of the pulmonary artery. *Pediatrics, 19*:399–410, 1957.

Higbee, D. R., Calcigerous metaplasia of the auricular cartilage. *Arch. Otolaryngol., 14*:70–79, 1931.

Keutel, J., Jörgensen, G., and Gabriel, P., Ein neues autosomal-rezessiv vererbbares Syndrom. *Dtsch. Med. Wschr., 96*:1676–1681, 1971.

Keutel, J., Jörgensen, G., and Gabriel, P., A new autosomal recessive syndrome: peripheral pulmonary stenoses, brachytelephalangism, neural hearing loss, and abnormal cartilage calcifications/ossifications. *Birth Defects, 8*(5):60–68, 1972.

Kirsch, R., Vererbbare Verknocherung der Ohrmuschel. *Z. Laryng. Rhinol., 32*:729–734, 1953.

Martin, E., Knochenbildung in der Ohrmuschel und ihre Entstehungsursachen. *Arch. Klin. Exp. Ohren-, Nasen-, Kehlkopfhcilkd., 160*:23–31, 1951.

McCue, C. M., Robertson, L. W., Lester, R. G., and Mauck, H. P., Pulmonary artery coarctations. A report of 20 cases with review of 319 cases from the literature. *J. Pediatr., 67*:222–238, 1965.

Say, B., Balci, S., Pirnar, T., Israel, R., and Atasu, M., Unusual calcium deposition in cartilage associated with short stature and peculiar facial features. *Pediatr. Radiol., 1*:127–129, 1973.

van Epps, E. G., Primary pulmonary hypertension in brothers. *Am. J. Roentgenol., 78*:471–482, 1957.

Walbaum, R. E., Personal communication, Roubaix, France, 1974.

CARPAL AND TARSAL ABNORMALITIES, CLEFT PALATE, OLIGODONTIA AND STAPES FIXATION

Gorlin, Schlorf, and Paparella (1971) described a syndrome of cleft palate, oligodontia, carpal and, especially, tarsal anomalies, and stapes fixation in two sisters.

CLINICAL FINDINGS

Physical Findings. The findings in the 19- and 21-year-old sisters were virtually identical. Each had cleft soft palate which had been repaired at about 10 years of age. Each exhibited mild primary telecanthus. Neither girl had ever had more than 3 to 4 primary teeth and neither had permanent teeth. The halluces were short and dorsiflexed with a wide separation between the hallux and the rest of the toes (Fig. 5–31A).

Auditory System. Reduced hearing was noted prior to puberty. Audiometric testing demonstrated bilateral conductive deafness in both girls, being more marked in the right ear of one girl. Exploratory surgery revealed that each had bilateral congenital fixation of the footplate of the stapes.

Vestibular System. Vestibular studies were not carried out.

LABORATORY FINDINGS

Radiographic examinations of the hands, feet, and skull showed the following: the third toe was the longest on both feet; there was shortening of the first metatarsal, which was fused with the navicular; the second and third cuneiforms, the talus and navicular, and the talus and calcaneus were fused; the talus was malformed and showed a hump on the superior and medial surfaces; there was underdevelopment of the joint surface of the tibia with only the posterior two thirds being in articulation.

In the hands there was underde-velopment of the navicular bones bilaterally with small sesamoid bones associated with the distal facet of the navicular. The skull was normocephalic. No alveolar ridges were evident. The rest of the radiologic examination was negative.

HEREDITY

The syndrome occurred in sisters whose parents were second cousins. Two younger brothers were normal. Inheritance appears to be autosomal recessive.

DIAGNOSIS

The combination of abnormalities in this syndrome is unique.

TREATMENT

The hearing loss in each patient was satisfactorily corrected by stapedectomy.

PROGNOSIS

Prognosis is excellent. The stapes fixation can be corrected and dentures can be constructed. Neither girl experienced difficulty with the carpal or tarsal abnormalities.

SUMMARY

Characteristics of the syndrome include: 1) autosomal recessive inheritance, 2) dorsiflexion of halluces, talonavicular and talocalcaneal fusion, second and third cuneiform bone fusion, malformed talus, abnormal talotibial articulation, hypoplasia of the carpal navicular bones, 3) oligodontia, 4) cleft palate, and 5) conduction deafness due to stapes fixation.

REFERENCE

Gorlin, R. J., Schlorf, R. A., and Paparella, M. M., Cleft palate, stapes fixation, and oligodontia: a new autosomal recessively inherited syndrome. *Birth Defects,* 7(7):87–88, 1971.

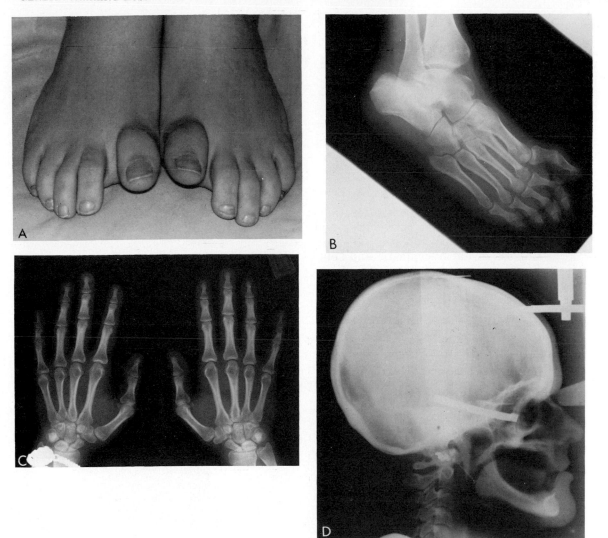

Figure 5–31 *Carpal and tarsal abnormalities, cleft palate, oligodontia, and stapes fixation. (A)* Shortening of dorsiflexed halluces with wide space between halluces and rest of toes. *(B)* Radiograph showing shortening of first metatarsal, talonavicular and talocalcancal fusions. Malformed talus with hump on superior surface. *(C)* Radiograph showing bilateral underdevelopment of navicular bones with small sesamoid bones at distal facet. *(D)* Cephalogram showing absence of alveolar processes. This demonstrates original lack of teeth since the alveolar process develops after the teeth are present.

Figure 5–32 *Hypoplasia of upper extremities, cardiac arrhythmia, malformed pinnae, and unilateral conduction deafness. (A, B)* Father and son with hypoplasia of the upper extremities. The humerus is hypoplastic on the left side, and the radius is missing bilaterally. The carpus consists of three bones; there are three metacarpals and a reduced number of digits. Bony alterations are limited to the upper extremities. Note also the malformed pinnae. *(C)* Radiograph showing bent and hypoplastic humerus. *(D)* Radiograph of hand showing the missing radius, the carpus consisting of three bones, and the three metacarpals. *(E)* Electrocardiogram showing cardiac arrhythmia. (From C. Stoll *et al., Arch. Fr. Pédiatr.,* 31:669, 1974.)

Illustration on the following page

HYPOPLASIA OF UPPER EXTREMITIES, CARDIAC ARRHYTHMIA, MALFORMED PINNAE, AND UNILATERAL CONDUCTION DEAFNESS

Stoll *et al.* (1974) reported an apparently unique syndrome of hypoplasia of the upper extremities, sinus arrhythmia, malformed pinnae, and conduction deafness in a father and son.

CLINICAL FINDINGS

Skeletal System. The bony alterations were limited to the upper extremities and were similar in father and son. The humerus was somewhat hypoplastic and bent. The radius was missing and the carpus consisted of three bones. There were three metacarpals. Each had two fingers on one side and three on the other.

Cardiac System. Both the father and son exhibited irregularity in cardiac rhythm, which was more pronounced in the son.

Auditory System. The pinnae were malformed. The external auditory meatus was reduced in size, and there was profound unilateral conduction deafness. In the son the stapes and oval window were absent.

Vestibular System. Vestibular studies apparently were not carried out.

HEREDITY

The occurrence of the syndrome in a father and his son suggests autosomal dominant inheritance.

REFERENCE

Stoll, C., Levy, J. M., Francfort, J. J., Roos, R., and Rohmer, A., L'association phocomelie-ectrodactylie, malformations des oreilles avec surdité, arythmie sinusale. *Arch. Franç. Pédiatr.,* *31:*669–680, 1974.

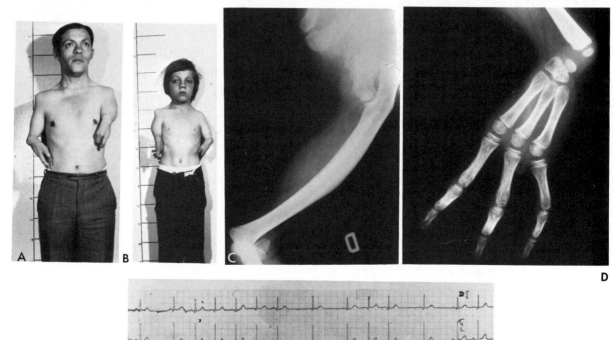

MISCELLANEOUS SKELETAL DISORDERS IN WHICH DEAFNESS IS INCONSISTENTLY ASSOCIATED

There are several skeletal disorders in which deafness is an inconsistent feature. Perhaps in some cases the association is aleatory. Nevertheless, there should be some documentation of the co-occurrence.

PROGRESSIVE DIAPHYSEAL DYSPLASIA (CAMURATI-ENGELMANN DISEASE)

From early infancy, leg pain is associated with a waddling gait, poor muscle mass (especially of the lower extremities), and easy fatigability. Puberty may be delayed. Radiologically, this autosomal dominantly inherited disorder is characterized by bilateral fusiform enlargement of the diaphyses of long bones, especially those of the tibia, femur, fibula, humerus, radius, and ulna (in that order) with normal epiphyses and metaphyses. Not uncommonly, the skull base is sclerotic with the increased density extending into the parietal bones (Sparkes and Graham, 1972).

We have reviewed over 50 case reports. Deafness has been rarely mentioned and when noted, poorly documented. Paul (1953) reported a "gradual impairment of hearing." Lennon et al. (1961) described mixed deafness with decreased vestibular function. Trunk et al. (1969) noted progressive sensorineural hearing loss in their 28-year-old patient. Nelson and Scott (1969) found conductive hearing loss, and Sparkes and Graham (1972) noted severe deafness (not otherwise characterized) and slitlike internal auditory canals.

MARFAN SYNDROME

Several hundred cases have been reported of this dominantly inherited disorder of connective tissue. Characteristic are arachnodactyly, scoliosis, joint hypermobility, dislocated lenses, and cardiac anomalies.

Rarely has deafness been associated. We suspect that the patients described by Brock (1929) and Bucklers (1935) had homocystinuria. Ganther (1972) found deafness but attributed it to numerous middle-ear infections in his patient. The deaf patients reported by Lloyd (1937) were poorly documented examples of the Marfan syndrome. Kelemen (1965) studied the temporal bone of an 11-month-old infant diagnosed as having this syndrome. A bony lip protruded from the external aperture of an abnormally narrowed vestibular aqueduct. In the cochlea, the round window bulged toward the scala. The utriculoampullary space and endolymphatic duct were dilated. Perhaps a number of these patients had the syndrome of *keratoconus, myopia, marfanoid habitus, and sensorineural deafness*.

FIBRODYSPLASIA OSSIFICANS PROGRESSIVA (MYOSITIS OSSIFICANS PROGRESSIVA)

Lutwak (1964), Ludman et al. (1968), and Letts (1968, 1969) described deafness in patients with fibrodysplasia ossificans progressiva, a disorder of connective tissue, transmitted by an autosomal dominant gene with reduced penetrance (McKusick, 1972). Usually, there is microdactyly of the great toes and thumbs and progressive ankylosis of the cervical spine followed by ossification of the paraspinal and limb girdle muscles. Deafness is sensorineural in some cases and conductive in others (Ludman et al., 1968; Letts, 1968, 1969). The cause of the deafness is unknown. Hearing loss, apparently, is not a common feature of the disorder.

CLEIDOCRANIAL DYSPLASIA (CLEIDOCRANIAL DYSOSTOSIS)

The syndrome of absence or hypoplasia of the clavicles and various other skeletal anomalies (wormian bones, delayed cranial suture and fontanelle and pubic symphysis closure, unerupted and supernumerary teeth, etc.) is inherited in an autosomal dominant manner. Rarely, there has been associated progressive conductive or mixed deafness and concentric narrowing of the external auditory canals (Nager and DeReynier, 1948; Davis, 1954; Gay, 1958; Jaffee, 1968; Føns, 1969). The mastoid cells are absent. Vestibular study by Gay (1958) showed somewhat reduced response to caloric stimulation, but those studies of Føns (1969) were normal. Tomography has demonstrated deformed ossicles (Føns, 1969).

DYSCHONDROSTEOSIS (MADELUNG'S DEFORMITY, LERI-WEILL DISEASE)

Dyschondrosteosis is characterized by deformity of the distal radius and ulna and proximal carpal bones and by mesomelic dwarfism (Herdman et al., 1966).

Nassif and Harboyan (1970) described brothers with 40 to 50 dB bilateral conductive hearing loss. The external auditory canals were narrow. The malleus was absent, and the incus was vestigial with no connection with the deformed stapes. In one ear, the chorda tympani could not be identified.

FAMILIAL OSTEOMA OF THE MIDDLE EAR

Osteomas of the middle ear are rare. Thomas (1964) described two examples in a 10-year-old boy and in his 6-year-old sister. Their parents and two older sibs were normal. Exploration of the boy's middle ears showed a smooth, broad-based osteoma arising in the region of the pyramid. The tumor extended forward to become adherent to the incudostapedial joint. The tympanic membranes were normal, and hearing was normal according to audiometric tests. A unilateral, but smaller, osteoma was found in the sister. Her reduced hearing returned to normal postoperatively. Exudative otitis, present in both sibs, was suggested as a possible cause of new bone formation in the middle ear.

Ombredanne (1966) described a similar growth in the middle ears of a 57-year-old male who had a 20-year history of bilateral progressive deafness. No other family members were affected, and there was no history of prior exudative otitis.

OCULODENTO-OSSEOUS DYSPLASIA AND CONDUCTION DEAFNESS

Oculodento-osseous dysplasia is a syndrome consisting of a narrow nose with hypoplastic alae, microcornea with iris anomalies, soft tissue syndactyly of the fourth and fifth fingers, poor modeling of long bones, and enamel hypoplasia.

The disorder has autosomal dominant inheritance (Reisner et al., 1969).

Among 45 cases, there have been three individuals who have manifested conduction deafness of variable degree (Gorlin et al., 1963; Gillespie, 1964; Reisner et al., 1969).

PFEIFFER SYNDROME AND CONDUCTION DEAFNESS

Pfeiffer syndrome consists of craniosynostosis, which results in turribrachycephaly, and broad thumbs and halluces. There may be partial soft tissue syndactyly of the first and second and second and third toes; less often the third and fourth fingers are involved. Intelligence is usually normal. Inheritance is autosomal dominant (Saldino et al., 1972). Hearing loss has been described in a few cases. It has not been severe. In three patients that we have personally examined the deficit was conductive.

SAETHRE-CHOTZEN SYNDROME AND CONDUCTION DEAFNESS

The Saethre-Chotzen syndrome is characterized by craniosynostosis, lowset frontal hair line, facial asymmetry, ptosis of one or both eyelids, deviated nasal septum, and variable cutaneous syndactyly. According to Pantke et al. (1975), about 85 examples have been published. They personally studied 31 cases. A good survey is that of Bartsocas et al. (1970).

Pantke (1975) reported that 15 per cent of the patients have mild conduction deafness—in some cases, unilaterally. He noted further that 11 of 22 published cases in which audiometric examination was carried out exhibited hearing defects. In most of these cases the type and/or degree of hearing loss was not specified. However, Chotzen (1932) and Hammar and Roggenkamp (1967) noted conduction deafness of moderate degree. Grebe (1940) found deafmutism, otherwise undefined.

Dolivo and Gillieron (1955) reported mixed hearing loss. The diagnosis in the case of Jorgenson (1971) is less certain, but the child had conductive hearing loss.

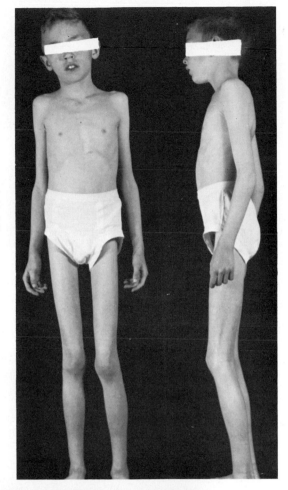

Figure 5-33 *Progressive diaphyseal dysplasia (Camurati-Engelmann syndrome).* Ten-year-old boy exhibiting general asthenic appearance, poor muscle mass, pronation of feet, and characteristic long limbs. (From R. S. Sparks and C. B. Graham, *J. Med. Genet., 9*:73, 1972.)

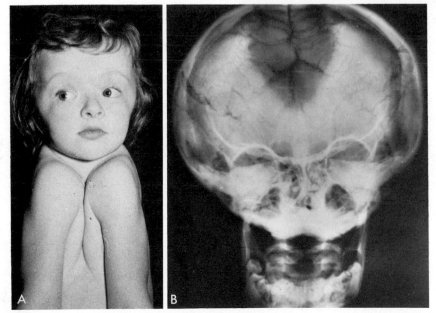

Figure 5-34 *Cleidocranial dysplasia. (A)* Child approximating the shoulders in front. *(B)* Wide open anterior fontanelle and numerous wormian bones. (From M. Forland, *Am. J. Med., 33*:792, 1962.)

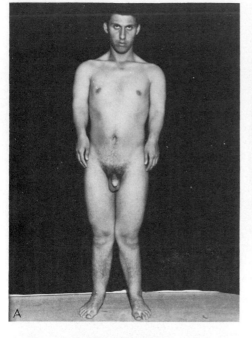

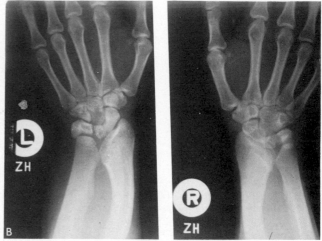

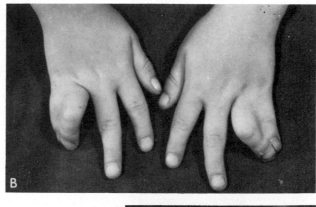

Figure 5-35 *Dyschondrosteosis (Madelung deformity; Leri-Weill disease).* (A) Note shortened forearms and lower extremities. There is posterior subluxation of the ulna and elbows with limited wrist motion. (B) Radiographs show increased distance between radius and ulna, which are curved and short. Note altered alignment of carpal bones. (From R. Nassif and G. Harboyan, *Arch. Otolaryngol., 91*:175, 1970.)

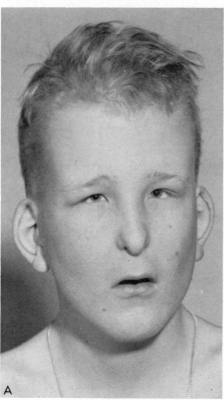

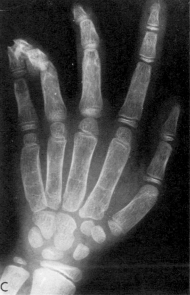

Figure 5-36 *Oculodento-osseous dysplasia and conduction deafness.* (A) Characteristic facies showing microcornea, lack of nasal alar flare. (B) Soft tissue syndactyly and ulnar deviation of the fourth and fifth digits. (C) Poor modeling of metacarpals, fusion of terminal phalanges of fourth and fifth fingers, hypoplastic middle phalanx of fifth finger. (A, C from R. J. Gorlin *et al., J. Paediatr. 63*:69, 1963; B, from S. H. Reisner *et al., Am. J. Dis. Child., 118*:600, 1969.)

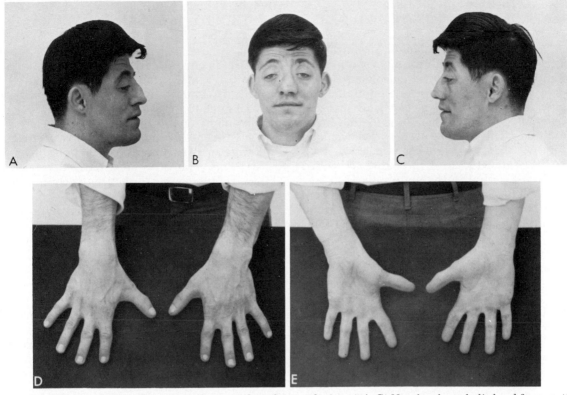

Figure 5-37 *Saethre-Chotzen syndrome and conduction deafness. (A–C)* Note brachycephalic head form, anti-mongoloid obliquity of palpebral fissures, ptosis of eyelids, and unusual nasal bridge. *(D, E)* Webbing between index and middle fingers. *(A–E* from S. Kreiborg *et al., Teratology,* 6:287, 1972.)

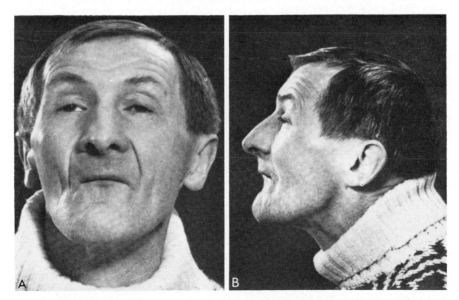

Figure 5-38 *Oculopharyngeal muscular dystrophy and sensorineural deafness. (A, B)* One of three affected sibs. Note ptosis of eyelids, wrinkled forehead, and sagging facial musculature. (From K. Graf, *Pract. Otorhinolaryngol. (Basel), 33:*203, 1971.)

FOCAL DERMAL HYPOPLASIA SYNDROME AND MIXED DEAFNESS

Focal dermal hypoplasia is characterized by atrophy and linear hyperpigmentation of the skin, localized cutaneous deposits of superficial fat, multiple papillomas of mucous membranes or periorificial skin, atrophy of nails, and a host of skeletal abnormalities. These have been reviewed by Goltz *et al.* (1970) and by Ginsburg *et al.* (1970). Inheritance is probably X-linked dominant, lethal in the male.

Perhaps 5 to 10 per cent of patients with this syndrome have hearing defects. No study has been carried out on the temporal bone. Holden and Akers (1967) reported mixed hearing deficit, noted at three years of age, in their patient. Stollman (1967) made brief note of sensorineural deafness in their patients. Goltz *et al.* (1970) also found mixed deafness. Daly (1968), Ginsburg *et al.* (1970), and Ferrara (1972) described a narrowed external auditory meatus.

OCULOPHARYNGEAL MUSCULAR DYSTROPHY AND SENSORINEURAL DEAFNESS

This is one of several disorders exhibiting a myopathic facies. Onset is late — usually in middle life. Facial musculature is weakened to the point of flaccid paralysis. Involvement of the masticatory muscles is reflected in hollowing of the temporal areas and sagging of the mandible. Blepharoptosis is striking. The brow is usually furrowed. There is increasing difficulty encountered in eating and drinking.

The disorder is characterized by autosomal dominant inheritance. A slowly progressive sensorineural deafness has been reported in a kindred (Graf, 1971). Conversely, Roberts and Bamforth (1968) noted no hearing loss among 26 patients with this disorder. Kuhn and Ey (1966) noted that eight of 23 patients with myotonic dystrophy exhibited hearing loss; of these, four were the result of chronic middle ear infections.

REFERENCES

Progressive Diaphyseal Dysplasia (Camurati-Engelmann Disease)

Lennon, E. A., Schechter, M. M., and Hornabrook, R. W., Engelmann's disease. *J. Bone Joint Surg., 43B*:273–284, 1961.

Nelson, M., and Scott, C. I., Engelmann's disease (a form of craniodiaphyseal dysplasia). *Birth Defects, 5*(4):301, 1969.

Paul, L. W., Hereditary multiple diaphyseal sclerosis (Ribbing). *Radiology, 60*:412–416, 1953.

Sparkes, R. S., and Graham, C. B., Camurati-Engelmann disease. Genetics and clinical manifestations with a review of the literature. *J. Med. Genet., 9*:73–85, 1972.

Trunk, G., Newman, A., and Davis, T. E., Progressive and hereditary diaphyseal dysplasia. *Arch. Intern. Med., 123*:417–422, 1969.

Wetzel, H., Progressive diaphyseal hyperostosis. *German Med. Mon., 9*:285–287, 1964.

Marfan Syndrome

Brock, J., Weiterer Beitrag zur Lehre von der Arachnodaktylie. *Z. Kinderheilkd., 47*:702–714, 1929.

Bucklers, M., Ectopia lentis und Marfanscher Symptomkomplex. *Klin. Mbl. Augenheilkd., 94*:109, 1935.

Ganther, R., Ein Beitrag zur Arachnodaktylie. *Z. Kinderheilkd., 43*:724–736, 1927.

Kelemen, G., Marfan's syndrome and hearing organ. *Acta Otolaryngol. (Stockh.), 59*:23–32, 1965.

Lloyd, R. I., A second group of cases of arachnodactyly. *Arch. Ophthalmol., 17*:66–77, 1937.

Fibrodysplasia Ossificans Progressiva (Myositis Ossificans Progressiva)

Letts, R. M., Myositis ossificans progressiva. *Can. Med. Assoc. J., 99*:856–862, 1968.

Letts, R. M., Mineral, metabolic and radioactive calcium studies of the effects of hormones. *Can. Med. Assoc. J., 100*:133, 1969.

Ludman, H., Hamilton, E. B., and Eade, A. W., Deafness in myositis ossificans progressiva. *J. Laryngol., 82*:57–64, 1968.

Lutwak, L., Myositis ossificans progressiva. *Am. J. Med., 37*:269–293, 1964.

McKusick, V. A., *Heritable Disorders of Connective Tissue*, 4th Ed. St. Louis, C. V. Mosby Company, 1972, pp. 689–706.

Cleidocranial Dysplasia (Cleidocranial Dysostosis)
Das, B. C., and Majumdar, N. K., An unusual case of congenital deafness associated with malformation of clavicle. *Calcutta Med. J., 66*:204–206, 1969.
Davis, P. L., Deafness and cleidocranial dysostosis. *Arch. Otolaryngol., 59*:602–603, 1954.
Føns, M., Ear malformations in cleidocranial dysostosis. *Acta Otolaryngol. (Stockh.), 67*:483–489, 1969.
Gay, I., A case of dysostosis cleidocranialis with mixed deafness. *J. Laryngol., 72*:915–919, 1958.
Jaffee, I. S., Congenital shoulder-neck-auditory anomalies. *Laryngoscope, 78*:2119–2139, 1968 (Case 1).
Nager, F. R., and DeReynier, J. P., Das Gehörorgan bei den angeborenen Kopfmissbildungen. *Pract. Otorhinolaryngol. (Basel), 10 (Suppl. 2)*:43–59, 1948.
Pou, J. W., Congenital anomalies of the middle ear. *Laryngoscope, 81*:831–839, 1971.

Dyschondrosteosis
Herdman, R. C., Langer, L. O., and Good, R. A., Dyschondrosteosis. *J. Pediatr., 68*:432–441, 1966.
Nassif, R., and Harboyan, G., Madelung's deformity with conductive hearing loss. *Arch. Otolaryngol., 91*:175–178, 1970.

Familial Osteoma of the Middle Ear
Ombredanne, M., Ostéome exceptionnel de l'orielle moyenne. *Ann. Otolaryngol. (Paris), 83*:433–436, 1966.
Thomas, T. R., Familial osteoma of the middle ear. *J. Laryngol., 78*:805–807, 1964.

Oculodento-osseous Dysplasia and Conductive Deafness
Gillespie, F. D., Hereditary dysplasia oculodentodigitalis. *Arch. Ophthalmol., 71*:187–192, 1964.
Gorlin, R. J., Meskin, L. H. and St. Geme, J. W., Oculodentodigital dysplasia. *J. Pediatr., 63*:69–75, 1963.
Reisner, S. H., Kott, E., Bornstein, B., Salinger, H., Kaplan, I., and Gorlin, R. J., Oculodentodigital dysplasia syndrome. *Am. J. Dis. Child., 118*:600–607, 1969.

Pfeiffer Syndrome and Conductive Deafness
Manns, K. J., and Bopp, K. P., Dysostosis craniofacialis Crouzon mit digitaler Anomalie. *Med. Klin., 60*:1899–1903, 1965.
Martsolf, J. T., Cracco, J. B., Carpenter, G. G., and O'Hara, A. E., Pfeiffer syndrome. *Amer. J. Dis. Child., 121*:257–262, 1971.
Saldino, R. M., Steinbach, H. L., and Epstein, C. J., Familial acrocephalosyndactyly (Pfeiffer syndrome). *Am. J. Roentgenol., 116*:609–622, 1972.

Saethre-Chotzen Syndrome and Conductive Deafness
Aase, J. M., and Smith, D. W., Facial asymmetry and abnormality of palms and ears: a dominantly inherited development syndrome. *J. Pediatr., 76*:928–930, 1970.
Bartsocas, C. S., Weber, A. L., and Crawford, J. O., Acrocephalosyndactyly type III: Chotzen's syndrome. *J. Pediatr., 77*:267–272, 1970.
Chotzen, F., Eine eigenartige familiäre Entwicklungsstörungen (Akrocephalosyndaktylie, Dysostosis craniofacialis und Hypertelorismus). *Mschr. Kinderheilkd., 55*:97–121, 1932.
Dolivo, G., and Gillieron, J. D., Une famille de "Crouzon-fruste" ou "pseudo-Crouzon." *J. Génét. Hum., 4*:88–101, 1955.
Grebe, H., Beitrag zur familiären Mikrocephalie. *Z. Menschl. Vererb. Konstitlehre, 24*:506–515, 1940.
Hammar, I., and Roggenkamp, K., Augenveränderungen bei Dysplasia renofacialis. *Klin. Mbl. Augenheilkd., 15*:534–539, 1967.
Jorgenson, R. J., Craniofacial dysplasia with features of the midface syndrome. *Birth Defects, 7(7)*:307, 1971.
Kreiborg, S., Pruzansky, S., and Pashayan, H., Saethre-Chotzen syndrome. *Teratology, 6*:287, 1972.
Pantke, O. A., Cohen, M. M., Jr., Witkop, C. J., Feingold, M., Schaumann, B., Pantke, H. C., and Gorlin, R. J., The Saethre-Chotzen syndrome. *Birth Defects, 11(2)*:190–225, 1975.

Focal Dermal Hypoplasia Syndrome and Mixed Deafness
Daly, J. G., Focal dermal hypoplasia. *Cutis, 4*:1354–1359, 1968.
Ferrara, A., Goltz's syndrome. *Am. J. Dis. Child., 123*:263, 1972.
Ginsburg, L. D., Sedano, H. O., and Gorlin, R. J., Focal dermal hypoplasia syndrome. *Am. J. Roentgenol., 110*:561–571, 1970.

Goltz, R. W., Henderson, R. R., Hitch, J. M., and Ott, J. E., Focal dermal hypoplasia syndrome. *Arch. Dermatol., 101*:1–11, 1970.

Holden, J. D., and Akers, H. A., Goltz's syndrome: focal dermal hypoplasia combined mesoectodermal dysplasia. *Am. J. Dis. Child., 114*:292–300, 1967.

Stollman, K., Bisher noch nicht beschriebene Befunde bei Incontinentia pigmenti. *Derm. Wschr., 153*:489–496, 1967.

Oculopharyngeal Muscular Dystrophy and Sensorineural Deafness

Graf, K., Myopathia oculo-pharyngealis tarda hereditaria. *Pract. Otorhinolaryngol. (Basel), 33*:203–208, 1971.

Kuhn, E., and Ey, W., Innenohrschwerhörigkeit bei Dystrophia myotonica und Dystrophia muscularis progressiva. *Dtsch. Med. Wochenschr., 91*:947–951, 1966.

Lewis, I., Late-onset muscle dystrophy: oculopharyngeal variety. *Can. Med. Assoc. J., 95*:146–150, 1966.

Roberts, A. H., and Bamforth, J., The pharynx and esophagus in ocular muscular dystrophy. *Neurology (Minneap.), 18*:645–652, 1968.

Chapter 6

GENETIC HEARING LOSS WITH INTEGUMENTARY SYSTEM DISEASE

Most of the syndromes considered in this chapter are associated with congenital deafness. They can be diagnosed rather easily because of skin, nail, or hair changes that occur along with the generally severe hearing loss.

Most of these disorders have been de-scribed in only one or perhaps a few fami-lies; the Waardenburg syndrome, however, accounts for about 2 per cent of the congeni-tally deaf. Knowledge of the basic features of these syndromes should bring to light many other cases of the rarer disorders dis-cussed in this chapter.

WAARDENBURG SYNDROME

The most characteristic features of pa-tients with this disorder are widely spaced medial canthi, flat nasal root, and confluent eyebrows. Frequently, patients have varia-bly colored irides as well as a white forelock (Fig. 6–1A). At least 20 per cent have some sensorineural hearing loss.

Although certain aspects of this dis-order were described by van der Hoeve (1916) and by Mende (1926), the syndrome was first well defined by Waardenburg (1948, 1961). Waardenburg (1951) esti-mated that 1.4 per cent of all deaf-mutes in the Netherlands had this syndrome. DiGeorge et al. (1960) suggested that about 2.3 per cent of the congenitally deaf have this disorder and estimated that there are some 400 affected children in the United States schools for the deaf. It is possible

that the actual frequency is twice this es-timate, since only about 50 per cent of af-fected individuals have pigmentation anom-alies.

CLINICAL FINDINGS

Facies. The facies is characterized by laterally displaced medial canthi, producing what appears to be widely spaced eyes (Fig. 6–2B). The maximal normal inner canthal distance in children up to 16 years of age is 34 mm.; in adult women, 37 mm; in adult men, 39 mm. (DiGeorge, 1960; Pryor, 1969). About 85 per cent of patients with the Waardenburg syndrome have inner canthal distances exceeding these measurements. However, the interpupillary distance is usually normal. True ocular hypertelorism has been found in about 10 per cent (Pantke and Cohen, 1971). Broad nasal root is found in 75 per cent of those affected, whereas about 50 per cent have confluent eyebrows (synophrys) (Fig. 6–1B). This characteristic may be less evident in women because they tend to pluck glabellar hairs. Hypoplasia of the nasal alar cartilages is usually present, but the degree of expression is quite variable.

Integumentary System. White forelock (poliosis) originating at the hairline in the middle of the forehead and continuing posteriorly is found in 20 to 40 per cent, varying from the width of only a few hairs to a large white forelock (Fig. 6–1C). In females, poliosis may not be evident as a result of dyeing of the hair. Premature graying of the hair, eyebrows, and eyelashes has been noted in several kindred (Waardenburg, 1951; Partington, 1959; DiGeorge et al., 1960).

In about 15 per cent of affected persons skin pigmentary changes ranging from small areas of vitiligo to depigmentation with patchy areas of pigmentation have been observed. In several patients described by Fisch (1959) the arms and face showed a patchy or freckled hyperpigmentation. Several Afro-American patients described by DiGeorge (1960) showed large areas of vitiligo.

Ocular System. In addition to the eye changes described above, heterochromia irides—more accurately termed hypoplasia irides—was found in about 25 per cent of the cases studied by Waardenburg (1961). The patterns of pigmentary changes involving the iris are varied. While some patients may have one brown and one blue iris, others may exhibit brown sectors in a blue iris or blue sectors in a brown iris. Still other patients may have brown or blue irides bilaterally (Goldberg, 1966; De Haas and Tan, 1966) (Fig. 6–1A, C).

Fundus pigmentation may vary as much as iris pigmentation in this disorder. Goldberg (1966) found a relationship between the pigmentation pattern of the iris and that of the fundus. In all cases in which a blue iris was present, the corresponding fundus was blond or albinoid. In patients having a brown iris the fundus was normal with brunet coloration. The fundus corresponding to bicolored irides was mottled, the pigment sector of the iris corresponding

to that of the fundus. Visual acuity was normal in all cases.

The inferior lacrimal points are displaced laterally, in most cases as far as the cornea. There is an increased susceptibility to dacrocystitis (Pantke and Cohen, 1971).

Auditory System. Over 20 per cent of those affected have some hearing loss. The extent of loss is quite variable, ranging from no measurable clinical deafness to severe congenital unilateral or bilateral sensorineural deafness.

Fisch (1959) divided the audiogram patterns of those affected with hearing loss into two types: Type I—almost total deafness with some residual hearing only at lower frequencies; Type II—moderate deafness with uniform hearing loss in the lower and middle frequencies but with improvement in higher tones.

Vestibular System. Although some authors (Zelig, 1961; DeHaas and Tan, 1966) described vestibular findings in the Waardenburg syndrome, the most complete survey of vestibular function was presented by Marcus (1968). He completed detailed vestibular tests in 16 affected members of a kindred. Only one individual had completely normal vestibular function. Three affected children had normal hearing. Rotation or caloric testing showed variable vestibular response in one or both ears. Of four children with mild to moderate sensorineural hearing loss a vestibular function abnormality was found either in rotation testing, in caloric testing, or in both. Sometimes only one side showed vestibular abnormalities. Six members of the family had bilateral congenital severe deafness. Five of these had no response to the vestibular function test, whereas one had completely normal function except for slightly reduced response to cold caloric stimulation. Thus, the number of patients showing abnormality in vestibular function exceeded the number having hearing loss. Although most sonographic studies of the inner ear have shown normal findings (Marcus and Valvassori, 1970; Nemansky and Hageman, 1975), a few investigators (Jensen, 1967; Kanzaki et al., 1971) have found abnormal labyrinthine development.

Other Findings. The mandible tends to be mildly prognathic, and the bigonial distance is often increased. Perhaps 3 per cent have cleft lip and/or cleft palate (Gorlin, 1971).

LABORATORY FINDINGS

Roentgenograms. Tomograms on two patients described by Marcus (1968) showed hypoplasia of the cochlea and of the superior and horizontal semicircular canal walls as well as complete absence of the posterior semicircular canal.

PATHOLOGY

The inner-ear pathology has been described in a 3-year-old girl (Fisch, 1959). The organ of Corti was found to be absent in all coils. The basal membrane was slightly thickened and smooth except for a small area covered by hydropic limbus-type cells (Fig. 6–1D). Only a few neurons remained in the spiral ganglion. Similar findings have been observed in white cats, dogs, horses, mice, mink, and other laboratory animals (Innes and Saunders, 1957; Hudson and Ruben, 1962; Hilding *et al.*, 1967; Deol, 1968; Bergsma and Brown, 1971), although the pathogenesis may be somewhat different in the various species.

HEREDITY

The syndrome exhibits autosomal dominant transmission with striking variation in the degree of expressivity of the various components.

Presumably, the mutant gene action affects the neural crest from which the melanocytes and ganglionic primordia are derived (Deol, 1968).

DIAGNOSIS

Klein (1950) described a female patient with primary telecanthus, synophrys, partial albinism of skin and hair, and blue irides. However, the patient also showed osseous dysplasia: aplasia of the first two ribs and carpal bones and cystic alteration of the sacrum. She exhibited cutaneous union of the thorax and upper arm and syndactyly (Fig. 6–1E). Wilbrandt and Ammann (1964) reported a similarly but less severely affected patient from a family stated to have Waardenburg syndrome; this case, however, was not documented. Amini-Elihou (1970) reported a syndrome of congenital sensorineural deafness, mental retardation, and hyperkeratosis of the palms and soles with what appears to us to have autosomal

recessive inheritance. We cannot accept this disorder as being a variant of Waardenburg syndrome.

Dystopia canthorum and hypertelorism may be seen in a variety of disorders (Peterson *et al.*, 1971). Synophrys is a feature of the deLange syndrome and may occur with pilonidal cyst (Sebrechts, 1961). Poliosis, vitiligo, and dysacousia may be seen in combination with alopecia and uveitis in the Vogt-Koyanagi syndrome (Johnson, 1963). Heterochromia irides may be acquired, may be inherited as an autosomal dominant trait, or may be associated with the Romberg syndrome (Fisch, 1959). Cases of heterochromia in combination with congenital deafness but without blepharophimosis have been reviewed by DeHaas and Tan (1966). One must exclude *dominant piebald trait, ataxia, and sensorineural hearing loss.* An autosomal recessive disorder similar to the Waardenburg syndrome but with black rather than white forelock was reported to occur in South America (Arias, 1971).

TREATMENT

Hearing aids may be used for those patients with moderate to severe hearing loss.

PROGNOSIS

There is no evidence of progression of the hearing loss in those cases with partial hearing.

SUMMARY

Major characteristics of this syndrome include: 1) autosomal dominant transmission with variable expressivity, 2) lateral displacement of medial canthi and lacrimal points in nearly all affected, 3) broad nasal root in about 75 per cent, 4) hyperplasia of medial eyebrows in about 50 per cent, 5) heterochromia (hypoplasia) irides and loss of pigment epithelium of optic fundus in about 25 per cent, 6) white forelock in about 20 per cent, 7) skin pigmentary changes, including vitiligo and spotty hyperpigmentation, in less than 15 per cent, 8) cleft lip and/or cleft palate in less than 5 per cent, 9) vestibular hypofunction in about 75 per cent, and 10) congenital mild to severe unilateral or bilateral sensorineural hearing loss in about 50 per cent.

REFERENCES

Amini-Elihou, S., Une famille Suisse atteinte du syndrome de Klein-Waardenburg associé à une hyperkératose palmo-plantaire et à une oligophrénie grave. *J. Génét. Hum., 18*:307–363, 1970.

Arias, S., Genetic heterogeneity in the Waardenburg syndrome. *Birth Defects, 7*(4):87–101, 1971.

Bergsma, D. R., and Brown, K. S., White fur, blue eyes, and deafness in the domestic cat. *J. Hered., 62*:171–185, 1971.

Brown, K. S., and Chung, C. S., *Genetic Studies of Deafness at the Clarke School for the Deaf, Northampton, Mass.* Doc. No. 106. Washington, D.C., U.S. Government Printing Office, 1964.

DeHaas, E. B. H., and Tan, K. E., Waardenburg's syndrome. *Doc. Ophthalmol., 21*:239–282, 1966.

Deol, M. S., Inherited diseases of the inner ear in light of studies in the mouse. *J. Med. Genet., 5*:137–157, 1968.

DiGeorge, A. M., Olmsted, R. W., and Harley, R. D., Waardenburg's syndrome. *J. Pediatr., 57*:649–669, 1960.

DiGeorge, A. M., Waardenburg's syndrome: a syndrome of heterochromia of the irides, lateral displacement of the medial canthi and lacrimal puncta, congenital deafness, and other characteristic associated defects. *Trans. Am. Acad. Ophthalmol., 64*:816–839, 1960.

Fisch, L., Deafness as part of an hereditary syndrome. *J. Laryngol., 73*:355–383, 1959.

Goldberg, M. F., Waardenburg's syndrome with fundus and other anomalies. *Arch. Ophthalmol., 76*:797–810, 1966.

Gorlin, R. J., Facial clefting and its syndromes. *Birth Defects, 7*(7):3–49, 1971.

Hilding, D. A., Sugiura, A., and Nakai, Y., Deaf white mink: electron microscopic study of the inner ear. *Ann. Otol., 76*:647–663, 1967.

Hudson, W. R., and Ruben, R. J., Hereditary deafness in the Dalmatian dog. *Arch. Otolaryngol., 75*:213–219, 1962.

Innes, J. R. M., and Saunders, L. Z., Diseases of the central nervous system of domesticated animals and comparisons with human neuropathology. *Adv. Vet. Sci., 3*:33–196, 1957.

Jensen, J., Tomography of inner ear in case of Waardenburg's syndrome. *Am. J. Roentgenol., 101*:828–833, 1967.

Johnson, W. C., Vogt-Koyanagi-Harada syndrome. *Arch. Dermatol., 88*:146–149, 1963.

Kanzaki, J., Suzuki, Y., Hommura, Y., Ito, T., and Nameki, H., Vestibular function and radiological findings in Waardenburg's syndrome. *Pract. Otorhinolaryngol. (Basel), 64*:1439–1444. 1971.

Klein, D., Albinisme partiel (leucisme) avec surdimutité, blepharophimosis, et dysplasia myo-ostéo-articulaire. *Helvet. Paediatr. Acta, 5*:38–58, 1950.

Marcus, R. E., Vestibular function and additional findings in Waardenburg's syndrome. *Acta Otolaryngol. (Stockh.), Suppl. 229*:5–30, 1968.

Marcus, R. E., and Valvassori, G., Cochleovestibular apparatus: radiologic studies in hereditary and familial hearing loss. *Int. Audiol., 9*:95–102, 1970.

Mende, I., Über eine Familie hereditär-degenerativer Taubstummer mit mongoloidem Einschlag und teilweisen Leukismus der Haut und Haare. *Arch. Kinderheilkd., 79*:214–222, 1926.

Nemansky, J., and Hageman, M. J., Tomographic findings in Waardenburg's syndrome. *Am. J. Roentgenol., 124*:250–255, 1975.

Pantke, O. A., and Cohen, M. M., Jr., The Waardenburg syndrome. *Birth Defects, 7*(7):147–152, 1971.

Partington, M. W., An English family with Waardenburg's syndrome. *Arch. Dis. Child., 34*:154–157, 1959.

Peterson, M. A., Cohen, M. M., Jr., Sedano, H. O., and Frerichs, C. T., Comments on frontonasal dysplasia, ocular hypertelorism and dystopia canthorum. *Birth Defects, 7*(7):120–124, 1971.

Pryor, H. B., Objective measurement of interpupillary distance. *Pediatrics, 44*:973–977, 1969.

Sebrechts, P. H., A significant diagnostic sign of pilonidal cyst. *Dis. Colon Rectum, 4*:56–59, 1961.

Smith, N. G., and Schulz, H., Partial albinism. *Arch. Dermatol., 71*:468–470, 1955.

Sundfor, H., A pedigree of skin-spotting in man. *J. Hered., 30*:67–77, 1939.

van der Hoeve, J., Abnorme Länge der Tränenröhrchen mit Ankyloblepharon. *Klin. Mbl. Augenheilkd., 56* 232–238, 1916.

Waardenburg, P. J., Dystopia punctorum lacrimalium, blepharophimosis, en partiele irisatrophia bij een doofstomme. *Ned. Tijdschr. Geneeskd., 92*:3463–3466, 1948.

Waardenburg, P. J., A new syndrome combining developmental anomalies of the eyelids, eyebrows, and nose root with pigmentary defects of the iris and head, hair, and congenital deafness. *Am. J. Hum. Genet., 3* 195–253, 1951.

Wilbrandt, H. R., and Ammann, F., Nouvelle observation de la forme grave du syndrome de Klein-Waardenburg. *Arch. Klaus Stift. Vererbungsforsch., 39*:80–92, 1964.

Zelig, S., Syndrome of Waardenburg with deafness. *Laryngoscope, 71*:19–23, 1961.

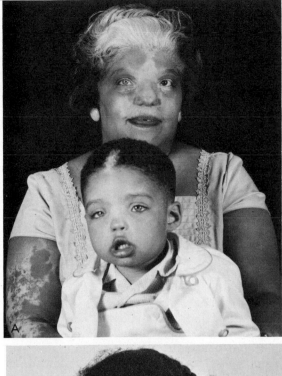

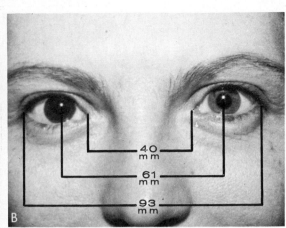

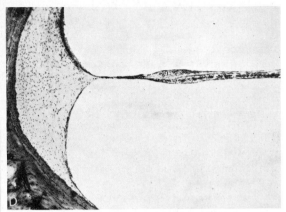

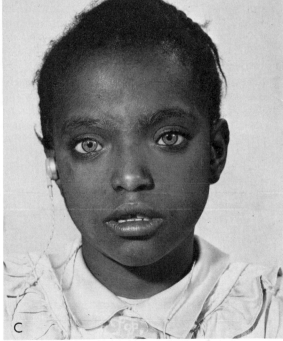

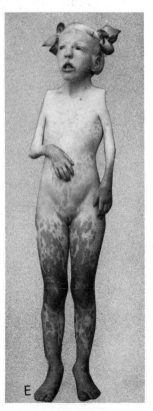

Figure 6-1 Waardenburg syndrome. (A) Mother and son exhibiting white forelock; mother displays heterochromia irides, son has blue irides. Eyes appear widely spaced. Mother has widespread vitiligo. (From V. Pinchazadeh and F . Char, *Birth Defects* 7(4):129, 1971.) *(B)* Note heterochromia irides, increased inter-inner canthal distance but normal interpupillary and inter-outer canthal distances; patient plucks glabellar hairs. *(C)* Note that white forelock is absent but that medial portion of eyebrows is white. Irides are bilaterally blue in this profoundly deaf girl. (From A. M. DiGeorge, R. W. Olmsted, and R. D. Harley, *J. Pediatr.,* 57:649, 1960.) *(D)* Section of cochlea showing absence of organ of Corti. (From L. Fisch, *J. Laryngol. Otol.* 73:355, 1959.) *(E)* Deaf girl with some of the stigmata seen in Waardenburg syndrome. In addition, however, she had bony anomalies, especially of the shoulder girdle and arms. (From D. Klein, *Helvet. Paediatr. Acta,* 5:38, 1950.)

OCULOCUTANEOUS ALBINISM AND CONGENITAL SENSORINEURAL DEAFNESS

A syndrome characterized by total oculocutaneous albinism and congenital severe deafness was found in four children in two sibships in a kindred and described by Ziprkowski and Adam (1964). However, only one sibship was examined.

CLINICAL FINDINGS

Integumentary System. Physical examination on two of the sibs showed classic albinism with totally white skin (Fig. 6–2A). The hair was white and the irides were translucent blue. Lacking pigment, the optic fundus was pink. The sibs had nystagmus and photophobia. In both sibs the medial portion of the eyebrows was absent.

Auditory System. Audiometric tests on the two sibs showed a response only at 500 Hz at 90 dB in one ear. There was a history of congenital severe deafness in two albino cousins. Audiograms of the parents were normal.

Vestibular System. No vestibular function tests were described.

LABORATORY FINDINGS

Urinary amino acid excretion was normal. Color vision was normal.

PATHOLOGY

Skin biopsy from the older affected sib showed no evidence of pigment in the basal layer of the epithelium. The dopa reaction was positive.

HEREDITY

From the pedigree (Fig. 6–2B) it is obvious that the parents in both sibships were closely related. The family was of Moroccan Jewish extraction. There were nine children, two of whom exhibited total albinism and deafness. Three of the children had congenital sensorineural deafness but no skin pigmentation abnormality, and four sibs were normal. Whether two separate genes are involved—one producing congenital

severe sensorineural deafness and the other producing deafness and albinism—or whether the syndrome was the pleiotropic effect of a single gene cannot be determined from this single sibship. When we consider the second sibship in which two of six sibs were affected with albinism and deafness, whereas the other four were completely normal, it would appear most likely that an autosomal recessive gene is responsible.

DIAGNOSIS

Male sibs with oculocutaneous albinism and sensorineural deafness were reported by Reed et al. (1967). They were also partially blind from hypoplasia of the fovea. Both were severely mentally retarded. Autosomal dominant oculocutaneous albinism and congenital deafness was reported by Tietz (1963). However, on re-examination of several members of the kindred Reed et al. (1967) cast doubt upon the validity of the findings. In all other syndromes that include deafness and pigmentary abnormalities, areas of hypo- and hyperpigmentation have been found, clearly separating the oculocutaneous albinism and congenital sensorineural deafness syndrome.

TREATMENT

In some cases, a hearing aid might be of help.

PROGNOSIS

There is no apparent change in the albinism or hearing loss throughout the life span of affected persons.

SUMMARY

The characteristics of this syndrome include: 1) autosomal recessive inheritance, 2) albinism of the entire body, including the optic fundi and irides, 3) deficient medial eyebrows, and 4) congenital severe sensorineural hearing loss.

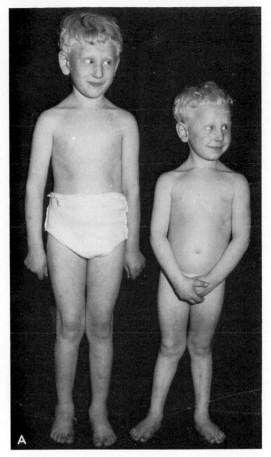

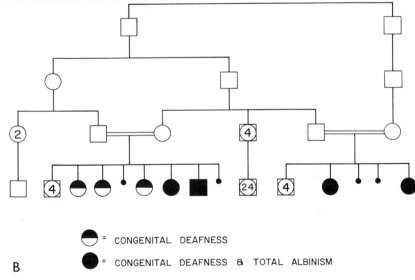

Figure 6-2 *Oculocutaneous albinism and congenital sensorineural deafness.* (A) Deaf-mute sibs exhibiting total albinism. (B) Pedigree of affected inbred kindred. (From L. Ziprkowski and A. Adam, *Arch. Dermatol., 89*:151, 1964.)

◐ = CONGENITAL DEAFNESS

● = CONGENITAL DEAFNESS & TOTAL ALBINISM

REFERENCES

Reed, W. B., Stone, V. M., Boder, E., and Ziprkowski, L., Pigmentary disorders in association with congenital deafness. *Arch. Dermatol., 95*:176–186, 1967.

Tietz, W., A syndrome of deaf-mutism associated with albinism showing dominant autosomal inheritance. *Am. J. Hum. Genet., 15*:259–264, 1963.

Ziprkowski, L., and Adam, A., Recessive total albinism and congenital deaf-mutism. *Arch. Dermatol., 89*:151–155, 1964.

MULTIPLE LENTIGINES (LEOPARD) SYNDROME

The term LEOPARD syndrome is an acronym derived from the following elements: *l*entigines, *e*lectrocardiographic defects, *o*cular hypertelorism, *p*ulmonary stenosis, *a*bnormalities of genitalia, *r*etardation of growth and sensorineural *d*eafness (Gorlin, Anderson, and Blaw, 1969). Earlier case reports were thoroughly reviewed by Gorlin, Anderson, and Moller (1971) and Voron *et al.* (1976).

CLINICAL FINDINGS

Facies. The face is usually triangular in shape and shows biparietal bossing, ocular hypertelorism, ptosis of the upper eyelids, epicanthal folds, and, commonly, pterygium colli.

Integumentary System. When present, dark-brown lentigines are striking. They are numerous, small (1 to 5 mm.), and spare only the mucosal surfaces. Most highly concentrated over the neck and the upper trunk, they may appear over the face, scalp, palms, soles, and genitalia (Fig. 6–3*A*). They may be present at birth or may appear shortly thereafter, rapidly increasing in number with age. One commonly finds a few large dark café-noir (if we may coin a term) spots scattered over the trunk. The lentigines differ from freckles in appearing earlier, having no relation to sun exposure, and microscopically having a greater number of melanocytes per unit skin area and prominent rete ridges. It now appears likely that some patients may lack lentigines; thus, identification of the syndrome will then depend upon the presence of other characteristics and familial occurrence.

Cardiovascular System. Valvular pulmonary stenosis, usually mild, appears to be the most common cardiac abnormality. In some patients, the stenosis is of the typical valvular type; in others, there is an unusual alteration in the pulmonary valve, which has been termed "pulmonary valvular dysplasia" by Koretzky *et al.* (1969). The pulmonary valve reveals three distinct cusps but no commissural fusion. The obstruction is based on thickening of the pulmonary valvular cusps by disorganized myxomatous tissue that renders the valve leaflets immobile. Clinically, patients with this type of valvular anomaly have a pulmonary systolic ejection murmur but no ejection click. Similar changes have been seen much less commonly in the aortic valves. Some patients have hypertrophic cardiomyopathy, involving primarily the interventricular septum, which results in both subaortic and subpulmonic stenosis (Polani and Moynahan, 1972; Somerville and Bonham-Carter, 1972). In other reports, associated atrial septal defect, infundibular or supravalvular pulmonary stenosis, or muscular subaortic stenosis has been described (Koretzky *et al.*, 1968; Lynch, 1970).

There is a unique and commonly present electrocardiographic anomaly that tends to characterize this syndrome regardless of the type of cardiac malformation. This feature is a superiorly oriented mean QRS axis in the frontal plane, generally located between −60° and −120° (S_1, S_2, S_3 pattern). This may not be demonstrable in every patient, but it may be present in other patients with the syndrome in whom there is no structural abnormality of the heart. Electrocardiograms in several patients have revealed complete heart block, hemiblock, or complete bundle branch block (Smith *et al.*, 1970).

Musculoskeletal System. Growth retardation is common, 85 per cent of the patients being below the twenty-fifth percentile for both height and weight, with the majority being below the tenth percentile for both parameters.

Pectus carinatum or excavatum, dorsal kyphosis, and hyperflexibility of metacarpophalangeal joints of fingers and thumbs as well as winging of the scapulae have been commonly observed.

Genitourinary System. Hypospadias has been present in about half of the male cases (Gorlin *et al.*, 1971). Cryptorchidism or descent of only one testicle has also been a common finding. In some females there has been absence or hypoplasia of an ovary. On the basis of published cases and unpublished material, it appears that since more cases have been transmitted through females, the gonadal hypoplasia has been of greater significance in the male. Late menarche has also been a common finding.

Nervous System. Mild mental retardation has been noted in about 20 per cent (Moynahan, 1962; Watson, 1967; Vickers and MacMillan, 1967; Pickering *et al.*, 1971).

Auditory System. Sensorineural hearing loss has been observed in about 25 per cent (Pickering *et al.*, 1971). There is marked variation in the degree of hearing loss in different affected persons, but in most it is mild. In contrast, the mother and daughter described by Capute *et al.* (1969) both had congenital severe sensorineural hearing loss with very poor speech development (Fig. 6–3*D*). Because of the severity of hearing loss, special audiometric tests could not be done. Lassonde *et al.* (1970) noted deaf-mutism in their patient.

Vestibular System. Vestibular testing was described by Capute *et al.* (1969). Caloric tests in these two patients showed no abnormalities.

LABORATORY FINDINGS

Electrocardiograms. The most common electrocardiographic abnormalities are conduction defects, although there may be bundle branch block, abnormal P waves, and prolongation of the PR interval, ST and T wave changes, and widening of the QRS complex (Matthews, 1968; Smith *et al.*, 1970; Somerville and Bonham-Carter, 1972) (Fig. 6–3*C*).

Roentgenograms. No radiographic abnormalities other than those described under skeletal changes have been noted.

PATHOLOGY

Skin biopsy taken from an area of hyperpigmentation shows elongated rete ridges, numerous melanocytes, and increased pigment in basal cells (Fig. 6–3*B*).

HEREDITY

Based on the range of manifestations in different affected persons, it is apparent that this syndrome is transmitted in an autosomal dominant manner with variable expressivity (Gorlin *et al.*, 1971) (Fig. 6–3*E*). The most clinically evident feature of this disease is the lentigines, usually absent at birth, but progressive thereafter. Selection is obviously biased by their presence.

DIAGNOSIS

Several disorders have findings somewhat similar to those in this syndrome. Noonan and Ehmke (1963) described several children with congenital cardiac disease who showed abnormal facies, pulmonary stenosis, and other extracardiac anomalies. The label "Noonan syndrome" has been applied to this cluster of anomalies. Patients with this syndrome have also been described as having a "Turner phenotype."

Noonan syndrome, occurring in both males and females, manifests many features in common with the multiple lentigines syndrome: hypertelorism, eyelid ptosis, small stature, pulmonary stenosis without an ejection click, abnormal QRS axis (frequently S_1, S_2, S_3), undescended testes and delayed development of secondary sex characteristics, skeletal anomalies of the chest, and possible autosomal dominant inheritance with incomplete penetrance. Patients with Noonan syndrome may occasionally show webbing of the neck, but they lack lentigines and deafness.

The relationship between the multiple lentigines syndrome and Noonan syndrome is unclear. Perhaps both result from the same pleiotropic gene, with emphasis being placed on different manifestations. Possibly they represent allelic mutations. In addition, both syndromes bear certain similarities to the rubella syndrome: pulmonary stenosis, abnormal QRS axis, small stature, delayed puberty, and deafness (in the case of the multiple lentigines syndrome). The angiographic appearance of the stenotic pulmonary valve in rubella syndrome is also strikingly similar to that observed in patients with dysplastic pulmonary valve.

Dominant piebald trait, ataxia, and sensorineural hearing loss with large depigmented areas is strikingly different from the lesions of multiple lentigines syndrome. The lentigines are also quite different from the striking pigmentary loss with areas of hyperpigmentation found in the syndrome of *X-linked pigmentary abnormalities and congenital sensorineural deafness.*

TREATMENT

Severe pulmonary stenosis requires cardiac surgery (Gorlin *et al.*, 1969). The lentigines have been treated by dermabrasion (Selmanowitz *et al.*, 1971). Patients with hearing loss may require hearing aids. The cryptorchidism should be corrected.

PROGNOSIS

Apparently the only progressive feature in this syndrome is the increasing number of lentigines throughout the first two decades of life. Some patients with severe obstructure cardiomyopathy have met early death (Somerville and Bonham-Carter, 1972), but most have experienced a normal life span.

SUMMARY

Characteristics of the syndrome include: 1) autosomal dominant transmission with variable expressivity, 2) lentigines developing after birth, 3) electrocardiographic defects exhibiting some combination of block in the bundle branch system, 4) pulmonary stenosis and/or hypertrophic cardiomyopathy, 5) ocular hypertelorism, 6) abnormalities of genitalia, including cryptorchidism and hypospadias, 7) somatic and mental retardation, 8) winged scapulae and various minor skeletal abnormalities, and 9) sensorineural deafness, variable in severity.

REFERENCES

Capute, A. J., Rimoin, D. L., Konigsmark, B. W., Esterly, N. B., and Richardson, F.: Congenital deafness and multiple lentigines. *Arch. Dermatol., 100*:207–213, 1969.

Cronje, R. E., and Feinberg, A., Lentiginosis, deafness, and cardiac abnormalities. *S. Afr. Med. J., 47*:15–17, 1973.

Gorlin, R. J., Anderson, R. C., and Blaw, M., Mutiple lentigines syndrome, complex comprising multiple lentigines, electrocardiographic conduction abnormalities, ocular hypertelorism, pulmonary stenosis, abnormalities of genitalia, retardation of growth, sensorineural deafness, and autosomal dominant hereditary pattern. *Am. J. Dis. Child., 117*:652–662, 1969.

Gorlin, R. J., Anderson, R. C., and Moller, J. H., The leopard (multiple lentigines) syndrome revisited. *Birth Defects, 7*(4):110–115, 1971.

Koretzky, E. D., Moller, J. H., Korns, M. E., Schwartz, C. J., and Edwards, J. E., Congenital pulmonary stenosis resulting from dysplasia of valve. *Circulation, 40*:43–53, 1969.

Lassonde, M., Trudeau, J. G., and Girard, C., Generalized lentigines associated with multiple congenital defects (leopard syndrome). *Can. Med. Assoc. J., 103*:293–294, 1970.

Lynch, P. J., Leopard syndrome. *Arch. Dermatol., 101*:119, 1970.

Matthews, N. L., Lentigo and electrocardiographic changes. *N. Engl. J. Med., 278*:780–781, 1968.

Moynahan, E. J., Multiple symmetrical moles, with psychic and somatic infantilism and genital hypoplasia. *Proc. R. Soc. Med., 55*:959–960, 1962.

Noonan, J., and Ehmke, O., Associated noncardial malformations in children with congenital heart disease. *J. Pediatr., 63*:469–470, 1963.

Pickering, D., Laski, B., MacMillan, D., and Rose, V., "Little leopard" syndrome. *Arch. Dis. Child., 46*:85–90, 1971.

Polani, P., and Moynahan, E. J., Progressive cardiomyopathic lentiginosis. *Q. J. Med., 41*:205–225, 1972.

Selmanowitz, V. J., Orentreich, N., and Felsenstein, J., Lentiginosis profusa syndrome (multiple lentigines syndrome). *Arch. Dermatol., 104*:393–401, 1971.

Smith, R. F., Pulicicchio, L. V., and Holmes, A. V., Generalized lentigo, electrocardiographic abnormalities, conduction disorders, and arrhythmias in three cases. *Am. J. Cardiol., 25*:501–506, 1970.

Somerville, J., and Bonham-Carter, R. E., The heart in lentiginosis. *Br. Heart J., 34*:58–66, 1972.

Vickers, H. R., and MacMillan, D., Profuse lentiginosis, minor cardiac abnormality, and small stature. *Proc. R. Soc. Med., 62*:1011–1012, 1969.

Voron, D. A., Hatfield, H. H., and Kalkhoff, R. K., Multiple lentigines syndrome. *Am. J. Med., 60*:447–456, 1976.

Watson, G. H., Pulmonary stenosis, café-au-lait spots and dull intelligence. *Arch. Dis. Child., 42*:303–307, 1967.

Figure 6–3 *Multiple lentigines (Leopard) syndrome.* *(A)* Lentigines involved entire body but were more marked over upper thorax and face. *(B)* Skin lesion showing elongated rete ridges and increased pigment in basal cells. There are numerous melanocytes (clear cells) in the basal layer of the epithelium. *(C)* Electrocardiographic anomalies including S_1, S_2, S_3 abnormality. *(D)* Audiograms from two cases showing marked neural hearing loss with preservation of only low tones. *(A–D* from A. J. Capute *et al., Arch. Dermatol., 100*:207, 1969.) *(E)* Pedigree of kindred showing variable expressivity of dominant gene. (From R. J. Gorlin *et al., Am. J. Dis. Child., 117*:652, 1969.)

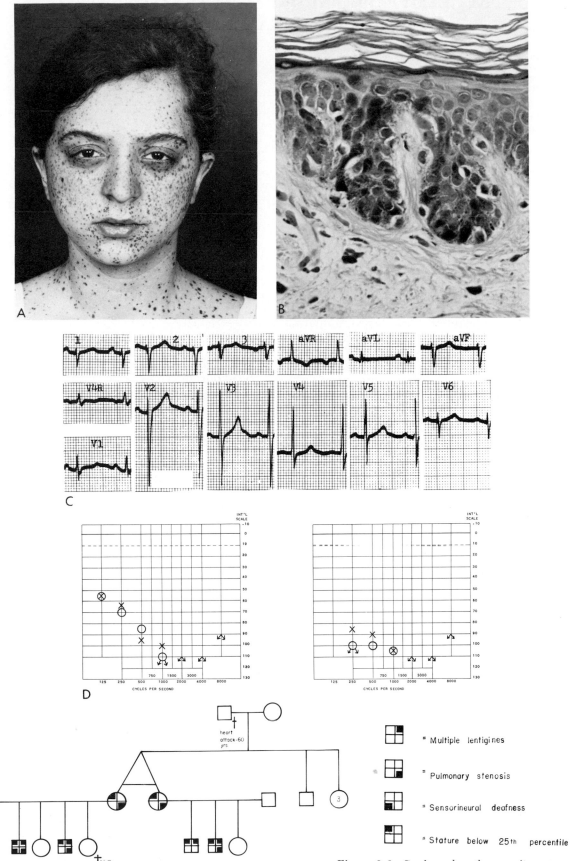

Figure 6–3 See legend on the opposite page.

RECESSIVE PIEBALDNESS AND CONGENITAL SENSORINEURAL DEAFNESS

A syndrome consisting of piebaldness and congenital sensorineural deafness was reported in two of three Hopi Indian brothers by Woolf, Dolowitz, and Aldous (1965).

CLINICAL FINDINGS

Integumentary System. The boys, 8- and 12-years-old, showed a similar pattern of depigmentation. Although the major part of their bodies (including the back and legs) showed normal pigmentation, the entire head and the hair as well as a strip across the upper chest and over both arms were depigmented (Fig. 6–4A, B). Within all of these depigmented areas were numerous small spots of hypopigmentation and hyperpigmentation.

Ocular System. The irides were blue with a pattern of very fine clumps of pigment closely and uniformly spaced throughout the retina. Vision was normal.

Auditory System. The brothers were congenitally deaf. They attended a school for the deaf but had not learned to speak. Audiograms showed a bilateral 60 to 100 dB sensorineural hearing loss. Hearing was normal in an unaffected male sib and in both parents.

Vestibular System. Caloric vestibular tests were normal.

LABORATORY FINDINGS

No roentgenograms, blood tests, or urine tests were described.

PATHOLOGY

Skin biopsies were not reported.

HEREDITY

Although both parents were Hopi Indians, no consanguinity was demonstrated. There was no history of pigmentary defects or of hearing loss in either parent's family. It is likely that this syndrome is transmitted by an autosomal recessive gene, although X-linked inheritance cannot be excluded.

DIAGNOSIS

This syndrome should be easily differentiated from *X-linked pigmentary abnormalities and congenital sensorineural deafness* in which large leopardlike spots of varying intensity of pigmentation are found. In the syndrome of recessive piebaldness and congenital sensorineural deafness, areas of depigmentation with speckled spots in these areas are the major skin findings. Also, vestibular responses in patients with X-linked pigmentary abnormalities and congenital sensorineural deafness are depressed or absent. In contrast, the caloric responses are normal in the syndrome considered in this section.

Piebaldness may be inherited as an isolated autosomal dominant trait (Sundfor, 1939; Smith and Schulz, 1955). Isolated cases of piebaldness and "profound deafness" were briefly mentioned by Reed, Stone, Boder, and Ziprkowski (1967). The patients, a 6-year-old girl and a 21-year-old man, had broad white forelocks and symmetric white spots over the arms, legs, and abdomen. Their condition was not otherwise documented.

Various authors (Mounier-Kuhn *et al.*, 1958; Fisch, 1959; Houghton, 1964) cited examples of piebaldness and deafness, but they did not document the cases sufficiently for us to judge whether they were examples of this syndrome. Probably, several of the cases were isolated examples of persons having the Waardenburg syndrome but in which dystopia canthorum was not present.

TREATMENT

No treatment other than use of a hearing aid appears to be necessary.

PROGNOSIS

Neither the pigmentary loss nor the deafness was progressive.

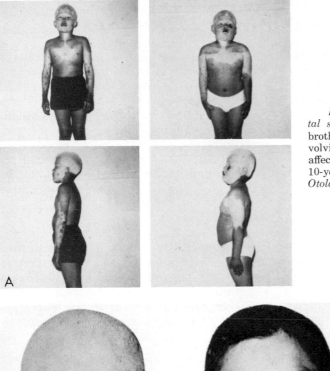

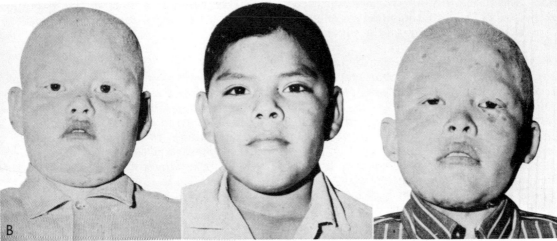

Figure 6-4 *Recessive piebaldness and congenital sensorineural deafness. (A)* Two Hopi Indian brothers showing similarity in depigmentation involving head, arms, and chest. *(B)* Facies of the two affected sibs (8- and 12-years-old) and their normal 10-year-old brother. (From C. M. Woolf *et al., Arch. Otolaryngol., 82*:244, 1965.)

SUMMARY

Characteristics of this syndrome include: 1) probable recessive transmission, 2) pigmentary changes, including depigmentation of head and portions of the arms, and hyperpigmented spots in depigmented areas, 3) normal vestibular responses, and 4) congenital sensorineural deafness.

REFERENCES

Fisch, L., Deafness as part of an hereditary syndrome. *J. Laryngol. Otol., 73*:355–382, 1959.

Houghton, N. I., Waardenburg's syndrome with deafness as the presenting symptom. Report of two cases. *N.Z. Med. J., 63*:83–89, 1964 (case 1).

Mounier-Kuhn, P., Gaillard, J., Chessebeuf, L., Robert, J., Persillon, A., and Morgan, A., Albinisme partiel et surdi-mutité. *J. Fr. Otorhinolaryngol., 7*:915–919, 1958.

Reed, W. B., Stone, V. M., Boder, E., and Ziprkowski, L., Pigmentary disorders in association with congenital deafness. *Arch. Dermatol., 95*:176–186, 1967.

Smith, N. G., and Schulz, H., Partial albinism. *Arch. Dermatol., 71*:468–470, 1955.

Sundfor, H., A pedigree of skin-spotting in man. *J. Hered., 30*:66–77, 1939.

Woolf, C. M., Dolowitz, D. A., and Aldous, H. E., Congenital deafness associated with piebaldness. *Arch. Otolaryngol., 82*:244–250, 1965.

X-LINKED PIGMENTARY ABNORMALITIES AND CONGENITAL SENSORINEURAL DEAFNESS

A Moroccan Jewish family having 14 congenitally profoundly deaf males appearing in three generations was described by Ziprkowski and coworkers (1962) and by Margolis (1962). Four of the affected persons were studied in detail and all showed similar clinical features. An isolated example was reported by Campbell *et al.* (1962).

CLINICAL FINDINGS

Integumentary System. At birth the skin was albinotic except for areas of light pigmentation over the gluteal and scrotal areas. Pigmentation gradually increased, particularly involving the arms, legs, buttocks, and face. Only a few spots appeared on the scalp. The hair remained completely white even when growing in the pigmented areas (Fig. 6–5*A*).

The skin changes ultimately involved the entire body and were characterized by large leopardlike spots of hypopigmentation and hyperpigmentation. Areas of the skin were sharply demarcated with rather symmetric distribution of pigmentary change. Nonpigmented areas were whitish-pink, whereas browned or pleomorphic hyperpigmented areas were mottled with shades of color varying from light brown to a deep brown-black; areas measured from a few millimeters to several centimeters in size.

Ocular System. Campbell *et al.* (1962) described partly albinotic retinas, myopia, and strabismus in their patient.

Auditory System. All affected persons were profoundly congenitally deaf. Otologic examination showed normal auricles, auditory canals, and ear drums. Puretone testing showed no response to frequencies above 500 Hz. No other audiometric tests were described. Female heterozygotes exhibited reduced hearing detectible on audiometry (Fried *et al.*, 1969).

Vestibular System. Caloric vestibular tests showed no vestibular responses in three patients tested. A fourth showed moderate depression of vestibular response, more marked on the left side.

LABORATORY FINDINGS

A series of skull roentgenograms in one patient showed apparently normal cochleas,

semicircular canals, and internal acoustic meatuses. Bone age was normal.

Electrocardiographic tests performed on five patients were found to be normal except for bundle branch block in one patient.

Other examinations, including hemoglobin level, electrophoresis, blood lipid levels, total blood protein, and urinalysis showed results that were all within normal limits.

PATHOLOGY

Histologically, the skin manifested areas of hypopigmentation and hyperpigmentation. The melanocytes in the hypopigmented areas were only weakly dopa-positive, whereas those in the hyperpigmented areas were strongly dopa-positive.

HEREDITY

Fourteen cases of this syndrome have been described in males in three generations of a single kindred (Fig. 6–5*B*). Transmission occurred through clinically unaffected mothers to half of their sons, a pattern characteristic for X-linked inheritance (Ziprkowski *et al.*, 1962).

DIAGNOSIS

This syndrome shows somewhat similar pigmentary skin changes to those found in *recessive piebaldness and congenital sensorineural deafness*. The melanotic pigmentary changes differ, however, in that there are large symmetric areas of depigmentation filled by small flecks of hyperpigmentation in the latter syndrome. This pattern of pigmentation is in contrast to the general lack of pigmentation over the entire body with large confluent pigmented areas appearing in certain sites in the syndrome considered in this section. Furthermore, depressed vestibular response has been noted in this disorder, whereas normal responses have been elicited in recessive piebaldness and congenital sensorineural deafness (Dolowitz, personal communication, 1970.)

TREATMENT

Therapy for hearing loss is symptomatic; a hearing aid may be used, if practical.

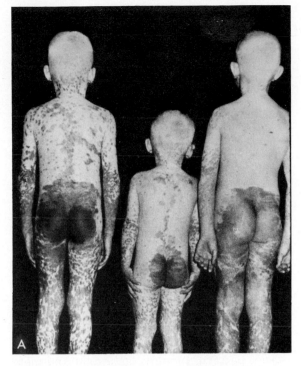

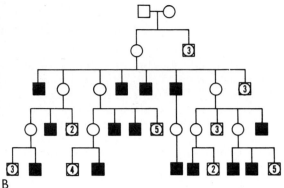

Figure 6–5 X-linked pigmentary abnormalities and congenital sensorineural deafness. (A) Three affected sibs exhibiting characteristic pigmentary pattern. Greatest pigment intensity is over the buttocks and gradually extends with age. Scalp hair is albinoid. (Courtesy of L. Ziprkowski, Tel-Hashomer, Israel.) (B) Pedigree showing 14 affected males in three generations of a family. (Adopted from L. Ziprkowski et al., Arch. Dermatol., 86:30, 1962.)

There is no known treatment for the pigmentary abnormalities other than use of covering creams.

PROGNOSIS

There is no evident change in hearing loss over the patient's life span. Pigmentary changes with increasing spotty pigmentation continue from infancy through the second decade of life but change little thereafter.

SUMMARY

Characteristics of this syndrome include: 1) X-linked transmission, 2) pigmentary changes of the skin beginning in infancy and characterized by large irregular spots of hypopigmentation and hyperpigmentation, 3) congenital profound sensorineural deafness, and 4) depressed vestibular responses.

REFERENCES

Campbell, B., Campbell, N. R., and Swift, S., Waardenburg's syndrome. *Arch. Dermatol.*, 86:718–724, 1962.

Fried, K., Feinmesser, M., and Tsitsianov, J., Hearing impairment in female carriers of the sex-linked syndrome of deafness with albinism. *J. Med. Genet.*, 6:32–134, 1969.

Margolis, E., A new hereditary syndrome—sex-linked deaf-mutism associated with total albinism. *Acta Genet. (Basel), 12*:12–19, 1962.

Margolis, E., Sex-linked albinism associated with deafness. *Ala. J. Med. Sci.*, 3:479–482, 1966.

Ziprkowski, L., Krakowski, A., Adam, A., Costeff, H., and Sade, J., Partial albinism and deaf mutism due to a recessive sex-linked gene. *Arch Dermatol.*, 86:530–539, 1962.

DOMINANT PIEBALD TRAIT, ATAXIA, AND SENSORINEURAL HEARING LOSS

Although possibly described earlier by Hammerschlag (1908), this syndrome was well-defined by Telfer, Sugar, Jaeger, and Mulcahy (1971) in studies of two Pennsylvania kindreds. In the first family 11 persons in four generations were affected. In the second kindred a father and daughter manifested the disorder.

CLINICAL FINDINGS

Integumentary System. All affected persons had congenital absence of pigmentation particularly involving a white forelock, the pubic hair, and variable patterns of absent pigmentation of the forehead, trunk, arms, and legs (Fig. 6–6A–C).

Nervous System. Mental retardation ranging from an I.Q. of 56 to an I.Q. of 86 was found in seven of ten patients. The remaining three had normal intelligence. In all patients with retardation, either ataxia or poor coordination was ascertained by hand rotation testing.

Auditory System. Hearing loss was variable, in some being normal in one ear and showing moderate deafness in the other. Others exhibited mild loss in one ear and profound deafness in the other. Of ten patients examined, six had hearing loss ranging from mild high-frequency loss to profound sensorineural deafness. The hearing loss appeared to be progressive.

Vestibular System. Vestibular testing was not described.

LABORATORY FINDINGS

None were reported.

HEREDITY

Inheritance was clearly autosomal dominant (Fig. 6–6D).

DIAGNOSIS

Several other syndromes show pigmentary abnormalities and deafness. In the syndrome of *X-linked pigmentary abnormalities and congenital sensorineural deafness* the skin lacks pigment at birth but exhibits progressive pigmentation thereafter, and the hearing loss is congenital and profound, differing markedly from the congenital piebaldness and variable hearing loss in the present syndrome. *Waardenburg syndrome*, while being associated with white forelock and vitiligo, also includes broad nasal root, widely spaced medial canthi, synophrys, lack of nasal alar flare, and heterochromia (hypoplasia) irides – none of which are present in the syndrome under discussion.

Recessive piebaldness and congenital sensorineural deafness differs in the inheritance pattern. In addition, ataxia and mental retardation have not been noted in that disorder.

TREATMENT

A hearing aid should be used by patients when indicated.

PROGNOSIS

The hearing loss is progressive, whereas the pigment loss is not.

SUMMARY

This syndrome is characterized by: 1) autosomal dominant transmission, 2) congenital piebaldness, 3) ataxia or coordination difficulties in about 80 per cent, 4) mental retardation in about 80 per cent, and 5) variable, sometimes asymmetric, sensorineural hearing loss in about 60 per cent.

REFERENCES

Hammerschlag, V., Zur Kenntnis der hereditär-degenerativen Taubstummheit. VI. Über einen mutmasslichen Zusammenhang zwischen "hereditärer Taubheit" und "hereditärer Ataxie." *Z. Ohrenheilkd.*, 56:126–138, 1908.

Telfer, M. A., Sugar, M., Jaeger, E. A., and Mulcahy, J., Dominant piebald trait (white forelock and leukoderma) with neurologic impairment. *Am. J. Hum. Genet.*, 23:383–389, 1971.

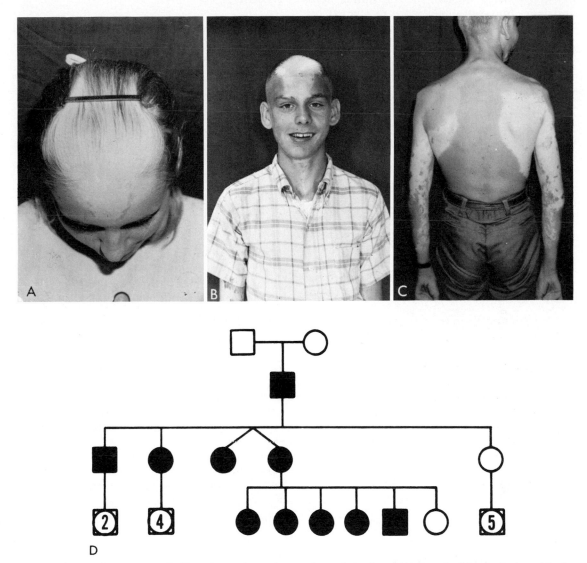

Figure 6-6 *Dominant piebald trait, ataxia, and sensorineural deafness.* (*A*) Broad white forelock and leuko-derma of forehead with hyperpigmented borders. (*B*) White forelock, depigmented forehead, and medial whitening of eyebrows. (*C*) Dorsal view of individual in *B*, exhibiting extensive leukoderma of arms and back. (*D*) Pedigree of kindred showing autosomal dominant inheritance. (From M. A. Telfer *et al.*, *Am. J. Hum. Genet.*, *23*:383, 1971.)

VITILIGO MUSCLE WASTING, ACHALASIA, AND CONGENITAL SENSORINEURAL DEAFNESS

A brother and sister with congenital severe sensorineural deafness, congenital depigmented areas on the neck and torso, marked muscle wasting in the hands, feet and legs, and achalasia were described by Rozycki, Ruben, Rapin, and Spiro (1971).

CLINICAL FINDINGS

Physical Findings. Height was reduced below the third percentile.

Integumentary System. Both patients had depigmented areas over the neck and torso. There were no hyperpigmented spots in these areas (Fig. 6–7*A*).

Nervous System. Marked muscle wasting was evident in the hands, feet, and legs (Fig. 6–7*B*). Both sibs had hyperreflexia with flexor plantar responses and normal sensation. A history of frequent vomiting and dysphagia was noted for both patients.

Auditory System. Both sibs had congenital severe sensorineural deafness (Fig. 6–7*C*).

Vestibular System. Caloric vestibular tests were normal.

LABORATORY FINDINGS

An anterior tibialis muscle biopsy in the male revealed grouped muscle atrophy, indicating neuropathy that was confirmed by electromyography in both patients. A barium swallow, esophageal pressure studies, and responses to methacholine indicated achalasia in both sibs. Extensive laboratory studies were essentially normal except for elevated thymol turbidity and possible cephalin-cholesterol flocculation.

HEREDITY

Since the parents were first cousins and clinically normal the syndrome probably has autosomal recessive inheritance (Fig. 6–7*D*).

DIAGNOSIS

In the syndrome of *recessive piebaldness and congenital sensorineural deafness* there are small, hyperpigmented spots in areas of depigmentation. Musculature and esophageal motility are normal, however, in contrast to the vitiligo, muscle wasting, and achalasia seen in the syndrome considered here.

TREATMENT

The male's achalasia was relieved by esophageal dilatation.

PROGNOSIS

The syndrome is not life-threatening. The deafness is not progressive.

SUMMARY

The syndrome is characterized by: 1) autosomal recessive transmission, 2) mild vitiligo, 3) short stature, 4) distal neuropathic muscle wasting, more marked in the legs, 5) abnormal esophageal motility, and 6) congenital severe sensorineural deafness.

REFERENCES

Rozycki, D. L., Ruben, R. J., Rapin, I., and Spiro, A. J., Autosomal recessive deafness associated with short stature, vitiligo, muscle wasting, and achalasia. *Arch. Otolaryngol., 93*:194–197, 1971.

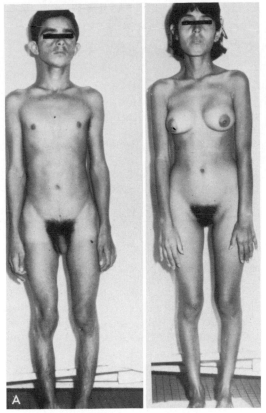

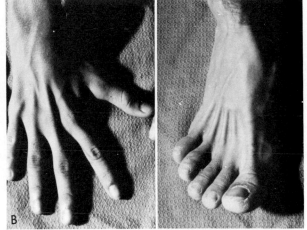

Figure 6-7 Vitiligo, muscle wasting, achalasia, and congenital sensorineural deafness. *(A)* Sibs having short stature and muscle wasting. *(B)* Muscle wasting of hands and feet. *(C)* Audiogram of the two sibs. *(D)* Pedigree of affected sibs. (*A–D* from D. A. Rozycki *et al.*, Arch. Otolaryngol., *93*:194, 1971.)

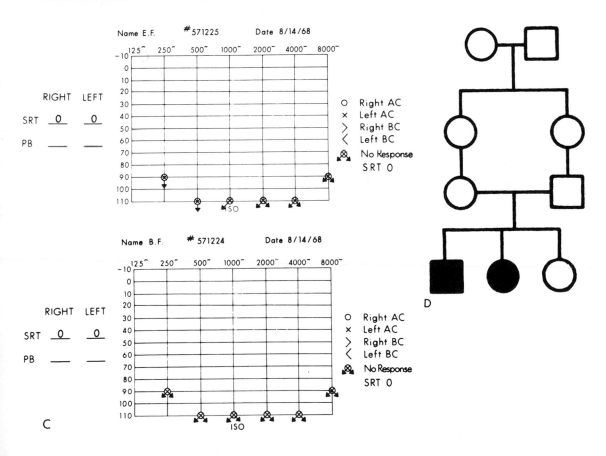

ATYPICAL ERYTHROKERATODERMA, SOMATIC RETARDATION, PERIPHERAL NEUROPATHY, AND CONGENITAL SENSORINEURAL DEAFNESS

Beare, Nevin, Froggat, Kernohan, and Allen (1972) reported an 8-year-old female with an atypical form of erythrokeratoderma, somatic retardation, neurologic disturbances and sensorineural deafness. Patients having similar features were reported by Haxthausen (1955), Pindborg and Gorlin (1962), Schnyder, Wissler, and Wendt (1968) and Rycroft et al. (1976). Possibly, the child reported by Lancaster and Fournet (1969) had the same disorder.

CLINICAL FINDINGS

Physical Findings. Height was reduced below the third percentile in the patient of Beare et al. (1972). From birth, all children had exhibited an erythematous rash, which was bilateral but not quite symmetric, on the face, limbs, and buttocks (Fig. 6–8A, B). The margins of the reddish patches changed slowly, becoming more extensive with time. The dorsa of the feet exhibited hyperkeratotic lesions (Fig. 6–8C). The palms manifested an orange-peel change (Fig. 6–8D). The nails were dystrophic, thickened, and yellow. Hyperplastic lesions about the mouth and keratosis have been documented (Rycroft et al., 1976).

Nervous System. At 2 years of age, the patient reported by Beare et al. (1972) began walking on her toes. This condition progressed until she was no longer able to put her heels on the ground. There was absence of tendon reflexes in the lower extremities.

Both psychic and somatic retardation were noted in the patient of Schnyder et al. (1968). Mild mental retardation was reported by Lancaster and Fournet (1969).

Auditory System. Profound bilateral congenital generalized sensorineural hearing loss with minimal residual low-tone retention in both ears and slight middle-tone retention in one ear were demonstrated by Beare et al. In the patient of Schnyder et al. (1968), deafness was unilateral (Fig. 6–8E). The patients of Haxthausen (1955) and Pindborg and Gorlin (1962) were congenitally deaf.

LABORATORY FINDINGS

Electromyograms and nerve conduction studies in the child described by Beare et al. (1972) demonstrated a neuropathy. Muscle biopsy showed small fibers with little variation in fiber size. A focal infiltrate of lymphocytes was noted around isolated fibers underlying dissolution. In the patient of Schnyder et al. (1968) an electromyogram, muscle biopsy, and nerve conduction studies were normal.

Histologic study of the skin showed hyperkeratosis and a mild chronic inflammatory infiltrate around blood vessels in the upper dermis. The oral mucosa exhibited marked intraepithelial edema throughout its entire thickness.

Carcinoma of the tongue developed in the child reported by Lancaster and Fournet (1969).

HEREDITY

All patients have been isolated cases. Parents and sibs have been normal. Although classic erythrokeratoderma variabilis is heritable as a dominant trait (see below), there is no evidence that the syndrome discussed here is genetic. Perhaps each child represents a new dominant mutation, but proof to confirm this is needed.

DIAGNOSIS

The syndrome under discussion shares several features with the syndrome of *gen-*

Figure 6–8 *Atypical erythrokeratoderma, somatic retardation, peripheral neuropathy, and sensorineural deafness.* (A) Nine-year-old female with generalized cutaneous thickening, more marked and pigmented over lower extremities. (B) Scalp and face involved with marked keratosis that is papillomatous in some areas, especially around mouth. (C) Dorsa of hands were pigmented and rough. (A–C from J. J. Pindborg and R. J. Gorlin, *Acta Derm. Venereol. (Stockh.),* 42:63, 1962.) (D) "Orange peel" changes on palms; similar changes on soles. (E) Audiogram indicating hearing loss in 11-year-old child. (D and E from U. M. Schnyder et al., *Helvet. Paediatr. Acta,* 23:220, 1968.)

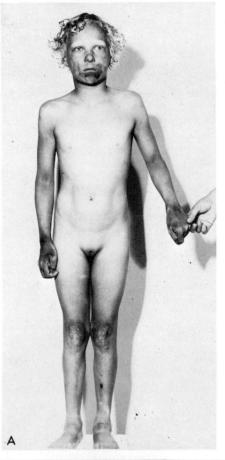

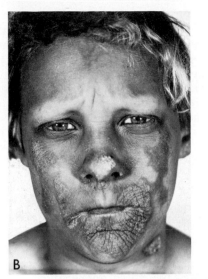

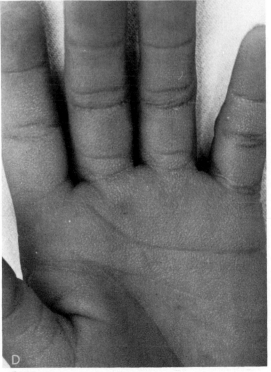

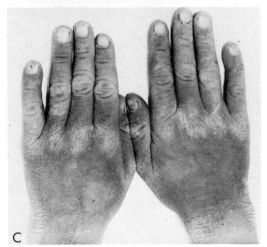

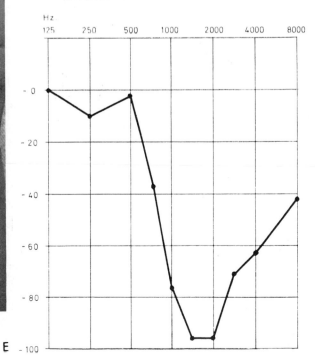

Figure 6-8 See legend on the opposite page

eralized spiny hyperkeratosis, universal alopecia, and congenital sensorineural deafness. Whether the conditions are the same disorder cannot be answered at this time but we suspect they are.

The skin lesions most closely resemble those of erythrokeratoderma variabilis, which is inherited as an autosomal dominant trait. However, the erythematous patches in that disorder, erratically outlined, alter in size and shape from day to day. The hyperkeratotic patches have a striking geographic outline; in contrast to the erythematous patches, however, they tend to be site-specific, involving particularly the face, buttocks, and extensor surface of limbs.

In the syndrome under consideration, the skin lesions are typical in appearance, but they fail to exhibit the marked fluctuation in size, location and shape.

Desmons *et al.* (1971) described congenital ichthyosiform erythroderma, congenital sensorineural deafness, and late-onset hepatomegaly in three of six children of consanguineous parents. There was mild growth retardation.

Other erythrokeratodermas have been reviewed by Beare *et al.* (1966), but none

were associated with deafness. Patients with ichthyosiform erythroderma and deafness have been briefly mentioned by Fraser (1971). Inheritance was not known.

An autosomal dominantly inherited syndrome of congenital sensorineural deafness, ichthyosis congenita, and mental retardation was reported in 20 members in three generations; documentation, however, was so scant that we are uncertain as to the nature of the disorder (Gryczynska and Omulecki, 1973).

TREATMENT

There is no therapy for the skin lesions. A hearing aid may be employed as needed.

PROGNOSIS

There is no evidence that the deafness or skin lesions are progressive.

SUMMARY

The characteristics of this syndrome include: 1) uncertain inheritance, 2) atypical erythrokeratoderma, 3) peripheral neuropathy, and 4) congenital sensorineural deafness.

REFERENCES

Beare, J. M., Froggatt, P., Jones, J. H., and Neill, D. W., Familial annular erythema. An apparently new dominant mutation. *Br. J. Dermatol.,* 78:59–68, 1966.

Beare, J. M., Nevin, N. C., Froggatt, P., Kernohan, D. C., and Allen, I. V., Atypical erythrokeratoderma with deafness, physical retardation, and peripheral neuropathy. *Br. J. Dermatol.,* 87:308–314, 1972.

Desmons, F., Bar, J., and Chevillard, Y., Érythrodermie icthyosiforme congénitale sèche, súrdimutité, hépatomegalia, de transmission récessive autosomique. *Bull. Soc. Fr. Dermatol. Syph,* 78:585–591, 1971.

Fraser, G. R., The role of genetic factors in the causation of human deafness. *Audiology (Basel)* 10:212–221, 1971.

Gryczyñska, D., and Omulecki, A., Syndrome of deafness, ichthyosis congenita and mental retardation with dominant inheritance. *Otolaryngologia Polska, 27:*647–652, 1973. (in Polish).

Haxtausen, H., Hyperkeratosis ichthyosiformis? – acanthosis nigricans? in a 4-year-old girl with congenital deafness. *Acta Derm Venereol. (Stockh.), 35:*191–192, 1955.

Lancaster, L., Jr., and Fournet, L. F., Carcinoma of the tongue in a child. *J. Oral Surg., 27:*269–270, 1969.

Pindborg, J. J., and Gorlin, R. J., Oral changes in acanthosis nigricans (juvenile type). *Acta Derm. Venereol. (Stockh.),42:*63–71, 1962.

Rycroft, R. J. G., Moynahan, E. J., and Wells, R. S., Atypical ichthyosiform erythroderma, deafness and keratosis. A report of two cases. *Br. J. Dermatol., 94:*211–218, 1976.

Schnyder, V. W., Wissler, H., and Wendt, G. G., Eine weitere Form von atypischer Erythrokeratoderma mit Schwerhörigkeit und cerebraler Schädigung. *Helv. Paediatr. Acta, 23:*220–230, 1968.

GENERALIZED SPINY HYPERKERATOSIS, UNIVERSAL ALOPECIA, AND CONGENITAL SENSORINEURAL DEAFNESS

Morris, Ackerman, and Koblenzer (1969) reported a syndrome of generalized hyperkeratosis, universal alopecia, and sensorineural deafness. In 1971 Myers, Stool, and Koblenzer reviewed the same patient and described another infant with the same disorder. Wilson, Grayson, and Pieroni (1973), and Šalomon et al. (1974) described other examples.

CLINICAL FINDINGS

Integumentary System. Soon after birth, the skin becomes thick and the few scalp hairs are lost. There are markedly diminished sweating and frequent episodes of hyperthermia in warm weather.

The skin exhibits marked, generalized hyperkeratosis, some sites having spinelike projections of heaped keratin, whereas other places, such as the periorbital, perioral, and groin areas, are less hyperkeratinized. Follicular plugging is evident on the extremities. The palms and soles are uniformly hyperkeratotic. There is universal alopecia with the exception of the eyelids having an occasional eyelash.

Acanthosis nigricans and nail involvement were noted by Wilson et al. (1973) and Šalomon et al. (1974).

Other Findings. Wilson et al. (1973) reported obstruction of the lacrimal puncta and vascularization of the cornea.

Auditory System. Congenital bilateral moderately severe sensorineural loss, more marked in the high tones, was noted. The external auditory canals were filled with hard, thick debris. When this was removed, the tympanic membranes were noted to be thickened.

Vestibular System. Vestibular testing was not mentioned.

LABORATORY FINDINGS

Šalomon et al. (1974) found low urinary levels of cystine, lysine, histidine and arginine.

PATHOLOGY

The temporal bones in one infant showed Scheibe's cochleosaccular abnormality (Myers et al., 1971).

Histopathologic study of the skin revealed basket-weave hyperkeratosis. The dilated orifices of the pilar units were plugged, and the hair follicles were atrophied.

HEREDITY

Affected children were isolated males. The parents and sibs did not have similar anomalies. Whether this syndrome represents a genetic entity requires documentation of additional cases.

DIAGNOSIS

This syndrome most closely resembles *atypical erythrokeratoderma, somatic retardation, peripheral neuropathy, and congenital sensorineural deafness.* There are several shared features and whether these represent separate entities is not known.

Ichthyosis in its many forms can be excluded on clinical and histologic grounds. Ichthyosiform erythroderma can also be excluded, since it is not associated with universal alopecia.

TREATMENT

The skin can be treated with topical lubricants. A hearing aid can be employed.

PROGNOSIS

One child died in infancy from aspiration. Whether this death resulted from the child's having the syndrome cannot be ascertained from the limited number of examples.

SUMMARY

Characteristics of this syndrome include: 1) generalized spiny hyperkeratosis, 2) universal alopecia, 3) hypohidrosis, 4) obstruction of lacrimal punctae and vascularization of cornea, and 5) congenital sensorineural deafness.

REFERENCES

Morris, J., Ackerman, A. B., and Koblenzer, P. J., Generalized spiny hyperkeratosis, universal alopecia, and deafness. *Arch. Dermatol., 100*:692–698, 1969.

Myers, E. N., Stool, S. E., and Koblenzer, P. J., Congenital deafness, spiny hyperkeratosis, and universal alopecia. *Arch. Otolaryngol., 93*:68–74, 1971.

Šalomon, T., Budai, V., Lazović, O., Macanović, K., and Volić, N., Erythrodermia ichthyosiformis congenita, mit Hypotrichose, Anhidrose, Taubstummheit und verminderten Ausscheidung einiger Aminosäuren im Harn. *Hautarzt, 25*:448–453, 1974.

Wilson, F. M., Grayson, M., and Pieroni, D., Corneal changes in ectodermal dysplasia. *Am. J. Ophthalmol., 75*:17–27, 1973.

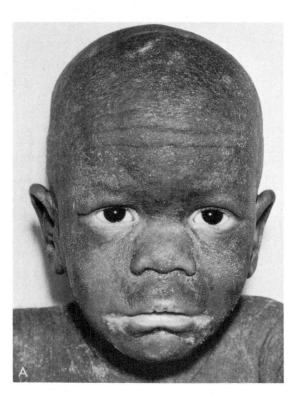 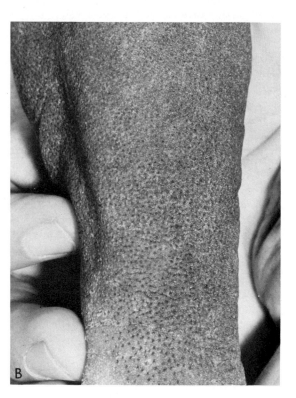

Figure 6–9 See legend on the opposite page

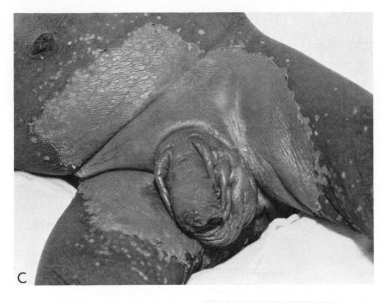

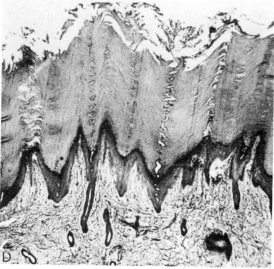

Figure 6–9 Generalized spiny hyperkeratosis, universal alopecia, and congenital sensorineural deafness. (A) Generalized hyperkeratosis and absence of hair. *(B)* Follicular plugging on extremities. *(C)* Peeling of stratum corneum in groin area. *(D)* Prominent stratum corneum; no hair present. *(E)* Puretone audiogram showing severe bilateral sensorineural impairment. *(A–C* from J. Morris *et al., Arch. Dermatol., 100*:692, 1969; *D* and *E* from E. N. Myers *et al., Arch. Otolaryngol., 93*:68, 1971.)

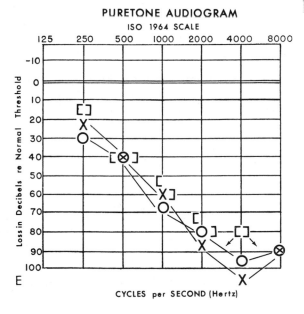

PURETONE AUDIOGRAM
ISO 1964 SCALE

KERATOPACHYDERMIA, DIGITAL CONSTRICTIONS, AND SENSORINEURAL DEAFNESS

Congenital sensorineural deafness, hyperkeratosis involving the palms, soles, knees, and elbows, and ringlike furrows developing on the fingers and toes were the major features of a syndrome affecting four members of a kindred described by Nockemann (1961). A similarly involved individual was reported by Drummond (1939). An affected father and daughter were documented by Gibbs and Frank (1966).

CLINICAL FINDINGS

Integumentary System. At about 2 years of age, thickening of the palmar and plantar skin began and was followed by involvement of the elbows and knees. At about 5 years of age, ring-shaped furrows developed in the skin and soft tissues of the middle phalanx of all fingers and toes. This condition was severe enough to require digital amputation in several of the affected persons (Nockemann, 1961).

Drummond's patients developed constricting bands about three fingers of each hand. The bands were about 1/8 to 1/4 inch in width and encircled each of the affected fingers. A marked hyperkeratosis of the palms and a thickening of the epidermis over the knuckles and knees were evident.

In the patient described by Gibbs and Frank (1966) the hyperkeratoses of the dorsa of the hands and feet were starfish-shaped; those on the knees and elbows tended to be linear. Diffuse alopecia of the scalp began at about 15 years of age. Ainhumlike constriction of all toes appeared near the posterior nail fold.

Auditory System. All individuals reported by Nockemann (1961) and Drummond manifested congenital profound deafness. No other audiometric information was presented. The female patient documented by Gibbs and Frank (1966) had bilateral mild high-frequency sensorineural deafness. Her father had been similarly affected.

Vestibular System. No mention was made of vestibular tests by any author.

LABORATORY FINDINGS

Roentgenograms. Radiographs of the feet of the proband described by Gibbs and

Frank (1966) showed constriction of the shaft of the distal phalanx of the right fourth toe. Other laboratory studies were normal.

PATHOLOGY

Histologic examination of one of the digits, which had been removed because of severe pain, showed marked thickening of the stratum corneum of the skin (Nockemann, 1961). In the area of the groove this layer was reduced to half this thickness. The remaining layers of the epithelium were normal, but somewhat thinner in the area of constriction. Elastic fibers were more abundant and interconnected in the area of the groove.

HEREDITY

Two pedigrees showed dominant transmission of this syndrome (Nockemann, 1961; Gibbs and Frank, 1966) (Fig. 6–10E). The patient presented by Drummond (1939) was an isolated example. Since there has not been male-to-male transmission in any case, X-linked dominant transmission cannot be excluded.

DIAGNOSIS

Ainhumlike constriction of the digits and hyperkeratosis of the palms and soles were described by Wigley (1929); deafness was not mentioned. Ringlike constriction of the digits, seen with a plethora of hereditary and nonhereditary conditions, has been extensively reviewed by Gibbs and Frank (1961). However, in none of these conditions was there associated deafness.

The syndrome of keratopachydermia, digital constrictions, and deafness can be distinguished from other isolated cases of annular constrictions of the fingers and toes because of the marked hearing loss and the dominant transmission of the syndrome.

TREATMENT

Treatment includes use of a hearing aid. The only therapy presently available

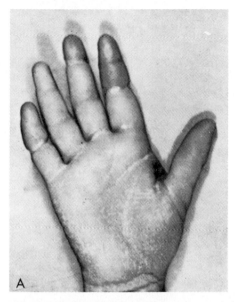

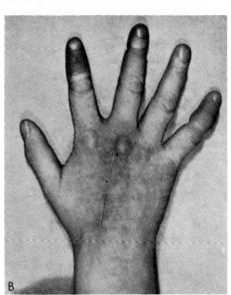

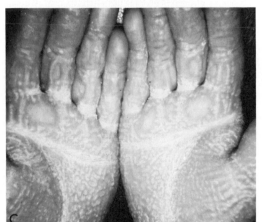

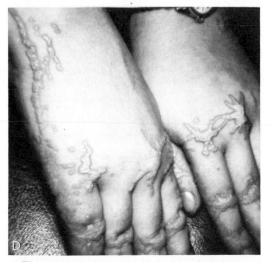

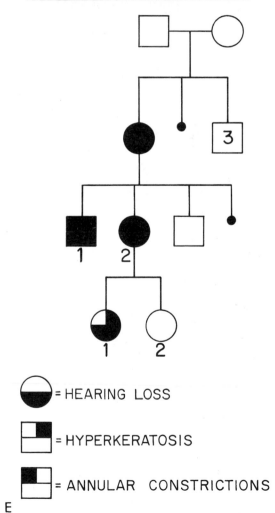

Figure 6–10 *Keratopachydermia, digital constrictions, and sensorineural deafness. (A and B)* Palm and dorsum of hand showing keratopachydermia and constriction of fifth digit. *(A and B* from M. Drummond, *Ir. J. Med. Sci.,* 8:56, 1939.) *(C and D)* Keratopachydermia of palms. Linear and starfishlike excrescences over the knuckles. *(C and D* from R. C. Gibbs and S. B. Frank, *Arch. Dermatol.,* 94:619, 1966.) *(E)* Pedigree of affected kindred. (Modified from P. F. Nockemann, *Med. Welt,* 2:1894, 1961.)

for the constricted fingers is surgical amputation, if necessary.

PROGNOSIS

There is no apparent change in hearing loss with age. The prognosis for the involved digits is poor, since there is usually continuing constriction of the phalanges and eventual loss of some digits.

SUMMARY

Characteristics of this syndrome include: 1) dominant transmission, probably autosomal, 2) hyperkeratosis of the palms, soles, elbows, and knees, 3) ringlike constrictions of the soft tissues of the middle phalanges of the fingers and toes, and 4) congenital mild to severe sensorineural deafness.

REFERENCES

Bitici, O. O., Familial hereditary progressive sensorineural hearing loss with keratosis palmaris and plantaris. *J. Laryngol. Otol., 89*:1143–1146, 1975.

Drummond, M., A case of unusual skin disease. *Ir. J. Med. Sci., 8*:85–86, 1939.

Gibbs, R. C., and Frank, S. B., Keratoma hereditaris mutilans (Vohwinkel). *Arch. Dermatol., 94*:619–625, 1966.

Nockemann, P . F., Erbliche Hornhautverdickung mit Schnürfurchen an Fingern und Zehen und Innenohrschwerhörigkeit. *Med. Welt., 56*:1894–1900, 1961.

Wigley, J. E. M., A case of hyperkeratosis palmaris et plantaris associated with ainhum-like constriction of the fingers. *Br. J. Dermatol., 41*:188–191, 1929.

ANHIDROSIS AND PROGRESSIVE SENSORINEURAL HEARING LOSS

Congenital anhidrosis is one of many ectodermal dysplasias. It may occur as an isolated finding, but usually it is associated with other skin defects—most frequently, oligodontia and hypotrichosis. In 1946, Helweg-Larsen and Ludvigsen described a syndrome characterized by congenital anhidrosis and progressive sensorineural hearing loss. The authors examined six affected family members and diagnosed eight other cases by history.

CLINICAL FINDINGS

Integumentary System. Patients exhibited a marked inability to sweat; onset was at about 1 year of age. During heavy exertion or hot weather the patients felt very uncomfortable and frequently were unable to work because of headache, dyspnea, and palpitation. Instead of sweat, granules of salt appeared on the skin of the axillae, neck, and nasal bridge. A starch-iodine test performed on one patient showed little evidence of sweating except on the bridge of the nose, axillae, forearms, neck, and pectoral regions (Fig. 6–11A). In each of these areas, 6 to 28 sweat spots appeared. During muscular work, no increase in the number of sweat points was noted. The proband was placed in a hot room (52° C) for 50 minutes, and in another test was given 0.3 mg. of pilocarpine subcutaneously. In this individual, sweating was limited to only a few sweat points. By contrast, a normal control individual sweated profusely in both tests.

Auditory System. Five individuals with impaired sweat secretion also suffered from progressive sensorineural hearing loss, which had been noticed first at 35 to 45 years of age. Audiograms obtained on two affected members showed severe high-tone sensorineural hearing loss. No further description of the deafness was made.

Vestibular System. Vestibular tests were not mentioned.

LABORATORY FINDINGS

Complete blood count and urinalysis were normal in the proband.

PATHOLOGY

Skin biopsies from the forearms of two affected persons showed normal hair follicles and blood vessels but no sweat glands or sebaceous glands. Skin biopsy from the axilla of one patient showed a marked lack

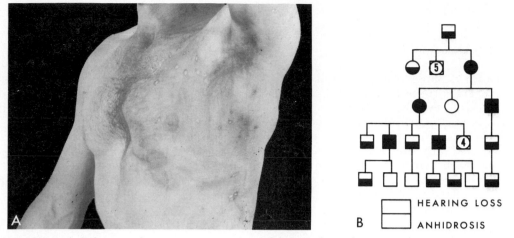

Figure 6–11 Anhidrosis and progressive sensorineural hearing loss. (A) Scattered sweat points in pectoral area indicated by starch-iodine test. *(B)* Pedigree showing 14 affected persons in five generations. *(A* and *B* from H. F. Helweg-Larsen and K. Ludvigsen, *Acta Derm. Venereol. (Stockh.), 26*:489, 1946.)

of sweat glands and only a single hypertrophic sweat gland. No sebaceous glands were seen.

HEREDITY

The diagnosis of anhidrosis was well established in six affected persons tested. Eight additional cases were diagnosed by history. Five of those affected with anhidrosis also had progressive hearing loss, which was confirmed by audiometric tests in two individuals.

The pedigree of the family thus showed 14 affected persons in five generations, a pattern compatible with autosomal dominant inheritance (Fig. 6–11*B*).

DIAGNOSIS

Several types of anhidrosis have been described. An autosomal recessively transmitted form characterized by anhidrosis but without abnormalities of teeth, face, or brain was presented by Mahloudji *et al.* (1967). Both the X-linked and the rare autosomal recessive types of hypohidrotic ectodermal dysplasia include anodontia and hypotrichosis (Gorlin *et al.*, 1970). Anhi-

drosis also occurs in association with congenital sensory neuropathy (Vassella *et al.*, 1968). These types of hereditary anhidrosis differ in mode of transmission and in associated defects from that described here.

TREATMENT

There is no treatment for the anhidrosis other than symptomatic. Patients should refrain from heavy exertion or exposure to hot temperatures since they are subject to hyperthermia. Treatment for the hearing loss is by use of a hearing aid.

PROGNOSIS

The hearing loss is apparently slowly progressive. More persons need to be studied to define clearly the progression of the hearing loss.

SUMMARY

Characteristics of this syndrome include: 1) autosomal dominant transmission, 2) congenital anhidrosis, and 3) onset of progressive sensorineural hearing loss in middle age.

REFERENCES

Gorlin, R. J., Old, T., and Anderson, V. E., Hypohidrotic ectodermal dysplasia in females. A critical analysis and argument for genetic heterogeneity. *Z. Kinderheilkd., 108*:1–11, 1970.

Helweg-Larsen, H. F., and Ludvigsen, K., Congenital familial anhidrosis and neurolabyrinthitis. *Acta Derm. Venereol. (Stockh.), 26*:489–505, 1946.

Mahloudji, M., and Livingston, K. E., Familial and congenital simple anhidrosis. *Am. J. Dis. Child., 113*:477–479, 1967.

Vassella, F., Emrich, H. M., Kraus-Ruppert, R., Aufdermaur, F., and Tonz, O., Congenital sensory neuropathy with anhidrosis. *Arch. Dis. Child., 43*:124–130, 1968.

GENERALIZED ALOPECIA, HYPOGONADISM, AND SENSORINEURAL DEAFNESS

Crandall, Samec, Sparkes, and Wright (1973) reported three affected brothers with short stature. Two had secondary hypogonadism, sensorineural deafness, and alopecia. A third brother was similarly involved but exhibited only minimal hypogonadism. They had been reported earlier by Reed *et al.* (1967) as persons having the Björnstad syndrome before they had been recognized as having hypogonadism.

CLINICAL FINDINGS

Integumentary System. The boys exhibited lanugo hair at birth but lost this and never developed body, axillary, or pubic hair. They had only very sparse head hair, which was broken about 0.5 cm. from the scalp. Eyelashes were short, curled, and deficient. The eyebrows were absent.

Genital System. Infrequent erections and/or ejaculations were experienced. The testes were markedly reduced in size in two of the boys.

Musculoskeletal System. Height ranged between the third and twenty-fifth percentile. The upper-to-lower segment ratio ranged from normal in two brothers to 1.22 in the other brother. Bone age was slightly decreased. The carrying angle was increased in two of the boys. Muscular development was generally poor.

Other Findings. Mental development was slightly retarded in two brothers. A high-pitched voice noted in all three boys was attributed to a prepubertal larynx.

Auditory System. A sensorineural hearing loss was detected at time of schooling. The deafness was described as being slowly progressive and ranged from 65 to 85 dB at the time of testing at 18 to 21 years. The monotonous voice, however, suggests earlier onset.

Vestibular System. No studies were reported.

LABORATORY FINDINGS

Plasma-luteinizing hormone and testosterone levels were significantly reduced in two boys. Normal response to human chorionic gonadotropin indicated gonadotropin insufficiency. There was also diminished release of growth hormone.

Microscopic examination of the head hair showed twisting of the hair shaft, characteristic of pili torti.

Dermatoglyphic analysis exhibited low total ridge counts in two of the boys.

HEREDITY

The occurrence of the syndrome in three sons of normal parents suggests recessive inheritance. X-linkage cannot be completely ruled out, but there were none affected among seven children from the mother's second marriage, and she did not exhibit any stigmata of a possible carrier.

DIAGNOSIS

Pili torti as an isolated entity may be sporadic or may exhibit autosomal recessive inheritance (Appel and Messina, 1942). This disorder must be differentiated from the syndrome of *pili torti and sensorineural hearing loss,* which exhibits autosomal dominant inheritance. Growth hormone deficiency (Goodman *et al.,* 1968; Poskitt and Rayner, 1974) and luteinizing hormone deficiency (Ewer, 1968) occur as separate disorders, but they are not associated with deafness or with a total lack of body hair as in the syndrome considered here.

TREATMENT

Testosterone and growth hormone therapy is indicated. A wig may be worn for cosmetic purposes. A hearing aid may be of some benefit.

SUMMARY

The syndrome is characterized by: 1) recessive inheritance, probably autosomal, 2) generalized alopecia with pili torti, 3) growth retardation, 4) hypogonadism, and 5) severe sensorineural hearing loss.

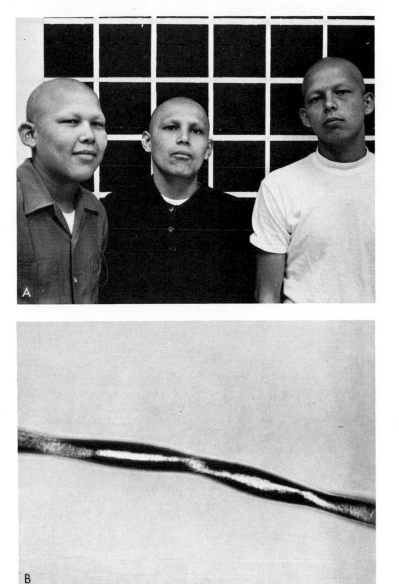

Figure 6–12 *Generalized alopecia, hypogonadism, and sensorineural deafness. (A)* Three male sibs affected with deafness and alopecia. The two brothers on the left also exhibit growth-hormone and luteinizing-hormone deficiency. *(B)* Scalp hair exhibiting characteristic twisting of hair shaft (pili torti). *(A* and *B* from B. F. Crandall *et al., J. Pediatr., 82*:461, 1973.)

REFERENCES

Appel, B., and Messina, S. J., Pili torti hereditaria. *N. Engl. J. Med., 226*:912–915, 1942.

Crandall, B., Samec, L., Sparkes, R. S., and Wright, S. W., A familial syndrome of deafness, alopecia, and hypogonadism. *J. Pediatr., 82*:461–465, 1973.

Ewer, R. W., Familial monotropic pituitary gonadotropin insufficiency. *J. Clin. Endocrinol. Metab., 28*:783–788, 1968.

Goodman, H. G., Grumbach, M. M., and Kaplan, S. L., Isolated growth hormone and multiple pituitary-hormone deficiencies. *N. Engl. J. Med., 278*:57–68, 1968.

Poskitt, E. M., and Rayner, P. H., Isolated growth hormone deficiency: two families with autosomal dominant inheritance. *Arch. Dis. Child., 49*:55–59, 1974.

Reed, W. B., Stone, V. M., Boder, E., and Ziprkowski, L., Hereditary syndromes with auditory and dermatologic manifestations. *Arch. Dermatol., 95*:456–461, 1967.

KNUCKLE PADS, LEUKONYCHIA, AND MIXED HEARING LOSS

A syndrome consisting of leukonychia, knuckle pads, and mixed hearing loss was described by Schwann (1963) and by Bart and Pumphrey (1967).

CLINICAL FINDINGS

Integumentary System. In the kindred studied by Bart and Pumphrey (1967), firm, thickened skin or knuckle pads had appeared over the interphalangeal joints of the fingers (Fig. 6–13*A–D*) and toes since early childhood. All fingernails and toenails exhibited leukonychia (white nails), obscuring the lunula (Fig. 6–13*C*). By history, spoon-nails (koilonychia) had developed in some deaf family members. Hyperkeratosis of the palms and soles appeared in middle life (Fig. 6–13*E*).

Schwann's (1963) 13-year-old male proband had hyperkeratosis of his palms and soles as well as leukonychia.

Auditory System. Audiometric findings in five patients were variable (Bart and Pumphrey, 1967). A 10 to 100 dB hearing loss, most marked in the higher frequencies, was found. In two cases a pure sensorineural hearing loss was present. However, in the remaining three cases mixed hearing loss was present in at least one ear. In another case the right ear showed a 10 to 70 dB sensorineural hearing loss, whereas the left ear had a 70 to 90 dB mixed hearing loss (Fig. 6–13*F*). Exploration of the left middle ear of one patient showed such disorganization of the middle ear structures that the ossicles and facial nerve could not be identified (Fig. 6–13*G*). Schwann (1963) noted congenital severe hearing loss, otherwise unspecified.

Vestibular System. Caloric vestibular tests were described in three individuals. One person showed normal response to caloric testing, whereas another showed no response, indicating vestibular paresis. A third patient had a hypoactive response on the left side and a normal response on the right side (Bart and Pumphrey, 1967).

LABORATORY FINDINGS

Urinalysis, urinary mucopolysaccharides and amino acid paper chromatography, complete blood count, and serum protein electrophoretic pattern were all normal. Roentgenograms of the temporal bones showed normal cochlear and labyrinthine structures.

HEREDITY

Bart and Pumphrey (1967) found a total of 21 affected persons in six generations with autosomal dominant transmission (Fig. 6–13*H*). Nine had only hearing loss, whereas the rest had both hearing loss and leukonychia. It is possible that leukonychia was not noted in those not carefully examined.

DIAGNOSIS

Two other syndromes exhibiting abnormalties of the nails and hearing loss: *dominant onychodystrophy, coniform teeth, and sensorineural hearing loss,* and *recessive onychodystrophy and congenital sensorineural deafness* must be excluded. Patients with the first disorder have several abnormalities, including small, misshapen nails, coniform crowned teeth, and, occasionally, polydactyly and/or syndactyly. Patients with the second disorder have no abnormalities other than small dystrophic nails, present from birth.

TREATMENT

A hearing aid should be employed as indicated. The knuckle pads are not sufficiently esthetically displeasing to merit surgical removal.

PROGNOSIS

The deafness was not progressive.

SUMMARY

Characteristics of the syndrome include: 1) autosomal dominant inheritance, 2) knuckle pads over the fingers and toes, 3) leukonychia, 4) hyperkeratosis of the palms and soles, and 5) mixed mild to severe hearing loss.

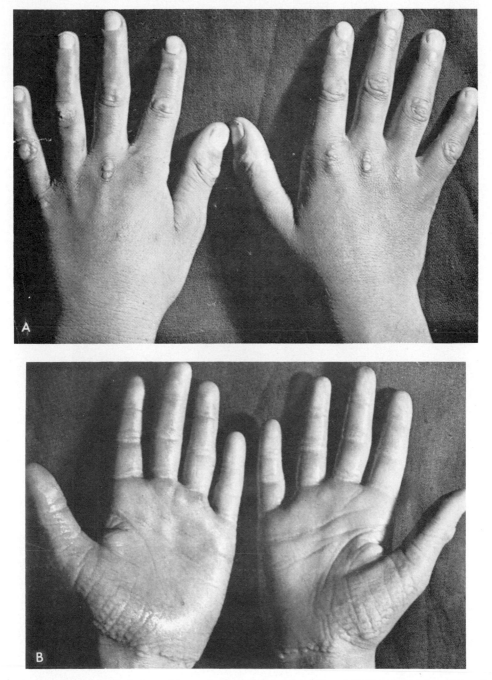

Figure 6–13   *Knuckle pads, leukonychia, and mixed hearing loss. (A and B)* Knuckle pads and keratosis palmaris.

Illustration continued on the following page

REFERENCES

Bart, R. S., and Pumphrey, R. E., Knuckle pads, leukonychia, and deafness: a dominantly inherited syndrome. *N. Engl. J. Med., 276*:202–207, 1967.

Schwann, J., Keratosis palmaris et plantaris cum surditate congenita et leukonychia totale unguium. *Dermatologica, 126*:335–353, 1963.

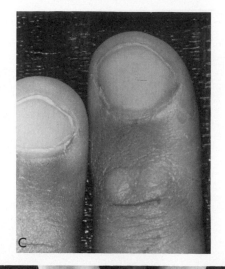

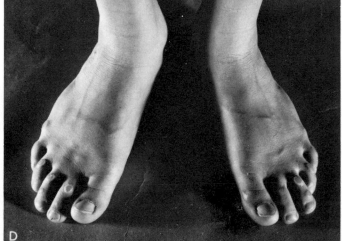

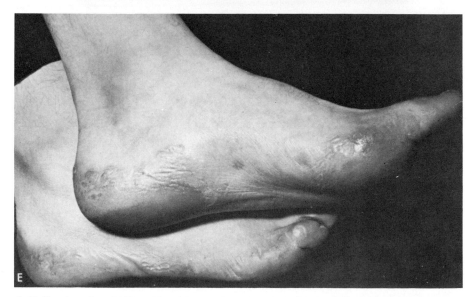

Figure 6–13 Continued. (C) Knuckle pads and leukonychia. (D) Knuckle pads resembling clavi over toes. (E) Hyperkeratosis of soles extending over sides of feet and heels.

Illustration continued on the opposite page

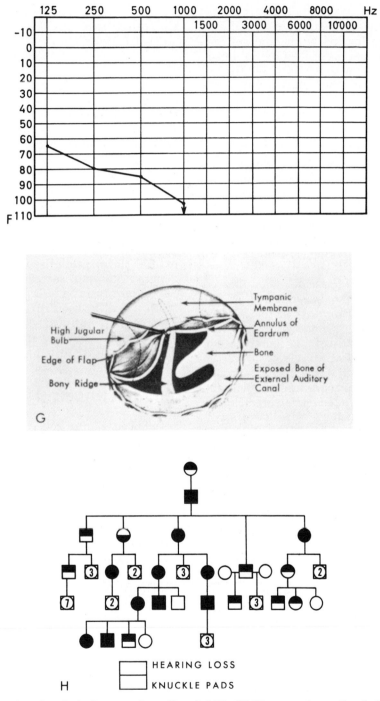

Figure 6-13 *Continued.* *(F)* Audiogram of an affected child. *(G)* Diagram of operative findings in middle ear. The vertical bony ridge is an abnormal structure. The ossicles were not present, but the bony projection on the right side of the drawing may represent a vestige of these structures. *(H)* Pedigree showing 21 affected members in six generations of a kindred. (*A, B, E,* and *H* from J. Schwann, *Dermatologica, 126:*335, 1963; *C, D, F,* and *G* from R. S. Bart and R. E. Pumphrey, *N. Engl. J. Med.,276:*202, 1967.)

DOMINANT ONYCHODYSTROPHY, CONIFORM TEETH, AND SENSORINEURAL HEARING LOSS

A syndrome consisting of small, fissured nails, malformed teeth, and sensorineural deafness was described by Robinson, Miller, and Bensimon in 1962. Of five affected members in the family, four were studied by the authors.

CLINICAL FINDINGS

Integumentary System. Fingernails and toenails were small and fissured (Fig. 6–14*B*), apparently being affected from birth. The hair and skin were normal.

Dental Findings. Each of those affected had coniform crowned teeth, many of which were missing (oligodontia) (Fig. 6–14*A*).

Musculoskeletal System. One affected individual had ulnar hexadactyly of the right hand, whereas another of the kindred exhibited soft tissue syndactyly of the first and second and the third and fourth toes of the right foot (Fig. 6–14 *C*).

Auditory System. A generally symmetric sensorineural hearing loss of 10 to 100 dB was found in all affected persons (Fig. 6–14*D*). Higher frequencies were more strikingly involved, particularly in one patient whose hearing was normal to 4000 Hz but showed profound 100 dB hearing loss at all higher frequencies. One sib showed a severe sensorineural hearing loss of over 70 dB in all frequencies, whereas another sib had almost normal hearing in the very low frequencies but a 60 dB loss in the higher frequencies. Apparently, the hearing loss was congenital, since no progression was noted to develop in later years. Other audiometric tests were not described.

Vestibular System. No vestibular tests were reported.

LABORATORY FINDINGS

Sweat electrolyte concentrations were elevated in two cases and near normal in the other two. No other laboratory tests were described.

HEREDITY

Since the affected persons included three sibs, their mother, and their maternal grandmother (Fig. 6–14*E*), transmission is probably autosomal dominant.

DIAGNOSIS

The syndrome of *recessive onychodystrophy and congenital sensorineural deafness* differs from this syndrome in that the teeth are not affected, the nails do not exhibit the striking fissuring, and transmission is autosomal recessive.

Oligodontia and/or coniform crowned teeth may be seen in a number of syndromes: hypohidrotic ectodermal dysplasia, chondroectodermal dysplasia, Rieger syndrome, incontinentia pigmenti, and others (Gorlin, Pindborg, and Cohen, 1976).

TREATMENT

There is no specific therapy for the onychodystrophy. The teeth may be crowned, and partial dentures may be constructed. The hearing loss can be treated symptomatically.

PROGNOSIS

The nail and tooth anomalies and the hearing loss do not change with time.

SUMMARY

Characteristics of this syndrome include: 1) autosomal dominant transmission, 2) onychodystrophy, 3) teeth with coniform crowns and oligodontia, 4) elevated sweat electrolyte concentrations, and 5) sensorineural hearing loss, varying from moderate to severe.

REFERENCES

Gorlin, R. J., Pindborg, J., and Cohen, M. M., Jr., *Syndromes of the Head and Neck,* 2nd Ed. New York, McGraw-Hill Book Company, 1976.
Robinson, G. C., Miller, J. R., and Bensimon, J. R., Familial ectodermal dysplasia with sensorineural deafness and other anomalies. *Pediatrics, 30*:797–802, 1962.

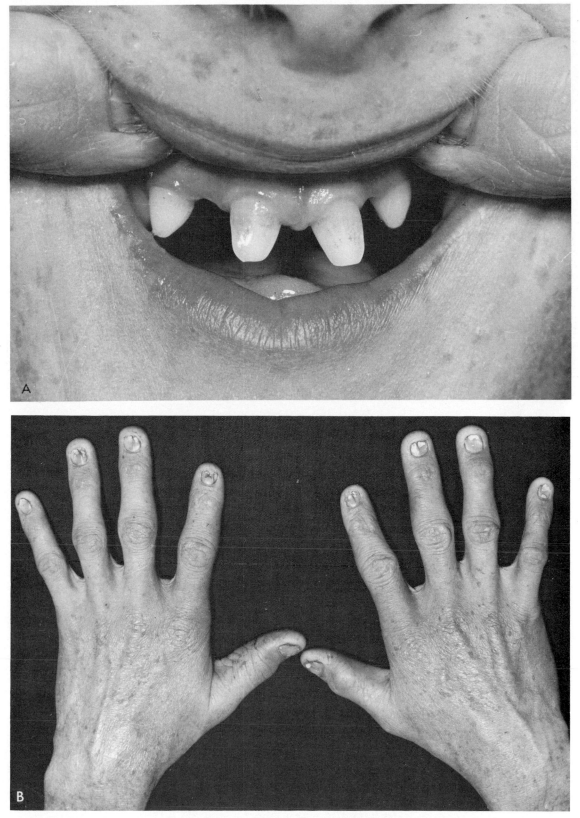

Figure 6–14 *Dominant onychodystrophy, coniform teeth, and sensorineural hearing loss. (A)* Absent and mis-shapen coniform crowned teeth. *(B)* Small dystrophic fingernails having furrows and cracks.

Illustration continued on the following page

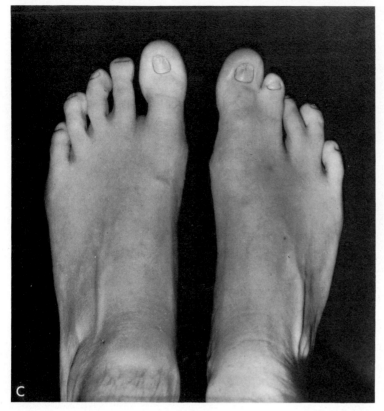

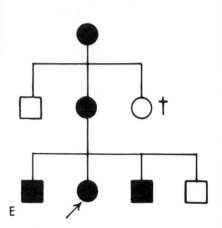

Figure 6-14 Continued. (C) Syndactyly and toenail hypoplasia. (D) Audiograms showing marked variation in degree of hearing loss in different affected persons. (E) Pedigree of family showing five affected persons in three generations. (A–E from G. C. Robinson *et al., Pediatrics, 30*:797, 1962.)

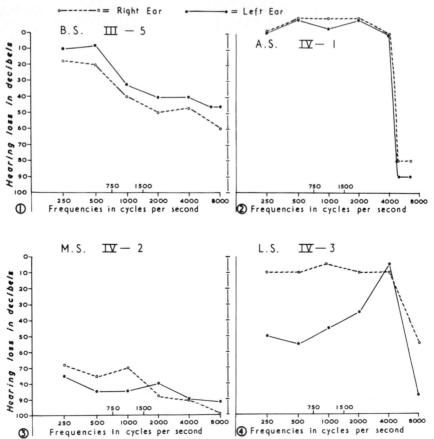

DOMINANT ONYCHODYSTROPHY, TRIPHALANGEAL THUMBS, AND CONGENITAL SENSORINEURAL DEAFNESS

This syndrome, characterized by rudimentary fingernails and toenails and congenital severe sensorineural hearing loss, was described by Goodman, Lockareff, and Gwinup (1969) and by Moghadam and Statten (1972).

CLINICAL FINDINGS

Integumentary System. Affected individuals had very similar abnormalities of their fingernails and toenails. The nails were rudimentary (about one-fourth normal size) but otherwise apparently normally formed (Fig. 6–15A). Hair and skin pigmentation and teeth were normal.

Musculoskeletal System. Triphalangeal thumbs were a characteristic finding. Bulbous swellings of the soft tissue about the terminal phalanges were evident in all, but varied in severity.

Auditory System. Both mother and son in the study of Goodman *et al.* (1969) had congenital severe sensorineural hearing loss. Otologic examination showed no abnormalities of the canals or drums. In the family studied by Moghadam and Statten (1972), the son had severe congenital sensorineural deafness, whereas the mother exhibited a bilateral low-tone moderate (30 to 40 dB) sensorineural deafness.

Vestibular System. Vestibular findings were not reported by either group of investigators.

LABORATORY FINDINGS

Roentgenograms. In the family reported by Goodman *et al.* (1969), roentgenograms of the mother's hands and feet showed an extra phalanx in the right thumb, an absence of a phalanx in both little fingers, and underdevelopment of the tufts of the distal phalanges of the hands (Fig. 6–15B). There was also absence of a phalanx in the second, third, and fourth toes of the left foot (Fig. 6–15C). Findings on the right foot were not noted, nor were roentgenographic findings in the son described. Other skeletal structures, including the mother's skull, pelvis, elbows, and knees were normal. In the family described by Moghadam and Statten (1972), each thumb had three phalanges and the fingers and toes showed pointed or rudimentary phalanges.

HEREDITY

Since this syndrome was found in a mother and son in two kindreds, the disorder appears to be transmitted by a dominant gene. Since there was no male-to-male transmission, X-linked dominant inheritance cannot be excluded.

DIAGNOSIS

This syndrome presumably can be differentiated from *recessive onychodystrophy, triphalangeal thumbs and halluces, mental retardation, seizures and congenital sensorineural deafness* because of its dominant hereditary transmission. Although genetic heterogeneity is possible, this syndrome may be transmitted via a dominant gene which may be incompletely penetrant.

This syndrome can also be distinguished from *dominant onychodystrophy, coniform teeth, and sensorineural hearing loss,* since the teeth in affected individuals were normal.

Sensorineural hearing loss and triphalangeal thumbs may also be seen in the syndrome of *lop ears, sensorineural deafness, imperforate anus, and triphalangeal thumbs.*

TREATMENT

There is no known treatment for the onychodystrophy. Affected persons should undergo a complete hearing evaluation to determine the necessity of using a hearing aid.

PROGNOSIS

The onychodystrophy and deafness are both congenital. There is no evidence of progression of the disease in later life.

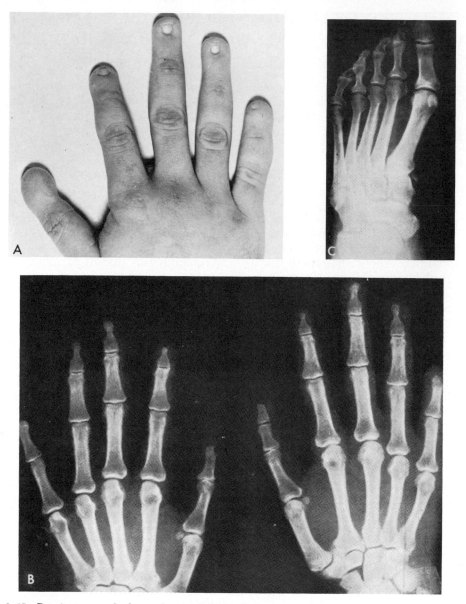

Figure 6–15 *Dominant onychodystrophy, triphalangeal thumbs, and congenital sensorineural deafness. (A)* Right hand of the proband's affected son showing nail and terminal digital changes. *(B)* Roentgenogram of the proband's hands showing underdevelopment of the tufts of the distal phalanges, especially of the index fingers and thumbs. In addition, there is an extra phalanx of the right thumb and absence of a phalanx in both little fingers. *(C)* Roentgenogram of the proband's left foot showing only two distal phalanges in all digits. The terminal tuft of the large toe is also underdeveloped. *(A–C from R. M. Goodman et al., Arch. Otolaryngol., 90:474, 1969.)*

SUMMARY

The major characteristics of this syndrome include: 1) autosomal dominant transmission, 2) onychodystrophy of fingernails and toenails, 3) triphalangeal thumbs, and 4) congenital severe sensorineural hearing loss.

REFERENCES

Goodman, R. M., Lockareff, S., and Gwinup, G., Hereditary congenital deafness with onychodystrophy. *Arch. Otolaryngol., 90:*474–477, 1969.

Moghadam, H., and Statten, P., Hereditary sensorineural hearing loss associated with onychodystrophy and digital malformations. *Can. Med. Assoc. J., 107:*310–312, 1972.

RECESSIVE ONYCHODYSTROPHY, TRIPHALANGEAL THUMBS AND HALLUCES MENTAL RETARDATION, SEIZURES, AND CONGENITAL SENSORINEURAL DEAFNESS

A syndrome characterized by congenital severe sensorineural deafness, rudimentary fingernails and toenails, and dysplastic terminal phalanges was reported by Walbaum, Fontaine, Lienhardt, and Piquet (1970) in male and female sibs. Similar cases were described by Qazi and Smithwick (1970) and by Cantwell (1975).

CLINICAL FINDINGS

Integumentary System. The nails were absent or severely hypoplastic on all fingernails and toenails. Dermatoglyphic studies of finger and toe prints have shown almost all to be arches.

Musculoskeletal System. The thumbs were long and had an extra phalanx and two flexion creases. The little fingers were short and clinodactylous in a few patients.

Neurologic System. All patients were mentally retarded and exhibited grand mal seizures from infancy.

Dental Findings. The teeth have been described as yellow or hypoplastic.

Auditory System. Severe congenital sensorineural hearing loss was evident in all affected.

Vestibular System. No tests of vestibular function have been reported.

LABORATORY FINDINGS

Radiographic examination showed an extra phalanx or greatly enlarged terminal phalanx in the thumbs and halluces. The terminal phalanx was hypoplastic in the remaining fingers and toes. In some patients, there were only two phalanges in the little fingers and fusion of the middle and distal phalanges of the third to fifth toes.

HEREDITY

Parental consanguinity was evident in the cases of Qazi and Smithwick (1970) and in those of Cantwell (1975). The syndrome exhibits autosomal recessive inheritance.

DIAGNOSIS

This syndrome shares many features with *dominant onychodystrophy, triphalangeal thumbs, and congenital sensorineural deafness*, but differs in that it is associated with mental retardation and seizures. The syndrome of *recessive onychodystrophy and congenital sensorineural deafness* does not exhibit digital anomalies.

TREATMENT

Use of a hearing aid, if deemed possible.

PROGNOSIS

The deafness is profound.

SUMMARY

This syndrome is characterized by: 1) autosomal recessive transmission, 2) rudimentary fingernails and toenails, 3) digital abnormalities, including triphalangeal thumbs and halluces and hypoplastic terminal phalanges of the remaining digits, 4) mental retardation, 5) grand mal seizures, and 6) congenital profound sensorineural deafness.

REFERENCES

Cantwell, R. J., Congenital sensori-neural deafness associated with onycho-osteo-dystrophy and mental retardation (D.O.O.R. syndrome). *Humangenetik, 26*:261–265, 1975.

Qazi, Q. H., and Smithwick, E. M., Triphalangy of thumbs and great toes. *Am. J. Dis. Child., 120*:255–257, 1970.

Walbaum, R., Fontaine, G., Lienhardt, J., and Piquet, J. J., Surdité familiale avec ostéo-onychodysplasie. *J. Génét. Hum., 18*:101–108, 1970.

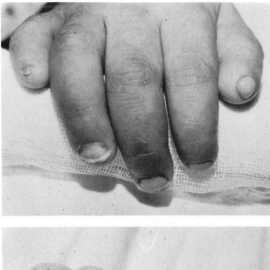

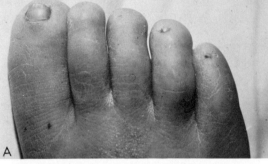

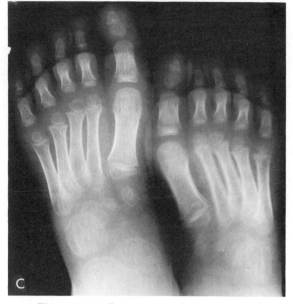

Figure 6–16 *Recessive onychodystrophy, triphal-angeal thumbs and halluces, mental retardation, seizures, and congenital sensorineural deafness. (A)* Hypoplasia of fingernails and toenails. *(B)* Triphalangy of thumbs and hypoplasia of distal phalanges of other digits. *(C)* Triphalangy of halluces and agenesis of terminal phalanges of other toes. *(A–C* from Q. H. Qazi and E. M. Smithwick, *Am. J. Dis. Child., 120:* 255, 1970.)

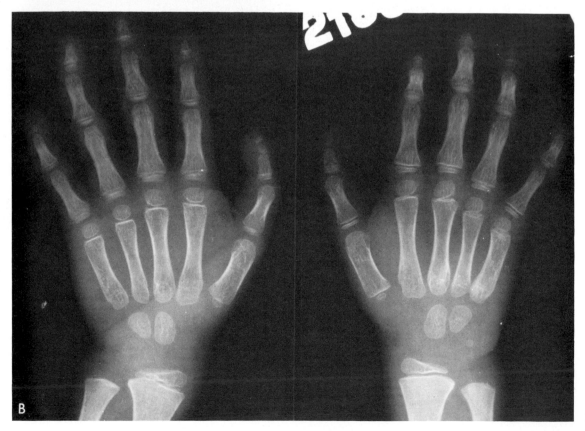

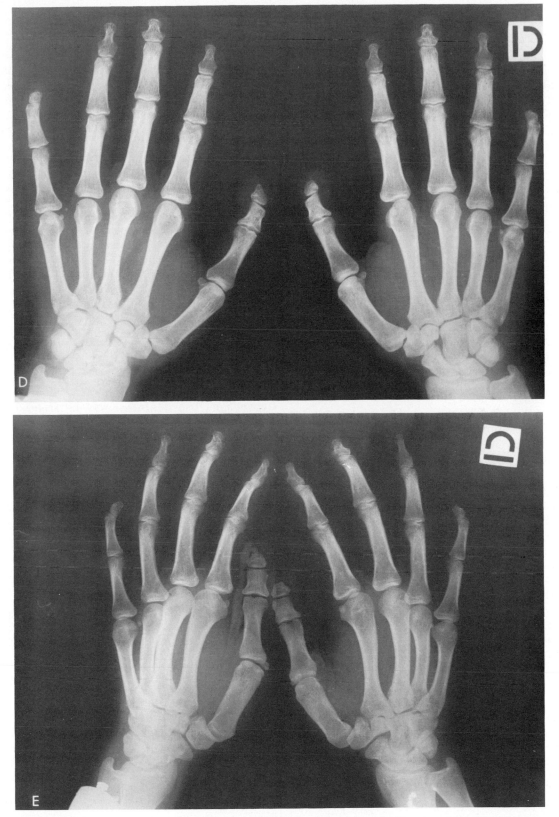

Figure 6–16 Continued. (*D*) Radiograph showing triphalangeal thumbs and blunting of terminal phalanges of third and fifth fingers. (*E*) Radiograph showing similar but less severe changes in another patient. (From R. Walbaum *et al., J. Génét. Hum., 18*:181, 1970.)

RECESSIVE ONYCHODYSTROPHY AND CONGENITAL SENSORINEURAL DEAFNESS

A syndrome characterized by congenital deafness and onychodystrophy occurring in two of five sibs was described by Feinmesser and Zelig (1961).

CLINICAL FINDINGS

Integumentary System. The finger and toenails of the two female sibs showed similar abnormalities. The nails had been short and malformed from birth (Fig. 6–17A). Hair and teeth were normal.

Auditory System. History revealed that the sisters had been congenitally deaf. Audiograms of both girls showed a 60 to 100 dB sensorineural hearing loss, most marked in the higher frequencies. Although otoscopic examination of the older sister showed a normal right ear, evidence of old otitis media was found on the left side. Audiometric testing of the younger sib also showed severe bilateral sensorineural hearing loss.

Vestibular System. Caloric vestibular testing showed hypoactivity of the labyrinth in the older girl and normal vestibular reaction in the younger sib.

LABORATORY FINDINGS

Roentgenograms of the skull and extremities showed no abnormalities. Blood chemistry examinations and urine tests were normal.

HEREDITY

The normal parents were first cousins on the paternal and second cousins on the maternal side (Fig. 6–17B). There was no family history of hearing loss or nail dystrophy. The syndrome appears to be transmitted by an autosomal recessive gene.

DIAGNOSIS

Patients with the nail-patella syndrome have defective nails of the thumbs and index fingers and rudimentary or absent patellae with deformities of the elbows and the presence of iliac horns. However, they do not have associated hearing loss. The syndrome of *dominant onychodystrophy, coniform teeth, and sensorineural hearing loss* has dominant transmission and involves the teeth, in contrast to this syndrome, which has recessive transmission and normal teeth.

TREATMENT

There is no specific therapy for the nail dystrophy other than use of artificial nail coverage. The deafness may be treated in the same manner as other severe sensorineural hearing losses.

PROGNOSIS

There are too few cases for a definite statement on prognosis. There appears to be little change in the nail dystrophy over the years.

SUMMARY

This syndrome is characterized by: 1) autosomal recessive inheritance, 2) congenital onychodystrophy with small, short, fingernails and toenails, and 3) congenital severe sensorineural hearing loss.

REFERENCE

Feinmesser, M., and Zelig, S., Congenital deafness associated with onychodystrophy. *Arch. Otolaryngol.*, 74:507–508, 1969.

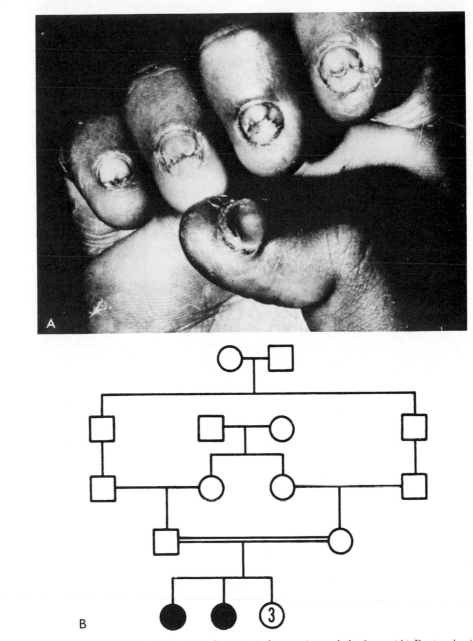

Figure 6-17 *Recessive onychodystrophy and congenital sensorineural deafness. (A)* Dystrophy involving all nails on the right hand of proband. *(B)* Pedigree showing two affected sisters in inbred kindred. *(A* and *B* from M. Feinmesser and S. Zelig, *Arch. Otolaryngol.,* 74:507, 1969.)

PILI TORTI AND SENSORINEURAL HEARING LOSS

A syndrome characterized by pili torti (flat, twisted hair) and sensorineural hearing loss has been described by Björnstad (1965), Reed *et al.* (1967), and Robinson and Johnston (1967).

CLINICAL FINDINGS

Integumentary System. The hair is untidy in appearance, dry, and brittle. Scalp hair, eyebrows and eyelashes are affected (Fig. 6–18*A*). The teeth, nails, and skin are normal. No other physical abnormalities were found in any affected patient.

Auditory System. Although 6 of the 7 reported patients had a 20 to 60 dB hearing loss, the patient described by Robinson and Johnston had severe bilateral sensorineural hearing loss. No other audiometric tests were described.

Vestibular System. Vestibular tests were not reported.

PATHOLOGY

Microscopic examination of the hair show markedly flattened, moderately twisted hairs.

HEREDITY

Although evidence suggests that the syndrome is hereditary, the type of transmission is not clear. Björnstad presented five patients with this disorder: two had affected sibs and one had an affected aunt. The two other patients were isolated examples. Of the four patients described by Reed *et al.,* three had another syndrome (see p. 258), and the fourth boy had a deaf mother who was not examined. Audiograms and physical examinations of the three sibs of the 5-year-old girl described by Robinson and Johnston were normal; there was no family history of hearing loss or hair defect.

It seems likely that these three authors have reported cases of the same syndrome. The only parent with possible involvement (described by Reed *et al.*) was not examined by the authors. Thus, the available data suggest that the syndrome is transmitted by an autosomal recessive gene.

DIAGNOSIS

Pili torti without hearing loss inherited as a dominant trait has been described. Björnstad presented eight patients, only five of whom had sensorineural hearing loss. Whether all had the same syndrome with variable hearing loss or whether there were two separate diseases (genetic heterogeneity)—both with pili torti but only one with hearing loss—is not yet clear. A number of conditions associated with short, brittle hair must be excluded (Menkes' disease, monilethrix, pseudomonilethrix, Netherton disease, trichorrhexis nodosa, argininosuccinic aciduria, etc.) but none has associated deafness (Levin, 1967; Pollitt *et al.,* 1968; Singh and Bresman, 1973; Bentley-Phillips and Bayles, 1973).

TREATMENT

A wig is useful for cosmetic purposes. A hearing aid should be employed.

PROGNOSIS

There is no evidence that the deafness is progressive.

SUMMARY

Characteristics of this disease include: 1) probable autosomal recessive inheritance, 2) congenital pili torti, and 3) congenital moderate to severe sensorineural hearing loss.

REFERENCES

Bentley-Phillips, B., and Bayles, M. A. N., A previously undescribed hereditary hair anomaly (pseudo-monilethrix). *Br. J. Dermatol., 89*:159–167, 1973.
Björnstad, R., Pili torti and sensory neural loss of hearing. *Proc. 17th Meeting Combined Scandinavian Dermatological Association.* Copenhagen, May, 1965.
Levin, B., Argininosuccinic aciduria. *Am. J. Dis. Child., 113*:162–165, 1967.
Pollitt, R. J., Jenner, F. A., and Davies, M., Sibs with mental and physical retardation and trichorrhexis nodosa with abnormal amino acid composition of the hair. *Arch. Dis. Child., 43*:211–216, 1968.

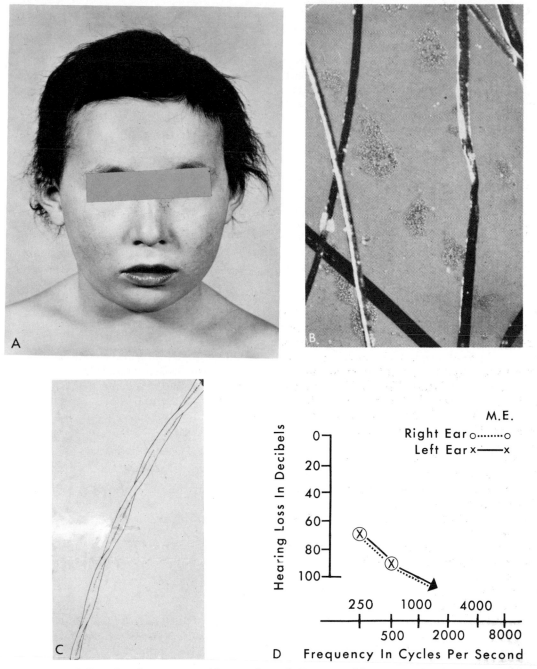

Figure 6–18   *Pili torti and sensorineural hearing loss. (A)* Five-year-old patient with pili torti. *(B)* Scalp hair showing flattening and twisting. *(C)* Drawing showing spiral twisting of hair shaft. (From S. J. Nechamin, *Am. J. Dis. Child.*, 95:612, 1958.) *(D)* Puretone audiogram showing profound bilateral sensorineural hearing loss. *(A, B,* and *D* from G. E. Robinson and M. M. Johnston, *J. Pediatr.*, 70:621, 1967.)

Reed, W. B., Stone, V. M., Boder, E., and Ziprkowski, L., Hereditary syndromes with auditory and dermatological manifestations. *Arch. Dermatol.*, 95:456–461, 1967.

Robinson, G. C., and Johnston, M. M., Pili torti and sensory neural hearing loss. *J. Pediatr.*, 70: 621–623, 1967.

Singh, S., and Bresman, M. J., Menkes' "kinky hair syndrome" (trichopoliodystrophy). *Am. J. Dis. Child.*, 125:572–578, 1973.

SCANTY HAIR, CAMPTODACTYLY, AND SENSORINEURAL HEARING LOSS

A syndrome characterized by congenital alopecia with later scanty, brittle hair, flexion contractures of the little fingers, and moderately severe sensorineural hearing loss was described in a brother and sister by Mikaelian *et al.* (1970).

CLINICAL FINDINGS

Integumentary System. The boy had alopecia until 10 years of age, when sparse and brittle hair developed on his scalp. The authors did not state whether pili torti was present. The girl had sparse hair from early childhood.

Musculoskeletal System. Since birth, the girl had not been able to extend her little fingers, and her brother had some difficulty in full extension of all fingers. Examination showed soft tissue contractures producing a constant flexion at the first interphalangeal joints. The girl had moderate kyphoscoliosis, but her brother had a normal spine. Both sibs were markedly retarded in height and the boy met his milestones late.

Auditory System. The hearing loss, which was probably congenital, was similar in both sibs. It was first noticed in early childhood, and although it was suggested that it was slowly progressive, this point was not documented. Recent hearing tests showed a 45 to 80 dB sensorineural hearing loss, more marked at higher frequencies with speech reception thresholds of about 60 dB bilaterally. A threshold tone-decay test showed no fatigue, and the SISI test was positive bilaterally, suggesting a cochlear locus for the hearing loss.

Vestibular System. Vestibular tests were normal.

LABORATORY FINDINGS

Radiographs showed the head of the proximal phalanx of the little finger to be rotated slightly forward. No bony changes other than the kyphoscoliosis in the girl were noted.

A battery of laboratory tests was normal.

HEREDITY

The two affected persons among ten sibs were the product of a first cousin mating. There was no family history of hearing loss or digital or hair abnormalities. Inheritance appears to be autosomal recessive.

DIAGNOSIS

These sibs may have had the syndrome of *pili torti and sensorineural hearing loss.* However, no microscopic description of the hair was presented. Moreover, in that syndrome, camptodactyly had not been reported.

TREATMENT

A hearing aid and wig may be used.

PROGNOSIS

There is poorly documented evidence that the deafness is slowly progressive.

SUMMARY

Characteristics of this syndrome are: 1) autosomal recessive inheritance, 2) sparse hair, 3) camptodactyly, and 4) sensorineural hearing loss.

REFERENCE

Mikaelian, D. O., Der Kaloustian, V. M., Shahin, N. A., and Barsoumian, V. M., Congenital ectodermal dysplasia with hearing loss. *Arch. Otolaryngol.,* 92:85–89, 1970.

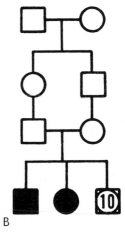

Figure 6-19 *Scanty hair, camptodactyly, and sensorineural hearing loss. (A)* The fingers could not be fully extended. *(B)* Pedigree of affected kindred showing consanguinity. (From D. O. Mikaelian *et al., Arch. Otolaryngol., 92:*85, 1970.)

ATOPIC DERMATITIS AND SENSORINEURAL HEARING LOSS

Two brothers and a sister from a sibship of four manifested nonprogressive sensorineural hearing loss and atypical atopic dermatitis (Konigsmark, Hollander, and Berlin, 1968).

CLINICAL FINDINGS

Integumentary System. Dermatitis was found in all affected sibs, with onset at about 10 years of age. The skin lesions consisted of mild ichthyosis with lichenified, excoriated erythematous areas involving the forearms, elbows, antecubital fossae, wrists, hands, and waist but sparing the legs (Fig. 6–20*A, B*). Because of the later onset and the lack of involvement of the legs, a diagnosis of atypical atopic dermatitis was made.

Auditory System. Hearing loss was first noted at 3 to 5 years of age. In no case was the hearing loss severe enough to cause difficulty in school. Hearing tests at 5 or 6 years of age showed a bilateral symmetric sensorineural hearing loss of 15 to 55 dB for both air and bone conduction. The speech reception threshold corresponded to the expected hearing loss. Speech discrimination was over 90 per cent in all three sibs. The SISI test was 100 per cent at 2000 and 4000 Hz, and tone decay tests were negative. Otologic examination showed no abnormalities except for the hearing loss. Hearing tests repeated over a 10-year period showed no progression of the deafness.

Vestibular System. Caloric vestibular tests administered to the three affected sibs exhibited no abnormalities.

PATHOLOGY

Biopsy of an active skin plaque in the antecubital fossa of the proband showed moderate acanthosis, hyperkeratosis, and a patchy lymphocytic infiltrate in the upper dermis (Fig. 6–20*C*).

HEREDITY

The parents were not related. The father's and mother's kindreds came from Poland and Czechoslovakia, respectively. There was no family history of hearing loss or dermatitis. Audiometric tests on both parents and on the fourth sib showed no abnormalities, suggesting autosomal recessive inheritance (Fig. 6–20*D*).

DIAGNOSIS

This syndrome must be separated from *recessive congenital moderate sensorineural hearing loss* noted by Konigsmark *et al.* (1970) in which no cutaneous abnormalities were found. Since the atopic dermatitis does not appear until about 10 years of age, diagnosis of this disorder cannot be made until that age, unless other family members are affected.

G. Frentz (personal communication, 1975) reported sensorineural hearing loss in male sibs with atopic dermatitis. Their mother and maternal grandfather had atopic dermatitis but no deafness.

TREATMENT

Treatment consists of local therapy for the atopic dermatitis and a hearing aid, when necessary, for the hearing loss.

PROGNOSIS

The hearing loss was apparently nonprogressive.

SUMMARY

The major characteristics of this syndrome include: 1) autosomal recessive inheritance, 2) atypical atopic dermatitis with onset at about 10 years of age and involvement of the trunk and arms, and 3) moderate nonprogressive sensorineural hearing loss beginning in early childhood.

REFERENCES

Konigsmark, B. W., Hollander, M. B., and Berlin, C. I., Familial neural hearing loss and atopic dermatitis. *J.A.M.A., 204*:953–957, 1968.

Konigsmark, B. W., Mengel, M. C., and Haskins, H., Familial congenital moderate neural hearing loss. *J. Laryngol., 84*:495–506, 1970.

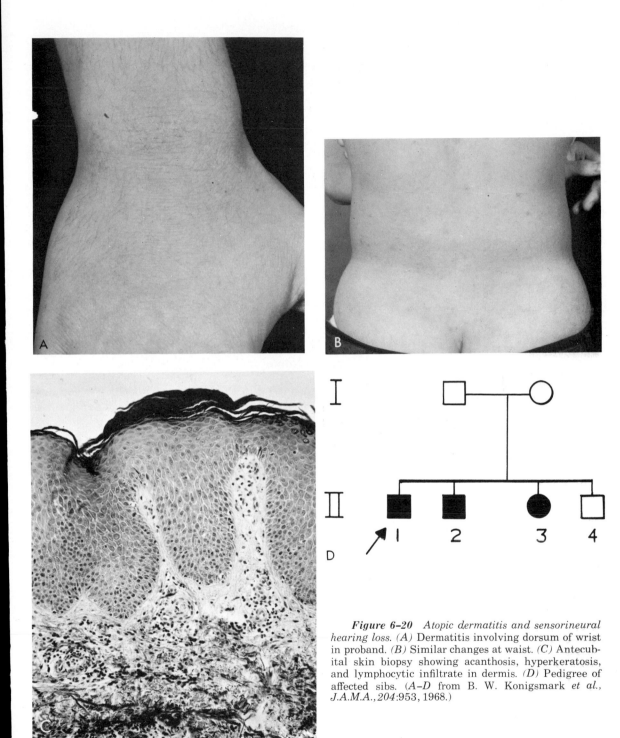

Figure 6–20 *Atopic dermatitis and sensorineural hearing loss. (A)* Dermatitis involving dorsum of wrist in proband. *(B)* Similar changes at waist. *(C)* Antecubital skin biopsy showing acanthosis, hyperkeratosis, and lymphocytic infiltrate in dermis. *(D)* Pedigree of affected sibs. *(A–D* from B. W. Konigsmark *et al., J.A.M.A.,204*:953, 1968.)

Chapter 7

GENETIC HEARING LOSS WITH RENAL DISEASE

NEPHRITIS AND SENSORINEURAL DEAFNESS

(Alport Syndrome)

Alport (1927) described a syndrome of chronic nephritis with intermittent or gross hematuria and progressive renal insufficiency, progressive sensorineural deafness, and a predilection for males. Since then, several hundred publications have appeared on Alport syndrome, which accounts for about 1 per cent of genetic deafness.

CLINICAL FINDINGS

Renal System. Hematuria is often the presenting sign. This remains pronounced for several years and then diminishes. It may appear during the first years of life ("red diapers") associated with asymptomatic albuminuria and pyuria, but more often it occurs during the first or second decade. Hypertension and renal failure occur, especially in males, during the teen years. Affected males usually die as a result of slowly progressive uremia before 30 years of age. Females have less severe renal disease but tend to have severe toxemia of pregnancy (Crawfurd and Toghill, 1968; Chiricosta *et al.*, 1970). Spontaneous abortion is not uncommon (around 15 per cent). However, the life span of affected females is usually normal.

Ocular System. About 10 per cent of patients with Alport syndrome have ocular abnormalities: lenticonus, spherophakia, and especially cortical cataracts (Sohar, 1956; Perrin, 1964; Arnott, Crawfurd, and Toghill, 1966; Arenberg *et al.*, 1967; Purriel *et al.*, 1970; Hauser, 1974).

Auditory System. There is marked variation in the degree of deafness. Symmetric progressive sensorineural hearing loss, more often in the middle to high frequencies, usually appears during the second decade, but it is relatively mild and rarely requires a patient's admission to a school for the deaf (Klotz, 1959; Johnson and Hagan, 1965; Gekle *et al.*, 1969).

The hearing loss occurs in most affected males but also in a smaller proportion of females. Cassidy *et al.* (1965), studying seven families with Alport syndrome, found hearing loss in about 55 per cent of the males and in about 40 per cent of the females. Similar findings were reported by Chiricosta *et al.* (1970). Slightly lower frequencies were noted by Ferguson and Rance (1972) and Hauser (1974).

Audiometric tests were carried out on 16 persons from four kindreds by Spear *et al.* (1970). Children below 10 years of age usually had normal hearing. Beginning in the second decade, a sensorineural hearing loss of about 50 dB, most marked in the higher frequencies, was found. Speech discrimination was usually normal. The SISI test was positive in three of seven cases, whereas the tone-decay test was positive in only one of nine cases. Similar findings by Miller et al. (1970) suggest that the hearing loss is cochlear in origin.

Vestibular System. Caloric stimulation shows decreased response (Miller et al., 1970; Celes-Blaubach et al., 1974).

LABORATORY FINDINGS

In patients with more severe renal disease, intravenous pyelography demonstrates atrophied, somewhat lobulated kidneys.

Urinalysis shows a variable degree of hematuria, proteinuria, and pyuria. Cellular casts containing red blood cells may be found. The level of blood urea nitrogen increases with the severity of the disease.

PATHOLOGY

The renal changes in Alport syndrome exhibit combined features of chronic glomerulonephritis, pyelonephritis, and interstitial nephritis but lack some characteristics of each one.

The kidneys are small and have a finely granular and pale texture. The cut surface of the cortex may show yellow linear streaks. The primary change occurs in the basement membrane of the glomeruli.

The earliest lesion is marked by epithelial proliferation in the glomeruli, interstitial fibrosis, or focal dilatation with atrophy of tubules occurring at about the same time. Lipid-laden foam cells, derived from tubular epithelial cells, are present in most cases. These foam cells may fill the interstitial tissues, particularly in the lower cortex, appearing as rows or nests. In most cases, plasma cells and lymphocytes as well as calcium deposits are found in the interstitial tissue. Tubular changes include epithelial atrophy and dilatation of some tubules. Occasionally, there is chronic interstitial nephritis in which the glomeruli are initially spared (White et al., 1964; Krickstein et al., 1966) (Fig. 7–1A–D). It should be emphasized that while these changes are suggestive of Alport syndrome, they are not specific for the condition. Ultrastructurally, however, there is evidence of a characteristic splitting of the glomerular basement membrane into many thin laminae, resulting in the accumulation of small, dense particles between the layers (Churg and Sherman, 1973; Sherman et al., 1974).

There are several reports concerning temporal bone pathology in Alport syndrome. Winter et al. (1968) found that all structures were intact except for about a 50 per cent loss of spiral ganglion cells in the basal turn of the cochlea. Gregg and Becker (1963) and Babai and Bettez (1968) described degeneration of the stria vascularis and hair cells of the organ of Corti, particularly in the basal turn of the cochlea. Fujita and Hayden (1969), Westergaard et al. (1972), Myers and Tyler (1972) and Bergstrom et al. (1972) were unable to find temporal bone changes characteristic of Alport syndrome.

PATHOGENESIS

The pathogenesis of Alport syndrome is not known. Quick et al. (1973) and Arnold and Weidaver (1975) noted similarity of the cochlea and kidney in several modalities (fluid and electrolyte balance, common ototoxic and nephrotoxic drugs) and demonstrated by immunochemistry and immunohistochemistry evidence for a shared antigen between the kidney and the cochlea.

HEREDITY

Several studies have suggested that heterozygote mothers transmit the gene to about 65 per cent of their offspring. Among children of affected males 75 per cent of their daughters have Alport syndrome as contrasted with 45 per cent of their sons. Cohen et al. (1961), Shaw and Glover (1961), and MacNeill and Shaw (1973) suggested that the syndrome is due to an autosomal gene that shows nonrandom segregation in females (going to the oocyte rather than to the polar body) and preferential segregation with the X chromosome in spermatogenesis. Preus and Fraser (1971) suggested that the unfavorable intrauterine milieu of an affected mother may cause increased penetrance of the gene in her sons. We agree with Mayo (1973) — Alport syndrome is probably a genetic heterogeneity.

DIAGNOSIS

Alport syndrome must be separated from all other causes of hematuria and proteinuria in childhood. Glomerulonephritis and glomerulitis are also associated with hematuria. Hereditary nephritis without deafness described by Dockhorn (1967) is probably a different disorder.

TREATMENT

The deafness is usually ameliorated by use of a hearing aid. Therapy should be directed toward the correction of biochemical disturbances associated with renal insufficiency.

Renal transplantation should be considered. In one patient seen by us hearing was improved following the procedure.

PROGNOSIS

Prognosis is variable. In some patients the disease may be mild and show practically no effect, whereas in other patients renal failure is severe, resulting in death at an early age.

SUMMARY

Characteristics of this syndrome include: 1) autosomal dominant inheritance, with males being more severely affected, 2) progressive nephritis with uremia, 3) ocular-lens abnormalities, including spherophakia, lenticonus, or cataracts in about 10 per cent of cases, 4) progressive sensorineural hearing loss beginning during the first or second decades and showing variable expressivity.

REFERENCES

Alport, A. C. Hereditary familial congenital haemorrhagic nephritis. *Br. Med. J.,* *1*:504–506, 1927.

Arenberg, K. K., Dodson, V. N., Falls, H. F., and Stern, S. D., Alport's syndrome. Re-evaluation of the associated ocular abnormalities and report of a family study. *J. Pediatr. Ophthalmol., 4*:21–32, 1967.

Arnold, W., and Weidauer, H., Experimental studies on the pathogenesis of inner ear disturbance in renal disease. *Arch. Oto-Rhino-Laryngol.,211*:217, 1975.

Arnott, E. J., Crawfurd, M. S. A., and Toghill, P. J., Anterior lenticonus and Alport's syndrome. *Br. J. Ophthalmol., 50*:390–403, 1966.

Babai, F., and Bettez, P., Lésions auditives du syndrome d'Alport (nephrite hématurique héréditaire). *Ann. Anat. Pathol. (Paris), 13*:289–302, 1968.

Bergstrom, L., Jenkins, P., Sando, I., and English, G. M., Hearing loss in renal disease: clinical and pathological studies. *Ann. Otol. Rhinol. Laryngol., 82*:555–576, 1973.

Cassidy, G., Brown, K., Cohen, M., and DeMaria, W., Hereditary renal dysfunction and deafness. *Pediatrics, 35*:967–979, 1965.

Celes-Blaubach, A., García-Zozaya, J., Pérez-Requejo, J., and Brass, K., Vestibular disorders in Alport's syndrome. *J. Laryngol. Otol., 88*:663–674, 1974.

Chiricosta, A., Jindal, S. L., Metuzals, J., and Koch, B., Nephropathy with hematuria (Alport's syndrome). *Can. Med. Assoc. J., 102*:396–401, 1970.

Churg, J., and Sherman, R. L., Pathologic characteristics of hereditary nephritis. *Arch. Pathol., 95*:374–379, 1973.

Cohen, M. M., Cassidy, G., and Hanna, B. L., A genetic study of hereditary renal dysfunction with associated nerve deafness. *Am. J. Hum. Genet., 13*:379–389, 1961.

Crawfurd, M., and Toghill, P., Alport's syndrome of hereditary nephritis and deafness. *Q. J. Med., 37*:563–576, 1968.

Dockhorn, R. J., Hereditary nephropathy without deafness. *Am. J. Dis. Child., 114*:135–138, 1967.

Ferguson, A. C., and Rance, C. P., Hereditary nephropathy with nerve deafness (Alport's syndrome). *Am. J. Dis. Child., 124*:84–88, 1972.

Fujita, S., and Hayden, R. C., Jr., Alport's syndrome. *Arch. Otolaryngol., 90*:453–466, 1969.

Gekle, D., Esser, H., and Brunner, H., Familiäre Nephropathie und Schallempfindungsschwerhörigkeit. *Arch. Kinderheilkd., 178*:290–302, 1969.

Gregg, J. B., and Becker, S. F., Concomitant progressive deafness, chronic nephritis, and ocular lens disease. *Arch. Ophthalmol., 69*:293–299, 1963.

Hauser, J., Néphropathie chronique héréditaire avec surdité et atteinte oculaire. *Schweiz. Med. Wochenschr., 104*:724–728, 762–772, 1974.

Johnson, W. J., and Hagan, P. J., Hereditary nephropathy and loss of hearing. *Arch. Otolaryngol., 82*:166–172, 1965.

Klotz, R. E., Congenital hereditary kidney disease and hearing loss. *Arch. Otolaryngol., 69*:560–562, 1959.

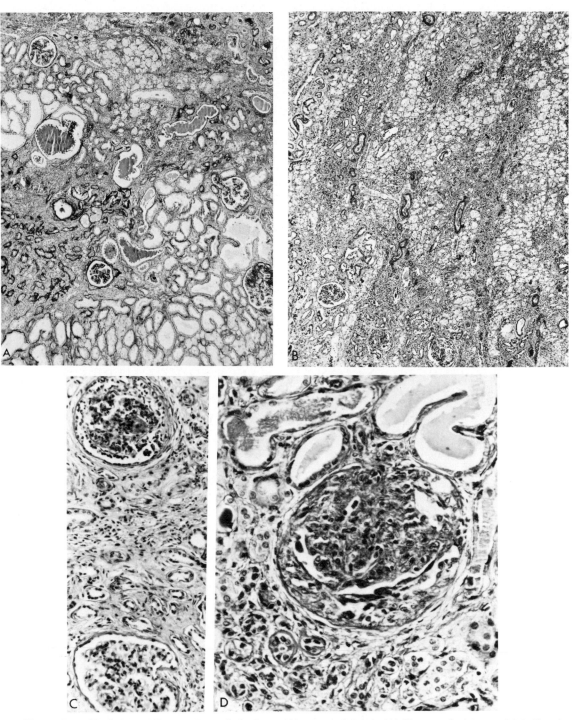

Figure 7–1 *Nephritis and sensorineural deafness (Alport syndrome).* *(A)* Note marked interstitial fibrosis with scattered lymphocytes and groups of foam cells surrounded by basement membrane. Hypertrophic tubules are dilated and contain proteinaceous casts. *(B)* Lower renal cortex with parallel rows of foam cells. *(C)* Glomerulus at top with thickened basement membrane and capsular adhesions. Contrast with nearly normal glomerulus at bottom. *(D)* Rare glomerulus showing crescent formation; dilated tubules containing proteinaceous casts. Thickened basement membrane surrounding atrophic tubules in fibrotic area. *(A–D* from H. I. Krickstein *et al., Arch. Pathol., 82*:506, 1966.)

Krickstein, H. I., Gloor, F. J., and Balogh, K., Renal pathology in hereditary nephritis with nerve deafness. *Arch. Pathol., 82*:506–517, 1966.

MacNeill, E., and Shaw, R. E., Segregation ratios in Alport's syndrome. *J. Med. Genet., 10*:23–26, 1973.

Mayo, O., Alport's syndrome. *J. Med. Genet., 10*:396–398, 1973.

Miller, G. W., Joseph, D. J., Cozad, R. L., and McCabe, B. F., Alport's syndrome. *Arch. Otolaryngol., 92*:418–432, 1970.

Myers, G. J., and Tyler, H. R., The etiology of deafness in Alport's syndrome. *Arch. Otolaryngol., 96*:333–340, 1972.

Perrin, D., Le syndrome d'Alport. *Ann. Ocul. (Paris), 197*:329–346, 1964.

Preus, M., and Fraser, F. C., Genetics of hereditary nephropathy with deafness (Alport's syndrome). *Clin. Genet., 2*:331–337, 1971.

Purriel, P., Drets, M., Pascale, E., *et al.*, Familial hereditary nephropathy (Alport's syndrome). *Am. J. Med., 49*:753–773, 1970.

Quick, C. A., Fish, A., and Brown, C., The relationship between cochlea and kidney. *Laryngoscope, 83*:1469–1482, 1973.

Shaw, R. F., and Glover, R. A., Abnormal segregation in hereditary renal disease with deafness. *Am. J. Hum. Genet., 13*:89–97, 1961.

Sherman, R. L., Churg, J., and Yudis, M., Hereditary nephritis with a characteristic renal lesion. *Am. J. Med., 56*:44–51, 1974.

Sohar, E., Renal disease, inner ear deafness, and occular changes; new heredofamilial syndrome. *A.M.A. Arch. Int. Med., 97*:627–630, 1956.

Spear, G. S., Whitworth, J. M., and Konigsmark, B. W., Hereditary nephritis with nerve deafness. *Am. J. Med., 49*:52–63, 1970.

Westergaard, O., Kluyskens, P., and John, H. D., Alport's syndrome. Histopathology of human temporal bones. *ORL, 34*:263–273, 1972.

White, R. H. R., Parson, V., and Walt, F. P., The renal disorder in Alport's syndrome. *Guy's Hosp. Rep., 113*:179–189, 1964.

Winter, L. E., Cram, B. M., and Banovetz, J. D., Hearing loss in hereditary renal disease. *Arch. Otolaryngol., 88*:238–241, 1968.

SEVERE HYPERTENSION, RENAL FAILURE, ABNORMAL STEROIDOGENESIS, HYPOGENITALISM, AND SENSORINEURAL DEAFNESS

Hamet *et al.* (1973) reported three sibs with severe hypertension, hypogenitalism, renal failure, and sensorineural deafness.

CLINICAL FINDINGS

Renal System. Progressive renal failure existed in all three sibs; death occurred in two sibs in the fourth decade. On autopsy, the male sib was found to have malignant nephrosclerosis, whereas his sister had focal nephritis.

Cardiovascular System. Marked hypertension was noted in all three sibs during late adolescence.

Endocrine System. Cryptorchidism was present in the male sib. The testes were decreased in size and there was reduced spermatogenesis. Both female sibs exhibited primary amenorrhea. The ovaries were fibrotic streaks, and the uterus was infantile. Breast development was deficient in one female sib. Axillary, pubic, and body hair was absent in the female sibs.

At autopsy, the zona glomerulosa of the adrenal glands was found to be hyperplastic—a possibly nonspecific result of the renal insufficiency.

Auditory System. In the male sib progressive deafness was first noted at the age of 5 years with total loss of hearing resulting within the next few years. A female sib had bilateral moderate sensorineural deafness. No information was available on the second female sib's hearing.

Vestibular System. No data were published.

LABORATORY FINDINGS

Bone age was delayed in the two female sibs. An adrenal biosynthetic defect compatible with incomplete 17-hydroxylation– and 11-hydroxylation–abnormalities was demonstrated.

HEREDITY

The three affected sibs, of French Canadian origin, had two normal sibs and healthy, nonconsanguineous parents. Inheritance of the syndrome is apparently autosomal recessive.

DIAGNOSIS

Alport syndrome may be excluded on the basis of absence of hypogenitalism, recessive inheritance, and hypertension, which occurs late in the course of this disorder. *XX gonadal dysgenesis and congenital sensorineural deafness,* an autosomal recessive syndrome, must be excluded (Josso et al., 1963; Christakos et al., 1969).

TREATMENT

The hypertension should be treated with antihypertensive drugs.

PROGNOSIS

Prognosis is poor. The male sib and one female sib died of cerebral hemorrhage at the age of 30 and 35 years, respectively.

SUMMARY

Characteristics of this syndrome include: 1) autosomal recessive inheritance, 2) progressive renal failure, 3) severe hypertension appearing during adolescence, 4) hypogenitalism manifested by cryptorchidism or primary amenorrhea, and 5) progressive sensorineural deafness appearing in childhood.

REFERENCES

Christakos, A. C., Simpson, J. L., Younger, J. B., and Christian, C. D., Gonadal dysgenesis as an autosomal recessive condition. *Am. J. Obstet. Gynecol., 104*:1027–1030, 1969.

Hamet, P., Kuchel, O., Nowaczynski, W., Rojo-Ortega, J. M., Sasaki, C., and Genest, J., Hypertension with adrenal, genital, renal defects, and deafness. *Arch. Intern. Med., 131*:563–569, 1973.

Josso, N., de Grouchy, J., Frézal, J., and Lamy, M., Le syndrome de Turner familiale. *Ann. Pédiatr.,10*:163–167, 1963.

CHARCOT-MARIE-TOOTH SYNDROME, NEPHRITIS, AND SENSORINEURAL DEAFNESS

(Lemieux-Neemeh Syndrome)

Lemieux and Neemeh (1967) described a syndrome appearing in two families and characterized by childhood onset of progressive distal muscle atrophy, nephropathy with proteinuria and hematuria, and progressive sensorineural hearing loss. A sporadic case was reported by Hanson et al. (1970).

CLINICAL FINDINGS

Renal System. Nephritis characterized by proteinuria and microscopic hematuria was present in all affected.

Renal function tests were essentially normal. Renal biopsies showed foci of atrophic tubules. In two, there were numerous hyalinized glomeruli (Fig. 7–2, *B*). Interstitial foam cells were seen in only one case (Lemieux and Neemeh, 1967).

Muscular System. Distal muscle atrophy began in childhood and was slowly progressive. This was associated with progressive weakness, which produced difficulty in walking and in holding objects. A clawhand slowly developed in later childhood. Neurologic examination showed marked atrophy and weakness of the distal musculature of the legs and of the intrinsic musculature of the hands. The proximal limb muscles remained normal (Fig. 7–2, *A*). Affected persons had an awkward gait with bilateral foot drop but no true ataxia. In the youngest patient triceps and biceps reflexes were active, but knee and ankle jerks were absent. In the three older patients, all of these reflexes were absent. Sensation was normal in all patients.

Auditory System. Hearing loss began in childhood and was slowly progressive. Two of the three patients reported by Lemieux and Neemeh as well as the patient described by Hanson et al. had progressive sensorineural deafness. In the latter patient there was moderate hearing loss more marked in the higher frequencies and first noted at 7 years of age. The 25- and 34-year-old patients of Lemieux and Neemeh both had hearing losses of about 50 dB. Audiometric tests apparently were not done on the 21-year-old sib.

Vestibular System. Caloric responses were absent bilaterally in the boy described by Hanson *et al.*

LABORATORY FINDINGS

Motor nerve conduction velocities in the ulnar and median nerves were about half normal speed (20 to 25 meters per second) (Hanson *et al.*, 1970). Electromyography showed no electrical activity at rest or with attempted voluntary contraction of the distal muscles. Proximal muscle showed normal potentials. The findings were diagnostic of a neurogenic lesion in the distal musculature.

Biopsy of the sural nerve showed no abnormalities. Muscle biopsies from the tibialis, gastrocnemius, and vastus lateralis exhibited changes compatible with both myopathy and neural atrophy.

HEREDITY

It is not clear whether the syndrome is transmitted in a recessive or dominant manner. Possibly, the condition described here is actually two different syndromes. In the first family described by Lemieux and Neemeh (1967), 4 of 11 sibs were affected. One had Charcot-Marie-Tooth syndrome, one had nephropathy, and two had both disorders. The remaining sib and mother were not examined. The father died of coronary heart disease at 55 years. In the sec-

ond family, the 21-year-old proband had distal muscle wasting and nephropathy but no hearing loss. A 12-year-old sister, a 13-year-old brother and their 46-year-old mother had distal muscle wasting. Urinalysis done on seven family members showed mild proteinuria. The patient described by Hanson *et al.* (1970) was the only affected member of a sibship of five. His parents were normal.

DIAGNOSIS

The nephropathy seems to be typical of that seen in *Alport syndrome*. However, Alport syndrome has not been described in association with Charcot-Marie-Tooth syndrome.

TREATMENT

A hearing aid is beneficial.

PROGNOSIS

It is difficult to give a prognosis on life span, since all affected with nephropathy were relatively young. The Charcot-Marie-Tooth syndrome seemed quite classic in its behavior.

SUMMARY

The syndrome is characterized by: 1) probable autosomal dominant inheritance, 2) nephropathy similar to that of Alport syndrome, 3) Charcot-Marie-Tooth syndrome, and 4) progressive sensorineural hearing loss, beginning in childhood.

REFERENCES

Hanson, P. A., Farber, R. E., and Armstrong, R. A., Distal muscle wasting, nephritis, and deafness. *Neurology (Minneap.)*, 20:426–434, 1970.
Lemieux, G.. and Neemeh, J. A., Charcot-Marie-Tooth disease and nephritis. *Can. Med. Assoc. J.,* 97:1193–1198, 1967.

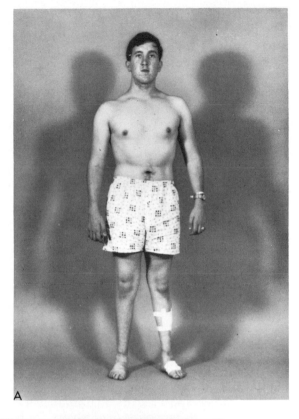

Figure 7-2 *Charcot-Marie-Tooth syndrome, nephritis, and sensorineural deafness (Lemieux-Neemeh syndrome). (A)* Sixteen-year-old patient showing tapering of extremities and claw hands. (From P. A. Hanson *et al., Neurology (Minneap.), 20*:426, 1970.) *(B)* Renal biopsy showing zone of tubular atrophy and hyalinization of glomerular tuft. (From G. Lemieux and J. A. Neemeh, *J. Can. Med. Assoc., 97*:1193, 1967.)

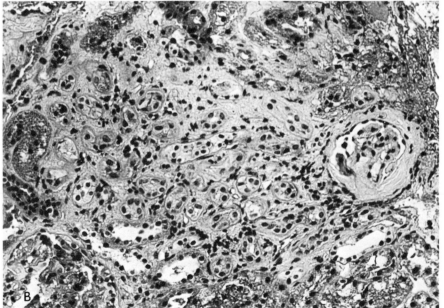

MACROTHROMBOCYTOPATHIA, NEPHRITIS, AND SENSORINEURAL DEAFNESS

Epstein *et al.* (1972) reported a syndrome consisting of giant platelets associated with thrombocytopenia, nephritis, and sensorineural deafness in two unrelated kindreds. Ekstein *et al.* (1975) documented a syndrome that affected another kindred in a similar manner. This syndrome contrasted with the first in that there was normal platelet function and different ultrastructural morphology.

CLINICAL FINDINGS

Physical Findings. The patients appear clinically normal except for occasional facial and/or periorbital edema and bruising following minor trauma.

Renal System. Renal involvement was noted in early childhood with the appearance of albuminuria and microscopic hematuria. Progressive renal deterioration and hypertension followed. Unlike classic Alport syndrome the disorder is clinically as severe in females as in males.

Hematopoietic System. Severe epistaxis and a mild bleeding tendency with easy bruising appeared during infancy or early childhood, becoming less severe with age. The 1-month-old daughter of an affected patient manifested ecchymoses; laboratory studies showed she had hypochromic anemia and platelet abnormalities.

Auditory System. Audiograms revealed bilateral moderate to severe sensorineural hearing loss, more marked in the higher frequencies. It was present as early as 3½ years of age in one patient. In the others the hearing loss was documented at ages 15, 12, and 9 years, but the time of onset was not stated. Ekstein *et al.* (1975) have suggested onset occurs between 5 and 10 years of age.

Vestibular System. No vestibular function tests were reported.

LABORATORY FINDINGS

Hypochromic anemia was noted in most patients. Thrombocytopenia (with platelet counts as low as 25,000 per cu. mm.) with giant platelets, prolonged bleeding time, and poor clot retraction were found. In addition to defective aggregation, adenine nucleotide release, impaired platelet factor III activity, and ultrastructural abnormalities of both platelets and megakaryocytes were found. Platelet function was normal, however, in the kindred of Ekstein *et al.* (1975). Bone marrow examination showed an increased number of megakaryocytes and promegakaryocytes.

Microscopic hematuria and albuminuria as well as granular red and white blood cell casts were found in the urine. Examination of the kidneys at autopsy revealed extensive hyalinization of the glomeruli, scarring, and crescent formation. The arterial and arteriolar walls were thickened and hyalinized, and interstitial fibrosis with focal and diffuse round cell infiltration was marked. The few remaining tubules were enlarged and dilated.

HEREDITY

The disorder appeared to be autosomal dominant, although there is yet no example of male-to-male transmission.

DIAGNOSIS

The microscopic changes in the kidney resemble those in *Alport syndrome.* However, the ultrastructural alterations shown in Alport syndrome have not been looked for. Furthermore, the severity of the syndrome discussed here is as marked in females as in males, quite unlike the circumstances in Alport syndrome. Moreover, giant platelets and thrombocytopenia are not a component of Alport syndrome.

TREATMENT

Although splenectomy was performed, the procedure failed to improve the thrombocytopenia. Intravenous plasma and prednisone were also ineffective. Renal transplantation was carried out in one patient.

PROGNOSIS

Prognosis was poor; death from uremia occurred in the third decade in some patients.

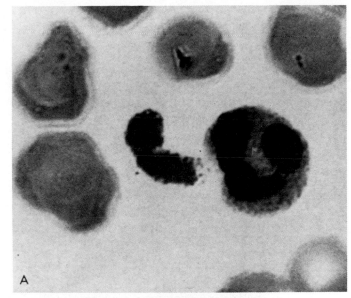

Figure 7-3 Macrothrombocytopathia, nephritis, and sensorineural deafness. (A) Blood smear showing large, irregularly shaped platelet. (B) Photomicrograph of kidney exhibiting interstitial fibrosis, focal glomerular proliferation, and sclerotic glomerulus. (A and B from C. J. Epstein et al., Am. J. Med., 52:299, 1972.)

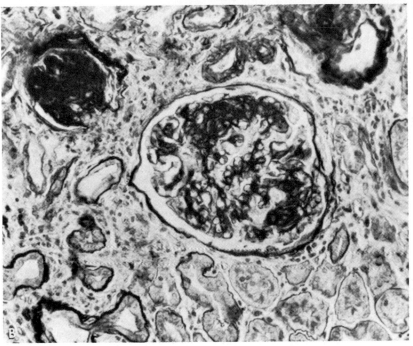

SUMMARY

This syndrome is characterized by: 1) dominant inheritance, probably autosomal, 2) nephropathy resembling that seen in Alport syndrome, 3) giant platelets with thrombocytopenia, and 4) moderate to severe sensorineural deafness.

REFERENCES

Ekstein, J. D., Filip, D. J., and Watts, J. C., Hereditary thrombocytopenia, deafness, and renal disease. *Ann. Intern. Med.*, 82:639–645, 1975.

Epstein, C. J., Sahud, M. A., Piel, C. F., Goodman, J. R., Bernfield, M. R., Kushner, J. H., and Albin, A. R., Hereditary macrothrombocytopathia, nephritis, and deafness. *Am. J. Med.*, 52:299–310, 1972.

INFANTILE RENAL TUBULAR ACIDOSIS AND CONGENITAL SENSORINEURAL DEAFNESS

Cohen *et al.* (1973) reported four children, all products of consanguineous matings in two separate sibships stemming from a large inbred kindred, who had congenital sensorineural deafness and infantile renal tubular acidosis. Other cases were documented by Nance and Sweeney (1971) and by Donckerwolcke *et al.* (1976).

CLINICAL FINDINGS

Physical 'indings. Growth retardation was marked, being below the third percentile in all affected.

Renal System. The children presented at birth or soon thereafter with vomiting, dehydration, polydipsia, polyuria, and hyposthenuria.

Auditory System. A marked sensorineural deafness, more pronounced at higher frequencies, was demonstrated in infancy.

Vestibular System. No studies have been published.

LABORATORY FINDINGS

An intravenous pyelogram revealed renal calcinosis in infancy. At 2 years of age, the affected individuals showed radiologic signs of rickets.

Hyperchloremic acidosis was confirmed by tests of blood pH and serum electrolytes. Following an ammonium chloride loading test, the carbon dioxide content of the blood decreased significantly, but the pH of the urine remained high. Specific gravity was low. Serum chloride levels were markedly elevated. The distal tubule has been implicated.

HEREDITY

Because of parental consanguinity, the sibs described by Cohen *et al.* (1973) were first cousins once removed as well as second cousins to each other. The boy documented by Nance and Sweeney (1971) was also the offspring of a consanguineous union. Inheritance is clearly autosomal recessive.

A specific deficiency of carbonic anhydrase B was demonstrated in affected individuals (Cohen *et al.*, 1973).

DIAGNOSIS

This disorder should be differentiated from *adolescent or young adult renal tubular acidosis and slowly progressive sensorineural deafness,* which also has autosomal recessive inheritance. Infantile renal tubular acidosis also exists as an isolated disorder with autosomal recessive heritability and has been seen in a large number of syndromal associations reviewed by Nance and Sweeney (1971).

TREATMENT

The children were maintained on an alkalizing solution and an increased level of fluids. A hearing aid was employed.

PROGNOSIS

Life expectancy does not seem to be reduced if the disorder is recognized and treated early. Growth retardation, however, is persistent.

SUMMARY

The syndrome is characterized by: 1) autosomal recessive inheritance, 2) infantile renal tubular acidosis manifested by hyperchloremia and an inability to acidify the urine normally, 3) growth retardation, and 4) congenital profound sensorineural deafness.

REFERENCES

Cohen, T., Brand-Auraban, A., Karshai, C., Jacob, A., Gay, I., Tsitsianov, J., Shapiro, T., Jatziv, S., and Ashkenazi, A., Familial infantile renal tubular acidosis and congenital nerve deafness: an autosomal recessive syndrome. *Clin. Genet.*, 4:275–278, 1973.

Donckerwolcke, R. A., Van Bierrliet, J. P., Koorevaar, G., Kuijten, R. H., and Van Stekelenburg, G. J. The syndrome of renal tubular acidosis and nerve deafness. *Acta Paediat. Scand.*, 65: 100–104, 1976.

Nance, W. E., and Sweeney, A., Evidence for autosomal recessive inheritance of the syndrome of renal tubular acidosis with deafness. *Birth Defects*, 7(4):70–72, 1971.

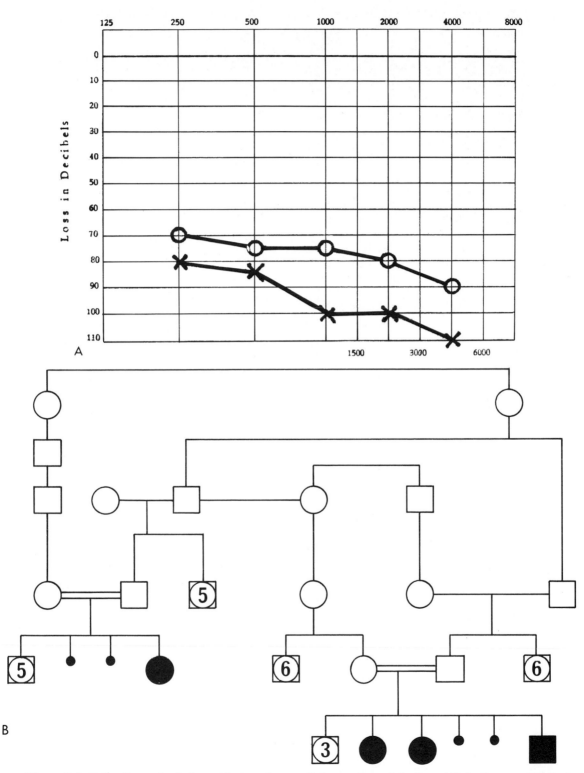

Figure 7–4 *Infantile renal tubular acidosis and congenital sensorineural deafness. (A)* Audiogram of patient at 6 years of age. *(B)* Pedigree of affected kindred. *(A* and *B* from T. Cohen *et al., Clin. Genet., 4*:275, 1973.)

ADOLESCENT OR YOUNG ADULT RENAL TUBULAR ACIDOSIS AND SLOWLY PROGRESSIVE SENSORINEURAL DEAFNESS

Konigsmark (1966) described a 17-year-old girl and her 20-year-old brother with renal tubular acidosis and slowly progressive sensorineural deafness that first became manifest during adolescence. Walker (1971, 1974) reported these same sibs several years later.

CLINICAL FINDINGS

Physical Findings. Growth and development are normal.

Renal System. The female sib observed by Konigsmark (1965) had bilateral renal calculi removed at 12 years of age. According to Walker (1971), she had recurrent bouts of renal colic and passed numerous small stones. The renal tubular acidosis, ascertained on laboratory study, was mild.

Auditory System. The sensorineural deafness was slowly progressive and moderate in degree, being more marked in the high frequencies. The hearing loss in the boy reported by Walker was first noted at 5 years of age. Speech discrimination was normal and the result of the SISI test was 100 per cent, suggesting a cochlear locus for the deafness.

Vestibular System. No studies have been reported.

LABORATORY FINDINGS

Radiographic studies showed renal calcinosis.

Hyperchloremic acidosis was demonstrated. Following ammonium chloride loading the urinary pH was not lowered.

HEREDITY

Inheritance is autosomal recessive.

DIAGNOSIS

This disorder should be differentiated from *infantile renal tubular acidosis and congenital sensorineural deafness* by time of onset.

TREATMENT

The patients should be administered an alkalizing solution and receive a high fluid intake.

PROGNOSIS

Prognosis is reasonably good. The renal tubular acidosis is mild, and although renal calcinosis is associated, it may be treated effectively.

SUMMARY

The syndrome is characterized by: 1) autosomal recessive inheritance, 2) mild renal tubular acidosis with onset in adolescence or early adulthood, and 3) slowly progressive sensorineural deafness.

REFERENCES

Konigsmark, B. W., Unpublished data, 1966.
Walker, W. G., Renal tubular acidosis and deafness. *Birth Defects*, 7(4):126, 1971.
Walker, W. G., Özer, F. L., and Whelton, A., Syndrome of perceptive deafness and renal tubular acidosis. *Birth Defects*, 10(4):163, 1974.

RENAL DISEASE, HYPERPROLINURIA, ICHTHYOSIS, AND SENSORINEURAL DEAFNESS

Goyer, Reynolds, Burke, and Burkholder (1968) found renal disease, hearing loss, hyperprolinuria and ichthyosis in various combinations in 23 members of a kindred.

CLINICAL FINDINGS

Physical Findings. The proband was admitted to the hospital when she was 12 years old because of progressive fatigue and failure to gain weight.

Renal System. Nephropathy of variable degree was present in eight individuals. The proband developed albuminuria and hematuria at 13 years of age. Her blood urea nitrogen gradually increased. Her 9-year-old brother had mild proteinuria, and another sib developed gross hematuria when he was 14-years-old. An intravenous pyelogram revealed a large cyst in the left kidney and a small calculus in a cortical cyst in the right kidney. The mother experienced gross hematuria at 22 years of age. Later, a renal calculus was found.

Integumentary System. Dry skin was present in many members of the kindred, and a brownish scaling ichthyosis was found in 6 of 23 individuals.

LABORATORY FINDINGS

The only radiographic abnormalities found in the kindred were the bilateral renal cysts noted in the proband's 15-year-old brother and the calculi noted above.

Plasma proline levels were elevated to approximately three times normal in the proband. Urinary proline and hydroxyproline levels were also elevated. Her sib had normal plasma levels but had developed elevated urinary levels of proline, suggesting decreased renal tubular reabsorption. Two other members of the kindred had elevated plasma proline levels.

PATHOLOGY

A renal biopsy done on the proband showed glomerular sclerosis. The interstitial tissue was infiltrated largely by lymphocytes. The arteries showed variable degrees of medial hypertrophy and subendothelial sclerosis. Electronmicrographs revealed a thickened mesangial basement membrane. Dense deposits were found in the matrix.

HEREDITY

The pedigree shows 23 persons in five generations of this kindred who were affected by different components of this syndrome (Fig. 7–5D). Two of three children, born of a consanguineous union of affected parents, showed all elements of the syndrome except deafness. One parent exhibited only hearing loss, and the other parent had only renal disease. The evidence suggests that this disease is transmitted by an autosomal dominant gene having variable expressivity.

DIAGNOSIS

Patients with the syndrome of *hyperprolinemia, renal anomalies, and hearing loss* (hyperprolinemia, type I) do not have ichthyosis, as occurs in the syndrome described above. Furthermore, the former is inherited in an autosomal recessive manner. A syndrome of hyperprolinemia and microscopic hematuria has been described as an autosomal dominant disorder in an Amerindian family; no deafness was demonstrable, however (Perry et al., 1968).

Ichthyosis, convergent strabismus, and sensorineural deafness were described in a girl who was the offspring of a consanguineous union. Among the 10 sibs in this kindred, 7 had a combination of 2 or more traits. No kidney anomalies or hyperprolinuria was found (Fishman and Crystal, 1973).

TREATMENT

A hearing aid may be employed. Treatment for the renal disease is not indicated except in case of uremia.

PROGNOSIS

This syndrome, in spite of the uremia, did not appear to decrease the life span. The hearing loss is probably slowly progressive, resulting in rather severe hearing loss in the later decades of life.

SUMMARY

Characteristics of the syndrome include: 1) autosomal dominant inheritance with variable expressivity, 2) nephropathy of variable degree, 3) hyperprolinuria, 4) ichthyosis, and 5) slowly progressive sensorineural deafness.

REFERENCES

Fishman, J. E., and Crystal, N., Sensorineural deafness: familial incidence and additional defects — study of a school for deaf children. *Am. J. Med. Sci.,* *266*:111–117, 1973.

Goyer, R. A., Reynold, J., Jr., Burke, J., and Burkholder, P., Hereditary renal disease with neurosensory hearing loss, prolinuria, and ichthyosis. *Am. J. Med. Sci.,* *256*:166–179, 1968.

Perry, T. L., Hardwick, D. F., Lowry, R. B., and Hansen, S., Hyperprolinemia in two successive generations of a North American Indian family. *Ann. Hum. Genet.,* *31*:401–408, 1968.

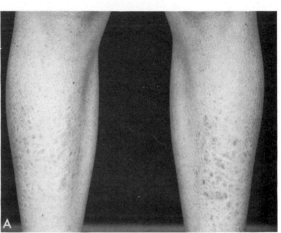

Figure 7–5 *Renal disease, hyperprolinuria, ichthyosis, and sensorineural deafness. (A)* Ichthyosis on ventral surface of legs of proband. *(B)* Photomicrograph showing sclerosis of renal parenchyma. *(C)* Note mild infiltration of lymphocytes and foam cells into scarred areas of the kidney.

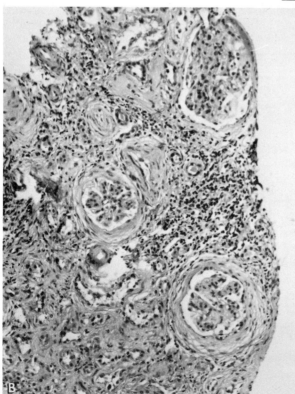

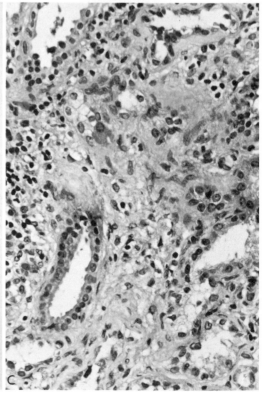

Illustration continued on the opposite page

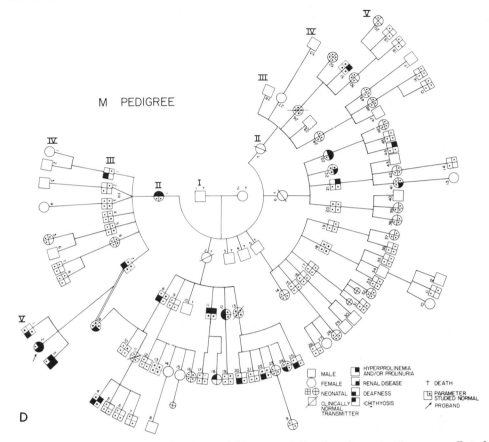

M PEDIGREE

☐ MALE	■ HYPERPROLINEMIA AND/OR PROLINURIA	
◯ FEMALE	■ RENAL DISEASE	† DEATH
⊕ NEONATAL	■ DEAFNESS	▣ PARAMETER STUDIED NORMAL
▨ CLINICALLY NORMAL TRANSMITTER	■ ICHTHYOSIS	↗ PROBAND

D

Figure 7–5 Continued. (D) Pedigree showing variable expressivity of syndrome in 23 persons affected in five generations of kindred. (A–D from R. A. Goyer *et al., Am. J. Med. Sci.,* 256:166, 1968.)

NEPHRITIS, URTICARIA, AMYLOIDOSIS, AND SENSORINEURAL DEAFNESS

(Muckle-Wells Syndrome)

A syndrome characterized by recurrent episodes of fever, urticaria, progressive sensorineural hearing loss, amyloidosis, and terminal uremia was described by Muckle and Wells (1962), Kennedy *et al.* (1966), Mamou *et al.* (1966, 1974), Andersen *et al.,* (1967), Van Allen *et al.* (1968), Black (1969), Lagrue *et al.* (1972), Perrottet *et al.* (1974), and Champion (1975). Less certain is the case of Campbell (1964).

CLINICAL FINDINGS

Physical Findings. The disease usually begins in adolescence with attacks of urticarial rash, fever, and aching limbs. Concurrently, progressive sensorineural hearing loss is noticed. In middle age, patients develop a nephrotic syndrome and die of uremia. However, there is considerable variability of time and mode of expression among families (Lagrue *et al.,* 1972).

Renal System. In the third and fourth decades, patients develop a nephrotic syndrome with proteinuria, uremia, anemia, and edema of the ankles.

Nervous System. Affected persons have limb pains that usually begin in the second decade of life. Arthralgias and fever accompany these bouts. An urticarial rash involving the entire body, but being more pronounced in the extremities, has been present in most patients. Pes cavus has occurred occasionally.

Auditory System. Hearing loss usually appears in childhood or adolescence, progressing slowly to severe loss in the third or fourth decades of life. Sensorineural deafness of moderate severity was found in six of nine persons described by Muckle and Wells (1962). Andersen et al. (1967) observed a moderately severe sensorineural hearing loss when the patient was 7-years-old and a very severe loss when he was 30-years-old (Fig. 7–6A). Progressive sensorineural hearing loss dating from the age of 12 years and 7 years was described by Black (1969) and Perrottet et al. (1974), respectively. Moderate bilateral sensorineural deafness was noted in the patient of Kennedy et al. (1966).

Vestibular System. No vestibular findings have been reported.

LABORATORY FINDINGS

In older patients the hemoglobin may be slightly decreased and the serum urea nitrogen may be elevated. Usually there is albuminuria, elevated erythrocyte sedimentation rate, and, in some individuals, increased serum globulin and hyperglycinuria.

PATHOLOGY

Three patients described by Muckle and Wells (1962) were autopsied. They ranged from 39 to 56 years of age. The kidneys were small with multiple surface adhesions. Histologic section of the kidneys showed amyloidosis throughout the parenchyma. Amyloid was noted in most glomeruli and in many tubules, as well as in vessel walls (Fig. 7–6C). Amyloid was also found throughout the parenchyma, follicles, and vessel walls of the spleen. The testes were small and had atrophic seminiferous tubules infiltrated by amyloid, both in tubules and vessel walls. In the liver and adrenal cortices, amyloid involved the vessels. Amyloid was also noted in the sciatic nerve and the dorsal root ganglia (Fig. 7–6D, E).

Histopathologic examination of the inner ear showed absence of the organ of Corti and vestibular sensory epithelium, atrophy of the cochlear nerve, and ossification of the basilar membrane. Amyloid was not present (Muckle and Wells, 1962).

HEREDITY

The family described by Muckle and Wells included eight affected persons in four generations. All eight suffered from recurrent urticaria. One developed nephropathy; another developed deafness, nephropathy, and hyperglycemia; five had both nephritis and deafness. Three became uremic; two showed amyloidosis at autopsy. In three generations of a kindred described by Black (1969), five members were affected.

This syndrome clearly has autosomal dominant inheritance with variable expressivity.

DIAGNOSIS

Systemic amyloidosis may be dominantly inherited in several syndromes: neuropathy with vitreous opacities, neuropathy with carpal tunnel syndrome, neuropathy with cutis laxa, cardiac form, visceral form, etc.) (McKusick, 1971; Meretoja, 1973). Patients with these conditions do not suffer from urticaria or hearing loss. Renal amyloidosis may be a complication of familial Mediterranean fever, occurring in about one fourth of those affected. These persons develop uremia but no hearing loss. Interestingly, Mamou and colleagues (1966, 1974) reported the co-occurrence of Muckle-Wells syndrome and familial Mediterranean fever. Amyloidosis may also occur with hypersensitivity as a dominantly inherited syndrome (McKusick, 1975). Although McKusick considers the disorder described by Van Allen et al. (1968) as a separate entity, we view this kindred as probably having the Muckle-Wells syndrome.

TREATMENT

The deafness may be helped by hearing aids. Andersen et al. (1967) reported relief from limb pains with 40 to 60 mg. of prednisone daily.

PROGNOSIS

Prognosis is poor. The hearing loss is slowly progressive, resulting in severe deafness in all patients. Affected individuals usually die of uremia in the third to fifth decades of life.

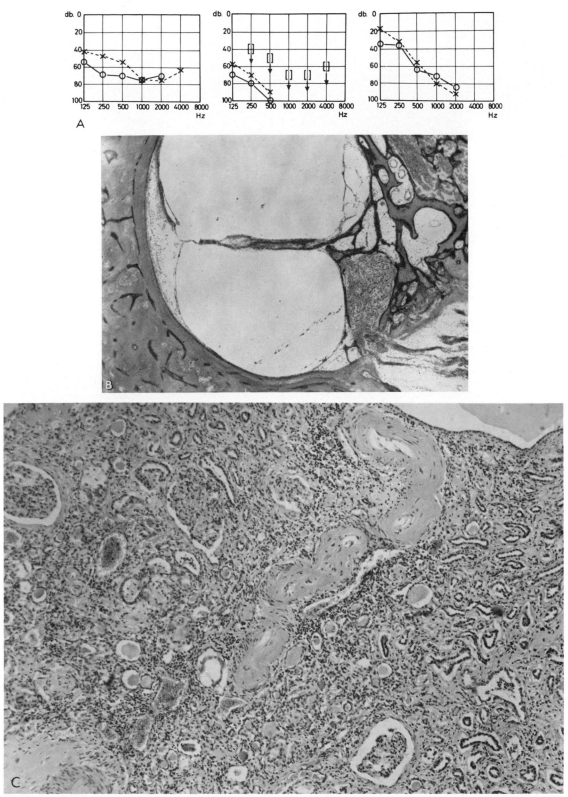

Figure 7–6 *Nephritis, urticaria, amyloidosis, and sensorineural deafness. (A)* Left: audiogram of patient at 7 years of age; center: audiogram of same patient at 30 years of age; right: audiogram of patient's brother at 10 years of age. (From V. Andersen *et al., Am. J. Med., 42*:449, 1967.) *(B)* Section of inner ear showing absence of organ of Corti and a line of ossification in the basilar membrane. *(C)* Section of kidney showing amyloid deposits primarily affecting large blood vessels. Renal parenchyma scarred and atrophic.

Illustration continued on the following page

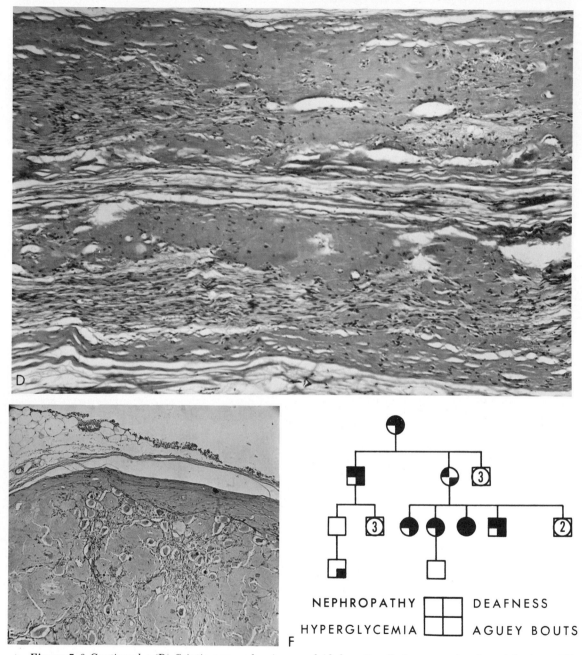

Figure 7-6 Continued. (D) Sciatic nerve showing amyloid deposits effacing nerve trunk architecture. (E) Dorsal root ganglion with dispersion of ganglion cells by amyloid masses. (C, D, and E from M. W. Van Allen *et al.,* *Neurology, 19*:10, 1969.) (F) Pedigree of affected kindred showing variable expressivity. (B and F from T. J. Muckle and M. Wells, *Q. J. Med.,* *31*:235, 1962.)

SUMMARY

Characteristics of this syndrome include: 1) autosomal dominant transmission with variable expressivity, 2) adolescent onset of recurrent episodes of urticaria, fever, and limb and joint pain, 3) amyloidosis resulting in nephropathy and uremia, and 4) childhood onset of progressive sensorineural deafness.

REFERENCES

Andersen, V., Buch, N. H., Jensen, M. K., and Killmann, S., Deafness, urticaria, and amyloidosis. *Am. J. Med.*, 42:449–456, 1967.

Black, J. T., Amyloidosis, deafness, urticaria, and limb pains: a hereditary syndrome. *Ann. Intern. Med.*, 70:989–994, 1969.

Campbell, A. M. G., The inherited amyloidoses. *Lancet*, 1:220, 1964.

Champion, R. H., Urticaria, amyloidosis, and deafness. Muckle-Wells syndrome. *Br. J. Dermatol.*, 93(Suppl. 11):46–48, 1975.

Kennedy, D. D., Rosenthal, F. D., and Sneddon, I. B., Amyloidosis presenting as urticaria. *Br. Med. J.*, 1:31–32, 1966.

Lagrue, G., Vernant, J. P., Revuz, J., Touraine, R., and Weil, B., Syndrome de Muckle et Wells. Cinquième observation familiale. *Nouv. Press Méd.*, 1:2223–2226, 1972.

Mamou, H., Maladie periodique familiale avec nephropathie et surdité. *Sem. Hop. (Paris), 54*: 3368–3370, 1966.

Mamou, H., Mamou, J. E., and de Regnault, D., Maladie periodique et syndrome de Muckle et Wells. *Nouv. Presse Méd., 3*:1363–1364, 1974.

McKusick, V. A., *Mendelian Inheritance in Man,* 4th Ed. Baltimore, Md., Johns Hopkins Press, 1975.

Meretoja, J., Genetic aspects of familial amyloidosis with corneal lattice dystrophy and cranial neuropathy. *Clin. Genet., 4*:175–185, 1973.

Muckle, T. J., and Wells, M., Urticaria, deafness, and amyloidosis: a new heredo-familial syndrome. *Q. J. Med., 31*:235–248, 1962.

Perrottet, C., Mach, R. S., and Fabre, J., Surdité, urticaire, arthrites, hypergonadisme et insuffisance rénale. Le syndrome de Muckle et Wells. *Praxis, 63*:651–659, 1974.

Van Allen, M. W., Frohlich, J. A., and Davis, J. R., Inherited predisposition to generalized amyloidosis. Clinical and pathological studies of a family with neuropathy, nephropathy, and peptic ulcer. *Neurology (Minneap.), 19*:10–25, 1968.

RENAL, GENITAL, AND MIDDLE EAR ANOMALIES

A syndrome characterized by renal hypoplasia, internal genital malformations, and malformations of the middle ear appearing in four female sibs was described by Winter *et al.* (1968). A second family with possibly the same syndrome was briefly reported by Turner (1970).

CLINICAL FINDINGS

Renal System. All four patients described by Winter *et al.* had renal anomalies. Both sibs who had died in infancy had bilateral renal agenesis, absent or hypoplastic ureters, and hypoplastic bladders. In both living sibs intravenous pyelograms revealed a normal kidney on one side and absence or hypoplasia of the kidney and ureter on the other side. Turner's patient had unilateral kidney agenesis and ipsilateral hemiaplasia of the bladder.

Genital System. The girls dying in infancy had variable genital anomalies, including normal ovaries but thin, coiled fallopian tubes in one and markedly hypoplastic ovaries and uterus, and vaginal atresia in the other. In the two living sibs the urethral opening was shifted posteriorly in one, and the vaginal opening was absent in both girls (Winter *et al.*, 1968). The girl reported by Turner had an anteriorly placed stenotic rectum and vaginal atresia.

Other Findings. Each of the sibs described by Winter *et al.* was born after a normal pregnancy and an uneventful delivery. One died at 2 hours and another died at 10 hours of age after episodes of dyspnea, apnea, and cyanosis. In both of these cases there was oligohydramnios. One of the living affected sibs had reduced intelligence. Her karyotype study revealed 47, XXX. The patient reported by Turner had a narrow nose.

Auditory System. The two living sibs had narrowed external auditory canals; the younger one had low-set ears. Deafness was suspected in the latter when she was 1 year old. Audiometric tests at 3 years of age showed a 50 dB bilateral conductive hearing loss. Unilateral endaural surgery revealed a malformed incus with fixation of the malleus and incus in the attic. Hearing loss was suspected in the older girl in early childhood. Otologic examination at 20 years of age showed a severe conductive loss in one ear and a moderate high-tone loss in the other. Tympanotomy revealed an absent incus. Hearing was considerably improved by repositioning the malleus to the stapes.

The girl reported by Turner had very narrow external auditory meatuses and mild deafness.

Vestibular System. Vestibular function tests were not reported.

LABORATORY FINDINGS

Intravenous pyelograms revealed renal anomalies in two sibs.

Autopsies were performed on two of the children. Renal and genital anomalies were found as noted above. In one child, interatrial septal defect and patent ductus arteriosus were also noted.

HEREDITY

Four children in a sibship of ten were affected. The remaining sibs and both parents were normal. There was no parental consanguinity (Fig. 7–7). Autosomal recessive inheritance is likely.

DIAGNOSIS

Patients with *renal disease, digital anomalies, and conductive hearing loss* (Braun and Bayer, 1962) have bulbous distal phalanges and cleft uvula, not described in the patients with the syndrome discussed above. However, until more cases are reported, the possibility of their being identical cannot be excluded.

TREATMENT

The hearing loss can be improved by middle ear surgery for the ossicular abnormalities. The vaginal aplasia should be corrected by plastic surgery.

PROGNOSIS

There is moderate variation in the degree of severity of the lesions in affected persons. If a single kidney is involved, a patient can live an essentially normal life.

SUMMARY

This syndrome is characterized by: 1) autosomal recessive transmission, 2) unilateral or bilateral renal hypoplasia or agenesis, 3) variable involvement of the genital system with occasional hypoplastic ovaries, tubes, or vagina, and 4) moderate to severe conductive hearing loss with malformation of the ossicles.

REFERENCES

Braun, F. C., Jr., and Bayer, J. F., Familial nephrosis associated with deafness and congenital urinary tract anomalies in siblings. *J. Pediatr., 60*:33–41, 1962.

Turner, G., A second family with renal, vaginal, and middle ear anomalies. *J. Pediatr., 76*:641, 1970.

Winter, J. S. D., Kohn, G., Mellman, W. J., and Wagner, S., A familial syndrome of renal, genital, and middle ear anomalies. *J. Pediatr., 72*:88–93, 1968.

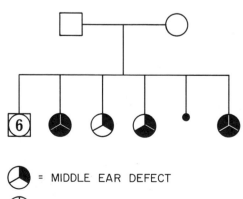

Figure 7–7 Renal, genital, and middle ear anomalies. Pedigree showing four affected persons among ten sibs. (From J. S. D. Winter *et al., J. Pediatr.,* 72:88, 1968.)

= MIDDLE EAR DEFECT

= RENAL DYSGENESIS

= VAGINAL ATRESIA

RENAL DISEASE, DIGITAL ANOMALIES, AND CONDUCTION HEARING LOSS

A syndrome characterized by renal anomalies, nephrosis, digital anomalies, cleft uvula, and conductive hearing loss was described by Braun and Bayer (1962) in five male sibs.

CLINICAL FINDINGS

Renal System. Several types of renal disease were noted. Two boys had nephrosis with severe proteinuria. Intravenous pyelograms done on all five affected sibs showed no abnormalities in two. In one patient, the pelvis and ureters were not visualized; in another, congenital ureterovesical obstruction and malfunction of one kidney were observed; in a third, unilateral duplication of the renal pelvis and upper ureter was noted.

Musculoskeletal System. The thumbs and great toes in three sibs had a short, broad, bulbous appearance.

Oral Findings. The uvula was bifurcated in two sibs.

Auditory System. Two of the boys had a 30 to 40 dB conductive hearing loss. One boy had a 60 to 80 dB mixed hearing loss; conductive loss was 20 to 40 dB bilaterally. Other audiometric tests were not reported.

Vestibular System. No vestibular findings were described.

LABORATORY FINDINGS

Radiographs of the abnormal digits of three of the boys showed short and rudi-

mentary distal phalanges, each exhibiting bifurcation of the distal ends.

Proteinuria was found in two sibs. Intravenous pyelograms were abnormal in three of the five sibs.

HEREDITY

Five brothers among a sibship of twelve had the same general features. The parents were normal and not related. A maternal cousin was born deaf but had no other abnormalities. From the pedigree it appears that the syndrome has X-linked or possibly autosomal recessive transmission.

DIAGNOSIS

This syndrome may be identical to that of renal, genital, and middle ear anomalies (Winter *et al.*, 1968). Other hereditary syndromes with renal disease and hearing loss must be distinguished from this disease. *Alport syndrome* is associated with a progressive sensorineural hearing loss in contrast to the rather stable conductive hearing loss found in the syndrome described here. Furthermore, Alport syndrome exhibits autosomal dominant transmission.

TREATMENT

Extensive medical care for the nephrosis is important. Diagnostic renal studies, including an intravenous pyelo-

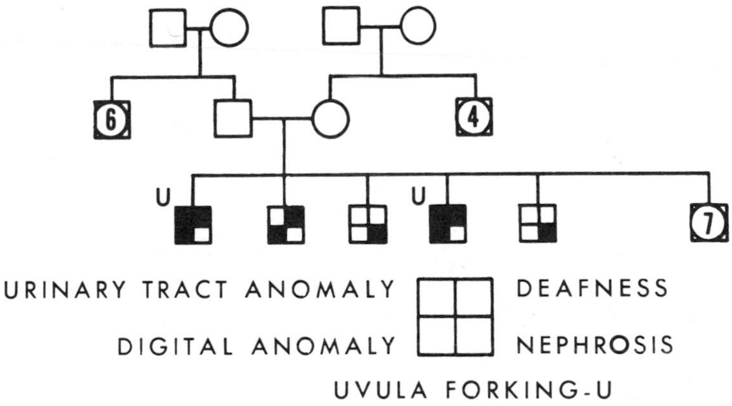

Figure 7–8 Renal disease, digital anomalies, and conductive hearing loss. Pedigree showing affected persons in kindred. (From F. C. Braun and J. F. Bayer, J. Pediatr., 60:33, 1962.)

URINARY TRACT ANOMALY   DEAFNESS

DIGITAL ANOMALY   NEPHROSIS

UVULA FORKING-U

gram, should be undertaken. Hearing aids may help the patient with hearing loss.

PROGNOSIS

Prognosis is rather poor because of the renal disease. The sibs with nephrosis had no other renal abnormalities. One died from the effects of the renal disease, whereas another sib at 5 years of age was in moderately good health.

SUMMARY

Characteristics of this syndrome include: 1) X-linked or autosomal recessive transmission, 2) shortened bulbous thumbs and halluces with bifurcation of the distal end of the terminal phalanx, 3) renal anomalies, including ureteral constrictions and duplication of the renal pelvis, 4) bifurcation of the uvula, and 5) congenital moderate to severe conductive hearing loss.

REFERENCES

Braun, F. C., Jr., and Bayer, J. F.: Familial nephrosis associated with deafness and congenital urinary tract anomalies in siblings. *J. Pediatr., 60*:33–41, 1962.
Winter, J. S. D., Kohn, G., Mellman, W. J., and Wagner, S., A familial syndrome of renal, genital, and middle ear anomalies. *J. Pediatr., 72*:88–93, 1968.

Chapter 8

GENETIC HEARING LOSS WITH NERVOUS SYSTEM DISEASE

ATAXIA, PES CAVUS, AND SENSORINEURAL DEAFNESS OF ADULT ONSET

Schimke (1974) reported an essentially "pure form" of progressive adult-onset cerebellar ataxia and sensorineural deafness in four sibs.

CLINICAL FINDINGS

Physical Findings. The findings are limited to pes cavus, ataxia, and sensorineural deafness.

Nervous System. All sibs began to exhibit cerebellar ataxia during their late 20s or early 30s. They were grossly ataxic with eyes either open or closed. Affected individuals walked with a wide stance and exhibited compensatory lumbar lordosis. Their speech was dysarthric, and they all manifested dysadiadochokinesia.

Ataxia was progressive. Intelligence was intact. Evidence of tremor, clonus, or spasticity never became apparent. Position and vibratory senses as well as deep tendon reflexes remained intact. Muscle strength was normal. Pes cavus preceded the occurrence of ataxia in all sibs.

Other Findings. Other systems and the fundi were normal. Cataracts were present, but they segregated independently in the family.

Auditory System. Progressive sensorineural deafness appeared during adolescence. This preceded the onset of the ataxia. The deafness slowly progressed and became profound in middle life.

Vestibular System. No tests were described.

LABORATORY FINDINGS

Extensive laboratory tests were carried out, but they showed nothing significant.

HEREDITY

The parents of the four affected sibs were normal except for cataract in the father. Inheritance appeared to be autosomal recessive.

DIAGNOSIS

This disorder is distinguished from the many syndromes of ataxia and deafness, pre-

303

sented in subsequent sections by the absence of associated anomalies. Although pes cavus was present, suggesting Friedreich ataxia, no other signs of spinocerebellar disease were evident.

TREATMENT

At present, only symptomatic therapy, such as surgical correction of the pes cavus, can be offered.

PROGNOSIS

Both the ataxia and the deafness are progressive.

SUMMARY

The syndrome is characterized by: 1) autosomal recessive transmission, 2) progressive adult onset of ataxia and dysarthria, 3) pes cavus, which precedes the ataxia, and 4) progressive sensorineural deafness with adult onset.

REFERENCES

Schimke, R. N., Adult-onset hereditary cerebellar ataxia and neurosensory deafness. *Clin. Genet.*, 6:416–421, 1974.

ATAXIA, HYPOGONADISM, MENTAL RETARDATION, AND SENSORINEURAL DEAFNESS
(Richards-Rundle Syndrome)

A syndrome consisting of slowly progressive ataxia, hearing loss, and mental deterioration beginning in childhood was found in two sibs described by Koennecke (1919) and in five sibs reported by Richards and Rundle (1959).

CLINICAL FINDINGS

Physical Findings. Affected persons in the family described by Richards and Rundle exhibited marked wasting of peripheral muscles.

Nervous System. Mental activity is normal for the first few years of life but deteriorates progressively thereafter. By the third decade, all affected persons were severely retarded, some having an I.Q. between 25 and 49.

Walking is sometimes late in onset. During the second year of life, ataxia markedly interferes with the development of gait. By 4 or 5 years of age, most affected individuals can walk but require support and are severely ataxic. Although deep tendon reflexes are present in the earlier years, patients generally become areflexic by the end of the first decade of life. A mild, horizontal nystagmus also develops during the second decade.

Reproductive System. The sibs described by Richards and Rundle lacked development of secondary sex characteristics. Axillary and pubic hair was scanty, the breasts were flat, menses were infrequent or absent, and the external genitalia were small.

Skeletal System. All affected persons had foot deformities, including pes varus, pes cavus, and pes equinovarus, which developed during the second decade. The 24-year-old patient described by Koennecke had cervical scoliosis and thoracic kyphosis. Some patients had clawhand.

Muscular System. Muscle wasting, particularly of the forearms and the small hand muscles and lower legs, was found in all cases. It was progressive, beginning in early childhood. Muscle tone was decreased.

Integumentary System. There was a general loss of subcutaneous fat.

Auditory System. Affected persons learned to say a few words in their first few years of life, and then their speech deteriorated. Hearing loss was noted at about 2 years of age, although partial hearing was maintained for several years before severe deafness supervened. In the two sibs described by Koennecke, hearing loss was

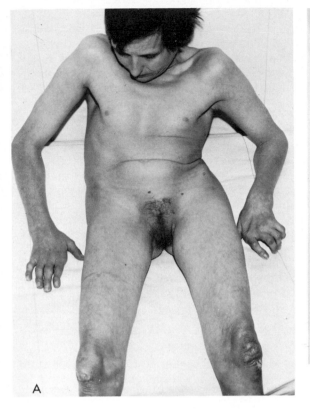

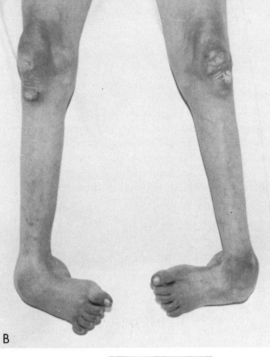

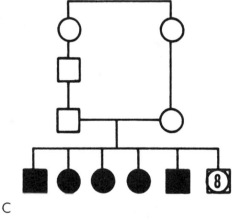

Figure 8–1 Ataxia, hypogonadism, mental retardation, and sensorineural deafness. (A) The patient, a deaf-mute, exhibits claw hands and wasting of peroneal muscles. The breasts are prepubescent, and the pubic hair is scanty. *(B)* Muscle atrophy and flexion deformities. *(C)* Pedigree showing five affected persons among 13 sibs of a consanguineous mating. *(A–C* from B. W. Richards and A. T. Rundle, *J. Ment. Defic. Res.,* 3:33, 1959.)

noted when the children were about 7 years old. Both became severely deaf during adolescence.

Vestibular System. No vestibular tests were described.

LABORATORY FINDINGS

There was marked reduction of urinary estrogen, pregnanediol, and total neutral 17-ketosteroid levels. Richards and Rundle (1959) suggested that there was a metabolic block in steroid metabolism. Urinary creatinine was low, but excretion of creatine was appreciable.

Excessive urinary excretion of β-aminoisobutyric acid was documented.

PATHOLOGY

Testicular biopsy of a 17-year-old patient showed decreased production of spermatozoa and arrest of development as well as desquamation of primary spermatocytes. Leydig cells showed no evidence of function (Richards and Rundle, 1959).

Sylvester (1972) studied two of the patients reported by Richards and Rundle and found the neuropathologic findings to be consistent with the Roussy-Levy syndrome, a form of spinocerebellar degeneration.

HEREDITY

In each of the two sibships, the parents were normal. Richards and Rundle (1959) noted parental consanguinity, which suggests autosomal recessive inheritance.

DIAGNOSIS

Progressive ataxia and hearing loss characterized the disorder in three brothers described by Matthews (1950). Sexual development and intelligence apparently were normal. In the syndrome described by Sylvester (1958) there was *optic atrophy, ataxia, and sensorineural hearing loss.* Inheritance was autosomal dominant.

TREATMENT

At present, only supportive therapy can be offered.

PROGNOSIS

The disease progresses from the first year through childhood and becomes fairly static during early adult life. It does not appear to shorten the life span.

SUMMARY

This syndrome is characterized by: 1) autosomal recessive transmission, 2) progressive severe mental deterioration, 3) early onset of progressive mild ataxia and horizontal nystagmus, 4) muscle wasting, particularly involving the distal extremities, 5) absent development of secondary sex characteristics, 6) reduced urinary estrogen, pregnanediol and total neutral 17-ketosteroids, and 7) early onset of severe progressive hearing loss.

REFERENCES

Koennecke, W., Friedreichsche Ataxie und Taubstummheit. *Z. Gesamte Neurol. Pathol., 53*:161–165, 1920.
Matthews, W. B., Familial ataxia, deaf-mutism, and muscular wasting. *J. Neurol. Neurosurg. Psychiatry, 13*:307–311, 1950.
Richards, B. W., and Rundle, A. T., A familial hormonal disorder associated with mental deficiency, deaf mutism, and ataxia. *J. Ment. Defic. Res., 3*:33–55, 1959.
Sylvester, P. E., Some unusual findings in a family with Friedreich's ataxia. *Arch. Dis. Child., 33*:217–221, 1958.
Sylvester, P. E., Spino-cerebellar degeneration, hormonal disorder, hypogonadism, deaf-mutism, and mental deficiency. *J. Ment. Defic. Res., 16*:203–214, 1972.

ATAXIA OLIGOPHRENIA MYOCARDIAL SCLEROSIS, AND SENSORINEURAL DEAFNESS

In 1963 Jeune, Tommasi, Freycon, and Nivelson described two Gypsy sibs who, at about 6 years of age, developed a syndrome that included cerebellar ataxia, progressive sensorineural hearing loss, mental deficiency, and skin pigmentation. Through personal communication (September, 1974) we have learned of a third affected sib (a male) and of other relatives with the same disorder.

CLINICAL FINDINGS

Nervous System. At about 6 years of age the sibs developed a mild cerebellar ataxia with intention tremor, adiadochokinesia, and hypotonia. The older sib, examined at 12 years of age, showed marked mental deterioration and increased severity

of the aforementioned changes. Reflexes, except extensor plantar response, were depressed.

Ocular System. The female sib exhibited minimal retinitis pigmentosa when she was about 12-years-old. She also had mild nystagmus.

Cardiovascular System. In all affected sibs the heart was moderately enlarged and showed an abnormal EKG with left ventricular hypertrophy. Terminally, the children developed an atrioventricular heart block.

Integumentary System. Numerous freckles or lentigines were noted over the face, arms, and legs.

Auditory System. Hearing loss was first noted when the children were about six years old. Hearing tests on one child at 6 years and on another at 11 years showed bilateral sensorineural deafness. According to the case history, the hearing loss was progressive.

Vestibular System. No vestibular tests were described.

LABORATORY FINDINGS

A chest radiograph of the older child showed cardiomegaly.

PATHOLOGY

An autopsy was performed on the 12-year-old child. Gross examination of the brain showed no abnormalities. There was mild pallor of the myelin in the cerebral white matter. The spinal cord exhibited moderate degeneration of the spinocerebellar tracts and fasciculis gracilis. The cerebellar cortex was normal.

The heart showed diffuse myocardial fibrosis.

HEREDITY

The disorder was quite similar in the affected sibs except for the presence of myocardial dystrophy in the older child.

The affected children had two normal younger sibs. The parents, who were normal, were first cousins. The syndrome appears to have autosomal recessive inheritance.

DIAGNOSIS

Friedreich ataxia, ataxia-telangiectasia, Wilson's disease, amaurotic family idiocy. *Refsum syndrome,* and *Usher syndrome* must be considered in a differential diagnosis. It is important to know whether retinitis pigmentosa is a consistent finding in this syndrome, or whether it is adventitious. Lentigines also occur in the *multiple lentigines (Leopard) syndrome.*

TREATMENT

The deafness may be ameliorated by a hearing aid. Mental deterioration, however, precludes much improvement.

SUMMARY

This syndrome is characterized by: 1) autosomal recessive transmission, 2) childhood onset of progressive oligophrenia, 3) progressive cerebellar ataxia, 4) skin pigmentary changes, including lentigo and achromatic nevi, 5) possible retinitis pigmentosa, 6) possible myocardial dystrophy, and 7) childhood onset of progressive sensorineural hearing loss.

REFERENCES

Jeune, M., Tommasi, M., Freycon, F., and Nivelon, J., Syndrome familial associant ataxie, surdité et oligophrénie. Sclérose myocardique d'evolution fatale chez l'un des enfants. *Pédiatrie,* *18*:984–987, 1963.

ATAXIA MENTAL RETARDATION, AND SENSORINEURAL HEARING LOSS

Berman, Haslam, Konigsmark, Capute, and Migeon (1973) reported infantile onset of progressive ataxia, hearing loss, and mental retardation as well as signs of both upper and lower motor neuron disease in three male sibs.

CLINICAL FINDINGS

Physical Findings. Each of the three sibs had a myopathic facies. Height was at the third percentile in two of the three sibs.

Nervous System. Walking was delayed in development, and gait was initially clumsy. Falling was frequent and became progressively worse, with truncal ataxia occurring within the next few years. The lower extremities became markedly atrophic. Muscle tone and deep-tendon reflexes were increased in the legs. Contractures developed at the heels and were accompanied by bilateral extensor plantar responses, suggesting upper motor neuron involvement. Marked horizontal nystagmus on lateral gaze was noted in all three sibs. Dysarthria was also present.

Intelligence was reduced to an I.Q. level of 50 to 60. The retardation appeared to be mildly progressive.

Auditory System. Audiometric testing during the first few years of life showed a hearing deficit. Within the next few years there was progressive hearing loss, terminating in severe sensorineural deafness.

Vestibular System. Normal caloric responses were elicited.

LABORATORY FINDINGS

Radiographs showed moderate osteoporosis of the lower limbs in one sib. All biochemical studies were normal. Nerve conduction velocity of the peroneal nerve was reduced in all three sibs. Sural nerve biopsy showed mild myelin degeneration. Fibrillations were noted on electromyography. These findings suggested anterior motor horn cell involvement.

HEREDITY

The parents of the three affected male sibs were nonconsanguineous. The pedigree is compatible either with autosomal recessive or with X-linked inheritance.

DIAGNOSIS

Several syndromes are characterized by hearing loss, ataxia, and mental retardation. However, they can be differentiated from the syndrome considered here by their inheritance pattern and/or associated anomalies. *Dominant piebald trait, ataxia, and sensorineural hearing loss* has white forelock, variable deafness, and mild retardation. Those patients with retardation exhibit incoordination and ataxia. *Ataxia, oligophrenia, myocardial sclerosis, and sensorineural deafness* can be excluded by the presence of pigmented spots on the face, arms and legs, and by myocardial sclerosis. The *Richards-Rundle syndrome* can be excluded, since patients with that condition have hypogonadism, elevated β-aminoisobutyric acid, and low ketosteroid levels in the urine. *Ataxia, hypotonia, depressed deep tendon reflexes, and progressive sensorineural deafness* differs in having later onset of ataxia, minimal mental changes, and milder hearing loss.

TREATMENT

A hearing aid is useful during the early stages of the disorder. Lengthening of the Achilles tendon is necessary for correction of the heel contractures.

PROGNOSIS

Prognosis is poor. All components of the syndrome were progressive in severity.

SUMMARY

Characteristics of the syndrome include: 1) autosomal recessive or X-linked transmission, 2) progressive ataxia, 3) mental retardation, 4) upper and lower motor neuron disease, and 5) profound sensorineural hearing loss. All findings are of infantile onset.

REFERENCES

Berman, W., Haslam, R. H., Konigsmark, B. W., Capute, A. J., and Migeon, C. J., A new familial syndrome with ataxia, hearing loss, and mental retardation. *Arch. Neurol.*, 29:258–261, 1973.

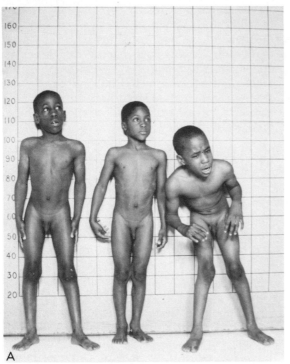

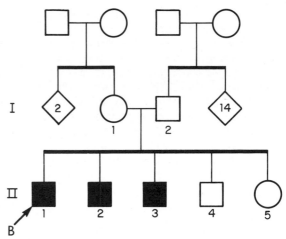

Figure 8–2 Ataxia, mental retardation and sensorineural hearing loss. (A) Two of the affected sibs and their normal brother. In the affected boys, note the myopathic facies, broad-based stance, and wasting of lower extremities. (B) Pedigree of affected kindred. (A and B from W. Berman et al., Arch. Neurol., 29: 258, 1973.)

ATAXIA HYPERURICEMIA RENAL INSUFFICIENCY, AND SENSORINEURAL DEAFNESS

A syndrome characterized by hyperuricemia, renal insufficiency, ataxia, and deafness was described in five members of three generations of a kindred (Rosenberg, Bergstrom, Troost, and Bartholomew, 1970). Six other members of the kindred had various components of the syndrome.

CLINICAL FINDINGS

Nervous System. Six patients had ataxic gait, first noted in the second or third decade, which progressed slowly thereafter and involved both arms and legs. Dysarthria was also a common finding. One patient had nystagmus on lateral gaze. Proximal muscle weakness or wasting was evident in five of the six ataxic patients. Reflexes were hyperactive. Sensory findings were normal, except for mild vibratory loss in the distal extremities in two patients.

Cardiovascular System. An electrocardiogram on the proband showed left atrial enlargement, left axis deviation, and Wolff-Parkinson-White syndrome. At 22 years of age the patient developed congestive heart failure and gallop rhythm. The condition was diagnosed as cardiomyopathy. The patient's 43-year-old mother had left ventricular hypertrophy.

Auditory System. Hearing loss was first noticed in the second or third decade. Younger affected persons had only high-tone sensorineural hearing loss, whereas the oldest affected patient had a severe sensorineural deafness with apparent progression. Speech discrimination varied markedly. Detailed audiometric testing on one patient suggested a cochlear locus for the hearing loss.

Vestibular System. All members with ataxia had electronystagmography examination. Two showed abnormal pendular thickening. One of these individuals had abnormal optokinetics, and the other had severe nausea and vomiting on caloric stimulation.

LABORATORY FINDINGS

Enzymatic studies carried out on all affected patients showed intact erythrocyte hypoxanthine-guanine phosphoribosyltransferase (HGPRT) and adenine phosphoribosyl-transferase (APRT) activities.

Nine members of the kindred had hyperuricemia. Renal function tests were done on seven of these patients. In five of these individuals the PAH, creatinine, and insulin clearance tests were borderline or decreased. On the basis of creatinine clearance tests four patients with hyperuricemia had normal renal function, suggesting that the hyperuricemia was not secondary to renal insufficiency.

HEREDITY

Affected persons were noted in each of three generations of the kindred. Expression varied, some individuals showing only hyperuricemia, others exhibiting deafness and ataxia. It appears that the hyperuricemia, ataxia, and hearing loss are different manifestations of the same pleiotropic gene. The syndrome has autosomal dominant inheritance.

DIAGNOSIS

In *Alport syndrome,* hyperuricemia is not a feature, and there is no ataxia. There are several hereditary syndromes that include ataxia and hearing loss as characteristics, but there are no others known to be associated with hyperuricemia or renal insufficiency. The syndrome discussed here differs from Lesch-Nyhan syndrome in that there is no self-mutilation, mental retardation, choreoathetosis, or absent HGPRT activity. There is also a different inheritance pattern. The syndrome described by Kelley *et al.* (1969), which is characterized by hyperuricemia, nephrolithiasis, and mild cerebellar ataxia with partial deficiency in the enzyme hypoxanthine-guanine phosphoribosyltransferase (HGPRT), differs from the syndrome considered here in that these patients have hearing loss and do not have HGPRT deficiency.

TREATMENT

Symptomatic treatment of the varying defects is necessary. For the hearing loss, a hearing aid may be necessary. Allopurinol may be given for the hyperuricemia. Little can be offered for the ataxia and weakness.

PROGNOSIS

Although there are variable manifestations of the ataxia and hearing loss, both become slowly progressive and severe. The hyperuricemia may lead to gout, as found in the oldest member of this kindred.

SUMMARY

Characteristics of this syndrome include: 1) autosomal dominant transmission with variable expressivity, 2) hyperuricemia, 3) ataxia, beginning in the second decade and progressing very slowly, 4) renal insufficiency, 5) sensorineural hearing loss, beginning in the second decade and progressing to severe deafness, and 6) vestibular abnormalities.

REFERENCES

Kelley, W. N., Greene, M. L., Rosenbloom, F. M., Henderson, J. F., and Seegmiller, J. E., Hypoxanthine-guanine phosphoribosyltransferase deficiency in gout. *Ann. Intern. Med.,* 70:155–206, 1969.

Rosenberg, A. L., Bergstrom, L., Troost, B. T., and Bartholomew, B. A., Hyperuricemia and neurologic defects. *N. Engl. J. Med.,* 282:992–997, 1970.

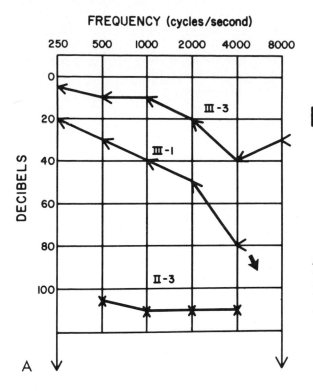

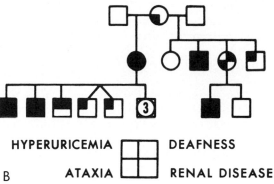

Figure 8–3 Ataxia, hyperuricemia, renal insufficiency, and sensorineural deafness. *(A)* Composite audiogram showing progression of hearing loss. III-3, age 18; III-1, age 22; II-3, age 38. *(B)* Pedigree showing variable expressivity of the syndrome. *(A* and *B* from A. L. Rosenberg *et al., N. Engl. J. Med.,282*:992, 1970.)

ATAXIA, HYPOTONIA, DEPRESSED DEEP TENDON REFLEXES, AND PROGRESSIVE SENSORINEURAL DEAFNESS

This combination of progressive severe hearing loss and ataxia described in two sibships may represent a syndrome distinct from Friedreich's ataxia (Lichtenstein and Knorr, 1930; Pires and de Carvalho, 1935).

CLINICAL FINDINGS

Nervous System. There was mild intention tremor and ataxia of gait, appearing between 10 and 20 years of age and progressing slowly. By 30 years of age patients were unable to walk. Hypotonia and depression of deep-tendon reflexes and flexion-plantar responses were noted. Speech was dysarthric and at times explosive. Several sibs developed kyphoscoliosis and pes cavus. In general, sensation was intact. Some mental deterioration was apparent in the 29- and 33-year old brothers (Pires and de Carvalho, 1935).

Ocular System. One patient had unilateral cataract, and another had bilateral cataract (Lichtenstein and Knorr, 1930).

Auditory System. One child reported by Lichtenstein and Knorr (1930) in early childhood had severe hearing loss that progressed to profound deafness by 20 years of age, when she died of heart failure. In the early school years the other two children had mild hearing loss that progressed to moderate deafness in their early 20s. Similar findings were noted by Pires and de Carvalho (1935) in two of the four affected brothers, two of whom had died prior to examination of the proband.

Vestibular System. Vestibular function was normal.

LABORATORY FINDINGS

No laboratory tests were reported.

HEREDITY

In one kindred there were three affected sibs; in the other, four affected sibs. The parents were healthy and in the case of

Lichtenstein and Knorr (1930) were consanguineous. The syndrome appears to have autosomal recessive inheritance.

DIAGNOSIS

In Friedreich's ataxia, which is inherited as an autosomal recessive disorder, there is involvement principally of the spinocerebellar and pyramidal tracts and dorsal columns with resultant limb incoordination, dysarthria, nystagmus, diminished or absent tendon reflexes, scoliosis, Babinski's sign, impairment of position and vibratory senses, and pes cavus. The disorder has preadolescent onset. Cardiac dysfunction and diabetes mellitus occur in about 25 per cent. Although hearing loss has been reported in Friedreich's ataxia, it is mild in degree and infrequent in occurrence. Several syndromes can be distinguished from this disorder because of retinal involvement. In *Richards-Rundle syndrome* mental deficiency and hypogonadism are present. *Myoclonic epilepsy, ataxia, and sensorineural deafness* may be excluded by the absence of myoclonus in the syndrome under discussion.

In the family described by Klippel and Durante (1892), affected individuals had mild hearing loss. Transmission was autosomal dominant, distinguishing it from the recessive transmission in the syndrome under discussion.

TREATMENT

Hearing aids may be used to assuage the hearing loss.

PROGNOSIS

The hearing loss progresses to severe deafness, and the ataxia worsens with age.

SUMMARY

This syndrome is characterized by: 1) autosomal recessive transmission, 2) adolescent onset of slow, progressive ataxia, 3) depression of reflexes, 4) dysarthric speech, 5) hypotonia, 6) pes cavus, and 7) childhood onset of progressive severe sensorineural hearing loss.

REFERENCES

Klippel, M., and Durante, G., Affectiones nerveuses familiales et héréditaires. *Rev. Méd. (Paris),* 12:745–785, 1892.
Lichtenstein, H., and Knorr, A., Über einige Fälle von fortschreitender Schwerhörigkeit bei hereditärer Ataxie. *Dtsch. Z. Nervenheilkd.,* 114:1–28, 1930.
Pires, W., and de Carvalho, A. H., Doença de Friedreich com surdez em dois irmãos. *Rev. Neuropsiquiatr. (São Paulo),* 1:435–441, 1935.

ATAXIA, CATARACT, PSYCHOSIS AND/OR DEMENTIA AND SENSORINEURAL DEAFNESS

Strömgren, Dalby, Dalby, and Ranheim (1970) reported the syndrome as occurring in nine members of five generations of a family.

CLINICAL FINDINGS

Nervous System. Cerebellar ataxia appeared in two of the kindred after the age of 40. There was intention tremor of the trunk and all four limbs with pendular reflexes. Gait was staggering and swaying. Speech was slurred; central-type nystagmus was noted. Pyramidal tract signs were normal. Paranoid psychosis developed in five patients after the age of 50. Increasing dementia starting a few years before death was found in four patients.

Ocular System. Posterior polar cataract was found in all affected persons, usually appearing between 20 and 30 years of age and slowly maturing over one or two decades. Intrabulbar hemorrhage was common. Nystagmus was present, as noted above. In some individuals the pupils did not react to light.

Other Findings. Ichthyosis and gastric achylia were variable findings.

Auditory System. Impaired hearing appeared some years after the ocular symptoms had started. After the age of 45 years, audiometry indicated severe or profound deafness in all patients.

Vestibular System. Vestibular reflexes were diminished or lost.

LABORATORY FINDINGS

None were described.

PATHOLOGY

Although autopsy studies were carried out on four patients, the findings were not revealed.

HEREDITY

The syndrome exhibits autosomal dominant inheritance.

DIAGNOSIS

The syndrome most closely resembles *Refsum syndrome,* but the latter has autosomal recessive inheritance.

TREATMENT

Treatment is apparently of no avail.

PROGNOSIS

Five affected members died between the ages of 57 and 60 years from bronchopneumonia, intractable diarrhea, and cerebrovascular disease.

SUMMARY

The syndrome is characterized by: 1) autosomal dominant inheritance, 2) cerebellar ataxia that appears after the age of 40, 3) intention tremor of the trunk and extremities, 4) slurred speech, 5) central-type nystagmus, 6) paranoid psychosis and dementia, 7) posterior polar cataract appearing during the third decade, 8) intrabulbar hemorrhage, 9) severe to profound sensorineural hearing loss after 45 years of age, and 10) loss of vestibular function.

REFERENCES

Strömgren, E., Dalby, A., Dalby, M. A., and Ranheim, B., Cataracts, deafness, cerebellar ataxia, psychosis, and dementia – a new syndrome. *Acta Neurol. Scand., Suppl. 43*:261–262, 1970.

PHOTOMYOCLONUS. DIABETES MELLITUS, NEPHROPATHY, AND SENSORINEURAL DEAFNESS

Herrmann, Aguilar, and Sacks (1964) described a syndrome in 3 generations of a family in which 13 members were affected with photomyoclonic seizures and progressive hearing loss appearing in the third decade. Mild diabetes mellitus and a progressive dementia began shortly thereafter.

CLINICAL FINDINGS

Nervous System. Photomyoclonic seizures began in the proband when she was 20 years old and in her two sisters and a cousin in early adult life. Occasional grand mal seizures occurred. In the fourth decade a moderately rapid deterioration characterized by progressive nervousness, memory

loss, and depression began; these changes eventually led to severe dementia within about ten years. The later course of the disease was characterized by slowing and slurring of speech, lateralizing signs, including progressive hemiparesis, hemihypesthesia, and hemianopsia as well as mild ataxia of the extremities.

Renal System. Four of the affected persons had renal disease. In three, no description other than "kidney trouble or Bright's disease" was given. Although urinalysis showed no abnormalities in the proband, interstitial nephritis was found on autopsy.

Endocrine System. All patients with this syndrome had evidence of diabetes mellitus, which in the proband was characterized by a fasting blood sugar of 200 mg. per cent. In three other cases, glucose tolerance curves indicated diabetes.

Auditory System. Progressive sensorineural hearing loss was first noticed in the fourth decade. It was found in 9 of 13 affected members. In one patient progression to severe hearing loss occurred within seven years. No audiometric findings were described.

Vestibular System. No vestibular function tests were reported.

LABORATORY FINDINGS

Pneumoencephalograms on the proband showed mild ventricular dilatation. Intravenous pyelograms on two patients revealed moderate to marked blunting of calyces.

As noted above, elevated blood sugar and abnormal glucose tolerance curves were demonstrated.

Urinalysis in four patients revealed no cells or proteinuria. Paper chromatographic study of the proband showed markedly elevated levels of valine and leucine; in three other patients, however, these were normal.

An electroencephalogram on the proband showed severe generalized disorganization (Fig. 8–4A). In two patients generalized spike-and-wave activity accompanied by myoclonic jerks and unconsciousness were produced by photic stimulation. Two other patients had marked myoclonic and convulsive response to photic stimulation, maximal at a flash rate of 15 per second.

PATHOLOGY

The kidneys were somewhat small and granular. Some glomeruli were atrophic and exhibited a capsular fibrosis. PAS-positive granules were present in the epithelium of the distal and collecting tubules. The lumina contained many casts. In the interstitium, small foci of lymphocytes and foamy macrophages were present; these changes were similar to those noted in Alport syndrome.

The brain manifested mild cortical atrophy. There was a cerebral neuronal loss and a possible loss in the cerebellar cortex, dentate nucleus, and inferior olivary nucleus (Fig. 8–4C).

HEREDITY

It seems likely that the affected persons in this kindred had the same disorder. All of the younger affected individuals had mild diabetes mellitus and photomyoclonus. The deafness and mental deterioration were found in all older affected persons. However, two sisters, aged 28 and 40 years, had normal intelligence and normal hearing. Males and females were affected in equal numbers. Inheritance appears to be autosomal dominant with complete penetrance and variability in expression (Fig. 8–4B).

DIAGNOSIS

Progressive renal failure and sensorineural hearing loss occur in *Alport syndrome*. However, there is neither mental deterioration nor epilepsy, except terminally, when they are accompanied by uremia. Myoclonic epilepsy is seen in (1) Lafora's disease, characterized by rapid mental deterioration and seizures; (2) Unverricht's myoclonic epilepsy, characterized by a very slow course, rigidity, cerebellar signs, and dementia; (3) subacute sclerosing panencephalitis with a rapid downhill course; and (4) neuronal storage disease, including curvilinear body disease. In none of these disorders is hearing loss a prominent feature. *Myoclonic epilepsy and congenital sensorineural deafness* can be distinguished from the syndrome considered here by its recessive mode of inheritance and severe congenital hearing loss. *Myoclonic epilepsy, ataxia, and sensorineural deafness* shows a very similar course to the present syndrome. However, mental deterioration is not a prominent part of that disorder.

TREATMENT

Anticonvulsant medication can be used for the myoclonus and the grand mal epilepsy. A hearing aid may be employed to compensate for the hearing loss.

PROGNOSIS

Prognosis appears to be rather good until the onset of mental deterioration, which portends death within a few years.

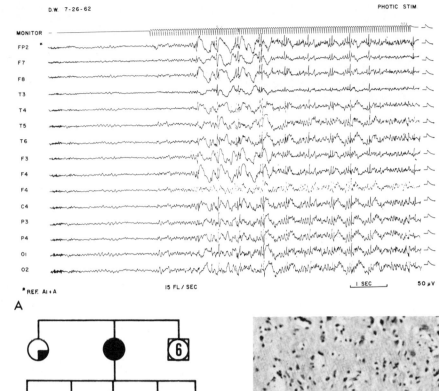

A

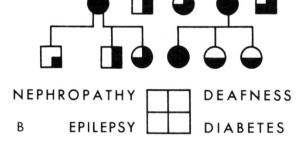

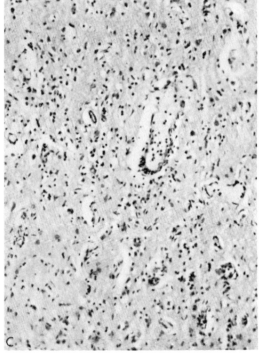

NEPHROPATHY — DEAFNESS

B EPILEPSY — DIABETES

Figure 8-4 Photomyoclonus, diabetes mellitus, nephropathy, and sensorineural deafness. (A) Electro-encephalogram of patient showing photomyoclonus. (B) Pedigree of kindred showing 13 persons affected in three generations. (C) Parietal cortex showing diffuse neuronal loss and astrocytosis. (A–C from C. Herrmann, Jr. et al., Neurology (Minneap.), 14:212, 1964.)

SUMMARY

This syndrome is characterized by: 1) autosomal dominant inheritance with variable expressivity, 2) photomyoclonic epilepsy beginning in early adult life, 3) adult onset of mild diabetes mellitus, 4) nephropathy with accumulation of PAS-positive material in renal tubular cells, and 5) progressive sensorineural hearing loss.

REFERENCES

Herrmann, C., Jr., Aguilar, M. J., and Sacks, O. W.: Hereditary photomyoclonus associated with diabetes mellitus, deafness, nephropathy, and cerebral dysfunction. *Neurology (Minneap.),* 14:212–221, 1964.

MYOCLONIC EPILEPSY, ATAXIA AND SENSORINEURAL DEAFNESS

In 1968 May and White reported a kindred in which six members in four generations were affected by a syndrome that included myoclonus, cerebellar ataxia, and sensorineural hearing loss.

CLINICAL FINDINGS

Nervous System. Four of the six patients had a history of grand mal epilepsy, and two of these four had myoclonus. The myoclonic movements began in the teens and included jerking motions that involved head, trunk, and limbs. Generalized seizures began shortly afterward, usually in the third decade. Two of the six patients had no evidence of grand mal seizures. Difficulty with arm and leg coordination, beginning in adolescence, occurred in three of the six. When present, the ataxia progressed slowly. Neurologic evaluation of the three patients studied showed an unsteady, broad-based gait, mild to moderate intention tremor, tremor on finger-to-nose or heel-to-knee test, and truncal ataxia. No nystagmus, cranial nerve abnormalities, sensory loss, or weakness were described, although speech was dysarthric in those patients with ataxia. There was no mental deterioration.

Auditory System. Hearing loss was first noted in childhood or in early adult life. It was slowly progressive, resulting in severe loss in the later years of life. An audiogram of one patient who was 32 years old showed about a 40 dB sensorineural hearing loss bilaterally. Another patient in her 50s had severe auditory loss, hearing only loud noises directed into the ear.

Vestibular System. No vestibular testing was described.

LABORATORY FINDINGS

Electroencephalograms on the three patients examined showed normal resting activity. In two patients with a history of seizures, photic stimulation induced continuous generalized spike discharges. In one case myoclonic jerks in the biceps muscle were associated with cortical spikes.

HEREDITY

Among the six affected persons the syndrome showed moderate variability. The proband and his mother had the complete syndrome, including hearing loss, myoclonus, epilepsy, and ataxia. A maternal uncle had hearing loss and ataxia without epilepsy. The maternal aunt and maternal grandfather had only epilepsy, and the maternal great-grandfather had only hearing loss; none of these three persons was examined. The syndrome appears to have autosomal dominant inheritance with variable expressivity.

DIAGNOSIS

Myoclonus is a characteristic of several different diseases. Benign essential myoclonus is characterized by autosomal dominant inheritance; however, there is no associated ataxia or hearing loss. Lafora's myoclonic epilepsy also exhibits dominant transmission; after onset of epilepsy in mid-adolescence there is rather rapid mental deterioration. In Unverricht's myoclonic epilepsy, transmission is recessive and there is only very slow mental deterioration after the onset of symptoms during adolescence. Myoclonic epilepsy appears in curvilinear body disease, a recessively transmitted condition; onset is in the first few years of life, with death by 10 years of age. Ramsey Hunt's myoclonic epilepsy is also recessively transmitted and consists of myoclonus and ataxia but no hearing loss.

TREATMENT

Diazepam (Valium) was found most effective in controlling the myoclonic movements. The grand mal seizures can be treated effectively with phenytoin (formerly diphenylhydantoin) (Dilantin) and by phenobarbital. A hearing aid may be used for the auditory loss.

PROGNOSIS

The illness is slowly progressive with deterioration in gait and in hearing.

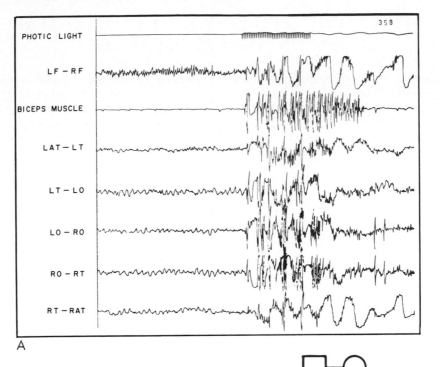

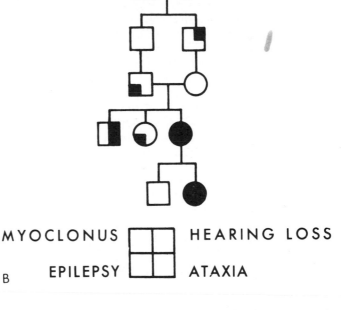

Figure 8-5 *Myoclonic epilepsy, ataxia, and sensorineural deafness. (A)* Electro-encephalogram of patient showing spike discharges and myoclonic jerks in response to photic stimulation. *(B)* Pedigree of kindred showing six affected individuals in four generations. *(A and B* from D. L. May and H. H. White, *Arch. Neurol., 19*:331, 1968.)

SUMMARY

Characteristics of this syndrome include: 1) autosomal dominant transmission with variable expression, 2) myoclonic and grand mal epilepsy beginning in the teens and occurring in about half the cases, 3) slowly progressive cerebellar ataxia beginning in adolescence, and 4) slowly progressive sensorineural hearing loss beginning in childhood.

REFERENCES

May, D. L., and White, H. H., Familial myoclonus, cerebellar ataxia, and deafness. *Arch. Neurol., 19*:331–338, 1968.

MYOCLONIC EPILEPSY AND CONGENITAL SENSORINEURAL DEAFNESS

The combination of congenital sensorineural deafness and childhood onset of myoclonic epilepsy was described in five of eight sibs by Latham and Munro (1937). The authors examined two of the five affected sibs and reviewed clinical histories on the remaining three.

CLINICAL FINDINGS

Nervous System. Each of the five affected sibs developed normally. Myoclonic epilepsy occurred in each between 10 and 12 years of age. The disorder was initiated by generalized shaking spells. The shaking became worse, resulting at times in falling. It occurred both during sleep and waking hours. Within the year, grand mal seizures followed bouts of shaking about once a week. The myoclonic jerking became more severe until the patient was helpless and confined to bed. There was marked muscle wasting. Although reflexes became depressed, there was neither spasticity nor sensory loss. Mental status generally remained intact with no evidence of memory loss or dementia.

Auditory System. Each of the affected persons was congenitally deaf and attended a school for the deaf. There was no history of ear disease. None of the patients developed speech; one could say his name, however. Audiometric testing was not described.

Vestibular System. No vestibular tests were mentioned.

LABORATORY FINDINGS

No laboratory findings were described.

HEREDITY

The hearing loss was complete in all affected persons. Although myoclonus and grand mal epilepsy had begun at about the same age in each case, there was much individual variation in the severity of the spells. The parents were second cousins and were apparently normal. Five of their eight children were affected. The syndrome exhibits autosomal recessive inheritance.

DIAGNOSIS

In *photomyoclonus, diabetes mellitus, nephropathy, and sensorineural deafness* the hearing loss has later onset and is slowly progressive. In addition, affected persons show renal involvement with uremia. The syndrome of *myoclonic epilepsy, ataxia, and sensorineural deafness* differs in that inheritance is autosomal dominant and the hearing loss and ataxia begin in childhood and are slowly progressive, in contrast to the deafness being congenital in the syndrome described here. Hearing loss is not a feature of benign essential myoclonus, Lafora's myoclonic epilepsy, or Unverricht's myoclonic epilepsy.

TREATMENT

Treatment was not described. Anticonvulsant medication is recommended in cases such as these.

PROGNOSIS

The prognosis is poor, since affected persons develop myoclonic and generalized epilepsy and possible mental deterioration secondary to prolonged seizures. Patients often require chronic hospitalization.

SUMMARY

This disease is characterized by: 1) autosomal recessive transmission, 2) myoclonus and grand mal epilepsy with onset at 10 to 12 years of age, 3) terminal neurologic deterioration, 4) occasionally mild, slow mental deterioration, and 5) congenital severe sensorineural deafness.

REFERENCES

Latham, A. D., and Munro, T. A., Familial myoclonus epilepsy associated with deaf-mutism in a family showing other psychobiological abnormalities. *Ann. Eugen.,* 8:166–175, 1937–38.

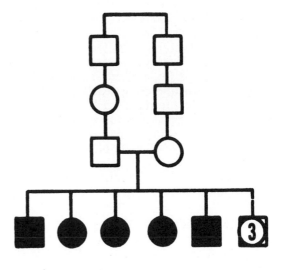

Figure 8–6 Myoclonic epilepsy and congenital sensorineural deafness. Pedigree of kindred showing five affected persons among eight sibs resulting from a consanguineous mating. (From A. D. Latham and T. A. Munro, *Ann. Eugen.*, 8:166, 1937–38.)

ACOUSTIC NEUROMAS AND NEURAL DEAFNESS

In 1930 Gardner and Frazier reported a family in which bilateral acoustic neuromas were transmitted through 5 generations and involved 38 members. Pathologic findings were described in four additional members of the family by Gardner and Turner (1940). Recent follow-up of this family by Young, Eldridge, and Gardner (1970) showed that almost 100 individuals now have definite or possible bilateral acoustic neuromas. An earlier report of three-generation involvement is that of Feiling and Ward (1920). Another kindred with bilateral acoustic neuromas occurring in 14 members in 4 generations was described by Moyes (1968). Several other kindreds have been reported (Hitselberger and Hughes, 1968; Lee and Abbott, 1969).

About 4 per cent of persons having acoustic neuromas have this syndrome.

CLINICAL FINDINGS

Nervous System. Young *et al.* (1970) had clinical data on 97 possibly or definitely affected persons. The average age of onset was 20 years. Rarely do the signs become manifest in infancy (Rosenberg *et al.*, 1974). Physical examination of affected persons showed no evidence of von Recklinghausen's neurofibromatosis.

Three types of nervous system signs developed: (1) those caused by encroachment on adjacent cranial nerves by the acoustic neuroma, (2) those caused by increased intracranial pressure, and (3) those occasionally caused by other nervous system tumors. In some affected persons palsies of the fifth, sixth, seventh, ninth, and tenth cranial nerves as well as cerebellar ataxia developed. Patients usually have rather severe headaches and progressive visual loss owing to increased intracranial pressure. Spinal root neuromas, ependymomas, astrocytomas, or meningiomas have also been found (Hitselberger and Hughes, 1968; Lee and Abbott, 1969; Perez De Moura *et al.*, 1969; Young *et al.*, 1970).

Ocular System. Progressive visual loss is common. Slightly over 50 per cent of those who died with known disease were blind, and 8 per cent had markedly decreased vision (Young *et al.*, 1969). Visual loss is due to increased intracranial pressure with papilledema. None of the postmortem studies indicated tumors involving the optic nerves.

Auditory System. Hearing loss was first noted in the second or third decade and consisted of progressive bilateral neural hearing loss, resulting in total deafness within 5 to 10 years. Hearing loss was the first symptom in about 50 per cent of the patients, tinnitus in about 30 per cent, imbalance in 10 per cent, and facial twitching in about 5 per cent. Audiograms generally show no or slow pure-tone change, progressive loss of discrimination, and more marked loss at higher frequencies (Hitselberger and Hughes, 1968; Perez De Moura *et al.*, 1969).

Vestibular System. Vestibular abnormalities are characteristic; they were evident in all seven patients tested by Gardner and Frazier. Young *et al.* noted that abnormalities of vestibular function generally occurred before audiometric change. Several persons in the family described by Young *et al.* nearly drowned because they had lost direction under water; three other members, not known to be affected, had drowned. It is possible that they were in the early stage of the disorder and had only vestibular involvement.

LABORATORY FINDINGS

The few radiographic studies described showed acoustic neuromas with enlarged internal auditory meatuses.

PATHOLOGY

Autopsy findings have been described in several patients (Gardner and Frazier, 1930; Gardner and Turner, 1940). Each showed similar findings, including bilateral acoustic tumors that measured from 1 to 6 cm. in diameter and encroached upon the basis pontis and adjacent cranial nerves.

Histologic sections of these tumors showed interlacing bundles of elongated cells forming palisades, characteristic of acoustic neuromas (Nager, 1964; Perez De Moura *et al.*, 1969).

HEREDITY

Males and females are equally affected, with about half of the offspring of an affected person having bilateral acoustic neuromas. The disorder has been described in at least five generations. No generations have been skipped. The syndrome has autosomal dominant inheritance.

DIAGNOSIS

This syndrome, with its dominantly transmitted bilateral acoustic neuromas, should be distinguished from neurofibromatosis. Patients with neurofibromatosis may occasionally have meningiomas, astrocytomas, or rarely bilateral acoustic neuromas. Neurofibromatosis also has autosomal dominant transmission and characteristically is associated with café-au-lait spots and cutaneous neurofibromatosis, which are not present in the syndrome under discussion.

Bilateral eighth nerve tumors differ in several ways from unilateral ones. The former are hereditary, the latter are not. The former can reach remarkable size, effecting severe distortion of the brain stem, enlarging and eroding the bony walls of the internal meatus, and finally extending extradurally into the middle cranial fossa. The tumors tend to invade the marrow spaces and mastoid air cells (Nager, 1969).

TREATMENT

Surgical removal of the tumor is the therapy of choice. However, Young *et al.* (1970) reported that surgical results on 12 patients in the kindred under study have not encouraged other affected family members to submit to surgery. One patient died immediately postoperatively, five died within one year, one within five years, and only three lived over five years following surgery. In only two cases had life been clearly prolonged. It is possible that surgical results would be better with current, improved techniques.

PROGNOSIS

The rate of growth of the neuromas in the syndrome is somewhat slower than that in patients who have sporadic acoustic neuromas. Patients live an average of about 20 years (with a range of 2 to 44 years) after the onset of symptoms.

SUMMARY

Characteristics of this syndrome include: 1) autosomal dominant transmission, 2) slow to rapid progression of neural hearing loss, 3) neurologic deficit due to acoustic neuromas beginning in early adult life, and 4) vestibular dysfunction.

REFERENCES

Feiling, A., and Ward, E., A familial form of acoustic tumour. *Br. Med. J., 1*:496–497, 1920.
Gardner, W. J., and Frazier, C. H., Bilateral acoustic neurofibromas: a clinical study and field survey of a family of five generations with bilateral deafness in thirty-eight members. *Arch. Neurol. Psychiatr., 23*:266–300, 1930.

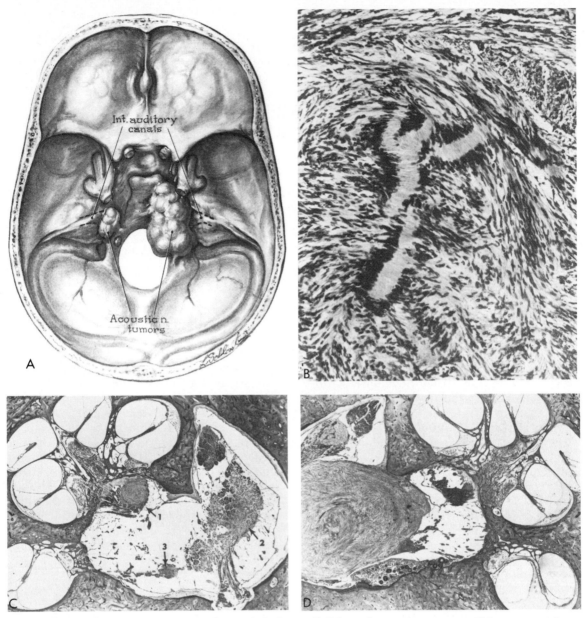

***Figure* 8-7** *Acoustic neuromas and neural deafness. (A)* Bilateral acoustic neuromas (Schwannomas) in a 20-year-old woman. *(B)* Marked palisading of cell nuclei in an area of fibrillary architecture. *(C)* Midmodiolar sections through cochlea showing three neurinomas in internal auditory canal. *(D)* Large vestibular neurinoma arising at inferior part of Scarpa's ganglion. Also note meningioma covering floor of internal acoustic meatus. *(A–D* from G. T. Nager, *Arch. Otolaryngol., 89:252,* 1969.)

Gardner, W. J., and Turner, O., Bilateral acoustic neurofibromas. Further clinical and pathologic data on hereditary deafness and von Recklinghausen's disease. *Arch. Neurol. Psychiatr., 44:* 76–99, 1940.

Hitselberger, W. E., and Hughes, R. L., Bilateral acoustic tumors and neurofibromatosis. *Arch. Otolaryngol., 88:*700–711, 1968.

Lee, D. K., and Abbott, M. L., Familial central nervous system neoplasia. *Arch. Neurol., 20:*154–160, 1969.

Moyes, P. D., Familial bilateral acoustic neuromas affecting 14 members from four generations. *J. Neurosurg., 29:*78–82, 1968.

Nager, G. T., Association of bilateral VIIIth nerve tumors with meningiomas in von Recklinghausen's disease. *Laryngoscope, 74:*1220–1265, 1964.

Nager, G. T., Acoustic neurinomas. Pathology and differential diagnosis. *Arch. Otolaryngol., 89:*252–279, 1969.

Perez De Moura, L. F., Hayden, R. C., Jr., and Conner, G. H., Bilateral neurinoma and neurofibromatosis. *Arch. Otolaryngol.*, *90*:28–34, 1969.

Rosenberg, D., Floret, D., Fischer, G., Kalifa, A., and Monnet, P., Le neurinome bilatéral de
l'acoustique chez l'enfant. *Ann. Pédiatr. (Paris)*, *21*:257–263, 1974.

Young, D. F., Eldridge, R., and Gardner, W. J., Bilateral acoustic neuroma in a large kindred.
J.A.M.A., 214:347–353, 1970.

SENSORY RADICULAR NEUROPATHY AND PROGRESSIVE SENSORINEURAL DEAFNESS

A syndrome that includes progressive peripheral sensory loss, perforating ulcers of the feet, shooting radicular pains, and progressive sensorineural hearing loss was described by Hicks (1922). Denny-Brown (1951) restudied this kindred. Isolated cases were described by van Bogaert (1953), Hallpike (1967), and Stanley *et al.* (1975). The patient reported by Blackwood (1952) may have been the same as that studied by Hallpike.

CLINICAL FINDINGS

Nervous System. All affected persons were normal, until they developed sensory loss, which appeared first in the distal legs and then in the arms; the onset was between 15 and 36 years of age (Hicks, 1922). The sensory loss was accompanied by large foot ulcers that penetrated to the underlying bone.

Neurologic examination showed normal cranial nerve function except for progressive sensorineural deafness. There was loss of pain, touch, and capacity to sense heat and cold appearing over the feet and later in the arms. Strength remained normal. Ankle and knee reflexes became depressed. Plantar responses remained flexor. Patients complained of severe radicular shooting pains involving the legs and at times the arms.

Auditory System. Ten persons who had been affected with perforating ulcers of the feet and who had been described by Hicks (1922) had sensorineural hearing loss beginning about the time of the peripheral sensory loss. Within a period of 10 to 20 years there was slow progression to severe deafness. Van Bogaert (1953) described a patient in a kindred with this disorder who had also had a sensorineural hearing loss. Hallpike's (1967) patient also manifested progressive sensorineural deafness.

Vestibular System. No vestibular tests have been reported.

LABORATORY FINDINGS

Radiographs of the feet showed severe deformities, including shortening of the phalanges, shortening of the foot, and displacement of the phalanges.

PATHOLOGY

Autopsy findings of a 53-year-old woman who was a member of the family described by Hicks showed a small brain. There was marked loss of ganglion cells in the sacral and lumbar dorsal root ganglia. The remaining ganglion cells showed proliferation of subcapsular dendrites. Clear hyaline bodies were seen in the involved ganglia (van Bogaert, 1953; Denny-Brown, 1954). At autopsy, Hallpike (1967) found that the posterior root ganglia, particularly in the lower thoracic and lumbar areas, showed neuronal loss. Sections of the temporal bone in another member of this family showed severe atrophy of the stria vascularis and loss of hair cells in the organ of Corti and the limbus.

HEREDITY

The syndrome has autosomal dominant transmission (Denny-Brown, 1951).

DIAGNOSIS

There are many published kindreds that exhibit the characteristic neurologic alterations but do not manifest deafness (Reimann *et al.*, 1958; Mandell and Smith, 1960). An autosomal recessive sensory radicular neuropathy apparently exists, since multiple sibs have been affected while their parents have been normal (Pallis and Schneeweiss, 1962; Kuroiwa and Murai,

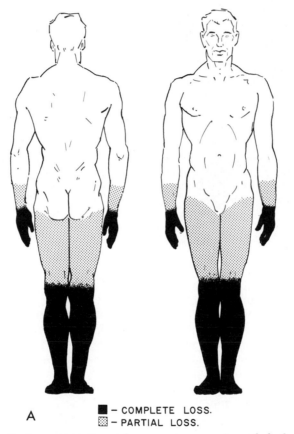

A

■ – COMPLETE LOSS.
▨ – PARTIAL LOSS.

Figure 8-8 *Sensory radicular neuropathy and progressive sensorineural deafness. (A)* Diagram showing areas of involvement.

Illustration continued on the following page

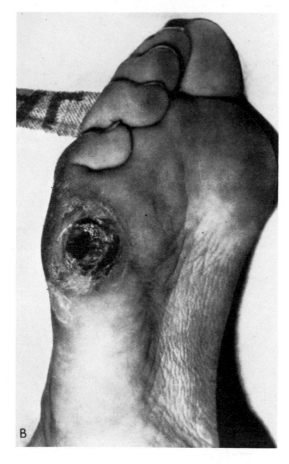

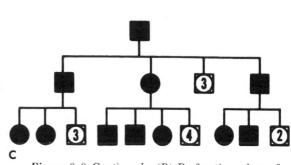

Figure 8–8 Continued. *(B)* Perforating ulcer of the foot. *(C)* Pedigree of affected kindred. (Adapted from D. Denny-Brown, *J. Neurol. Neurosurg. Psychiatry, 14*:237, 1951.)

1964; Schoene *et al.,* 1970). Munro (1956) and Ogden *et al.* (1959) reported a nonprogressive sensory radicular neuropathy in an 8-year-old child with congenital sensorineural deafness, especially marked in the lower tones. Vestibular function was abnormal. Congenital indifference to pain may be associated with sensorineural deafness.

Syringomyelia and leprosy may present with similar signs. In these disorders there is neither hearing loss nor family history of the condition.

TREATMENT

Treatment is symptomatic and, in general, is unsatisfactory.

PROGNOSIS

Each patient had a slowly progressive sensory loss with recurrent ulceration of the feet. The hearing loss was also slowly progressive, resulting in severe deafness.

SUMMARY

Characteristics of this syndrome include: 1) autosomal dominant transmission, 2) progressive sensory loss and lightning pains that involve the distal extremities and begin in the second or third decade, 3) loss of dorsal root ganglia, particularly in the lower thoracic and lumbar areas, and 4) progressive moderate to severe sensorineural hearing loss.

REFERENCES

Blackwood, W., Biopsy techniques in the diagnosis of peripheral neuropathies, especially hereditary and sensory neuropathy. *Proc. 1st Int. Cong. Neuropath., Rome, 3*:415–424, 1952.

Denny-Brown, D., Hereditary sensory radicular neuropathy. *J. Neurol. Neurosurg. Psychiatry, 14*:237–252, 1951.

Hallpike, C. S., Observations on the structural basis of two rare varieties of hereditary deafness. In CIBA Foundation Symposium: *Myotatic, Kinesthetic, and Vestibular Mechanisms.* de

Reuch, A. V. S., and Knight, J. (eds.), Boston, Little, Brown and Company, 1967, pp. 285–294.

Hicks, E. P., Hereditary perforating ulcer of the foot. *Lancet, 1*:319–321, 1922.

Kuroiwa, Y., and Murai, Y., Hereditary sensory radicular neuropathy. *Neurology (Minneap.), 14*:574–577, 1964.

Mandell, A. J., and Smith, C. K., Hereditary sensory radicular neuropathy. *Neurology (Minneap.), 10*:627–630, 1960.

Munro, M., Sensory radicular neuropathy in a deaf child. *Br. Med. J., 1*:541–544, 1956.

Ogden, T. E., Robert, F., and Carmichael, E. A., Some sensory syndromes in children: indifference to pain and sensory neuropathy. *J. Neurol. Neurosurg. Psychiatry, 22*:267–276, 1959.

Pallis, C., and Schneeweiss, J., Hereditary sensory radicular neuropathy. *Am. J. Med., 32*:110–118, 1962.

Reimann, H. A., McKechnie, W. G., and Stanisvaljevic, S., Hereditary sensory radicular neuropathy and other defects in a large family: reinvestigation after twenty years and report of a necropsy. *Am. J. Med., 25*:573–579, 1958.

Schoene, W. C., Asbury, A. K., Åström, K. E., and Masters, R., Hereditary sensory neuropathy. A clinical and ultrastructural study. *J. Neurol. Sci., 11*:463–487, 1970.

Stanley, R. J., Puritz, E. M., Briggaman, R. A., and Wheeler, C. E. J., Sensory radicular neuropathy. *Arch. Dermatol., 111*:760–762, 1975.

van Bogaert, L., Étude histopathologique d'une observation d'arthropathie mutilante symétrique familiale. *Acta Neurol. Belg., 53*:37–53, 1953.

PROGRESSIVE SENSORY NEUROPATHY, ABSENT GASTRIC MOTILITY, SMALL BOWEL DIVERTICULITIS, AND PROFOUND CHILDHOOD SENSORINEURAL DEAFNESS

Hirschowitz, Groll, and Ceballos (1972) reported a syndrome of progressive sensory neuropathy with trophic changes, progressive loss of gastric motility, multiple small inflamed intestinal diverticula, and profound sensorineural deafness in three female sibs.

CLINICAL FINDINGS

Nervous System. Tendon reflexes at knees and ankles were absent, but flexor plantar responses and other reflexes were normal in the oldest sib.

A younger sister had absent knee and ankle jerks at 16 years of age, and soon thereafter she experienced loss of sensation of the Achilles tendons and fingers and toes, decreased corneal reflex, and absent abdominal reflex. Eventually, she perceived pinprick but not touch in the fingers and thumbs; below the knees she did not perceive even pinprick. Sural nerve biopsy showed demyelinization.

The youngest sib exhibited only hypoactive deep tendon reflexes when first seen at 14 years of age, but she had lost her abdominal and corneal reflexes and pinprick sensation to the midcalf within the next six years. Bilateral pes cavus was noted in two of the affected sibs and in the father.

Sinus tachycardia was present in all three sibs within two years after the gastrointestinal symptoms. Eventually, there was normal pulse rate but loss of carotid sinus reflex and exercise-response tachycardia, suggestive of progressive damage to the cardiac autonomic innervation.

Gastrointestinal System. Abdominal cramps, vomiting, steatorrhea, and emaciation characterized the adolescent history of the three sibs. Ulcerated diverticulitis of the small bowel associated with massive mesenteric and retroperitoneal lymph node enlargement was found. The nodes showed only nonspecific lymphadenitis. The stomach was found to be atonic and distended. The vomiting and cramping were probably due to delayed gastric emptying, which had resulted from progressive loss of gastric motility, and, later, to intestinal ulceration.

Integumentary System. Acanthosis nigricans developed in two of the three sibs.

Auditory System. The ages of onset of bilateral sensorineural deafness were 8, 3, and 9 years of age, respectively; at 10, 5, and 18 years, respectively, the deafness became total. Examination of the temporal bones showed collapsed Reissner's membrane and destruction of the organ of Corti.

Although there was deafness in the father's family for three generations, it was of late onset, mild in degree, and probably otosclerotic in nature.

Vestibular System. Vestibular function was found to be normal in all three sibs.

LABORATORY FINDINGS

Serum proteins were low. Serum zinc levels were also depressed (personal communication, 1974).

HEREDITY

The occurrence of the syndrome in three sibs having normal parents suggests autosomal recessive inheritance.

DIAGNOSIS

In *sensory radicular neuropathy and progressive sensorineural deafness* loss of pain sensation was prominent. Mutilations, especially perforating ulcer of the foot, as well as shooting pains were prominent features. These findings are not part of the syndrome under consideration. The absence of progressive muscle wasting, of retinal changes (especially retinitis pigmentosa), and ataxia excludes *Refsum syndrome* and other forms of deafness associated with retinal disease.

TREATMENT

Oral antibiotic therapy, medium chain triglycerides, and methacholine chloride with meals are of benefit in regulating the level of the serum albumin and in controlling steatorrhea. Vitamin A acid is effective in treatment of the acanthosis nigricans (Montes *et al.*, 1974).

PROGNOSIS

Prognosis is poor because of the progressive nature of the disorder. One sib died; the second is now bedridden. Hearing loss was total in all three.

SUMMARY

The syndrome is characterized by: 1) autosomal recessive inheritance, 2) progressive sensory neuropathy without trophic changes, 3) small bowel diverticulitis, 4) progressive loss of gastric motility, 5) tachycardia, 6) acanthosis nigricans, and 7) progressive childhood profound sensorineural deafness.

REFERENCES

Hirschowitz, B. I., Groll, A., and Ceballos, R., Hereditary nerve deafness in three sisters with absent gastric motility, small bowel diverticulitis and ulceration, and progressive sensory neuropathy. *Birth Defects, 8*(2):27–41, 1972.

Montes, L. F., Hirschowitz, B. I., and Krumdieck, C., Acanthosis nigricans and hypovitaminosis A. Response of topical vitamin A acid. *J. Cutan. Pathol., 1*:88–94, 1974.

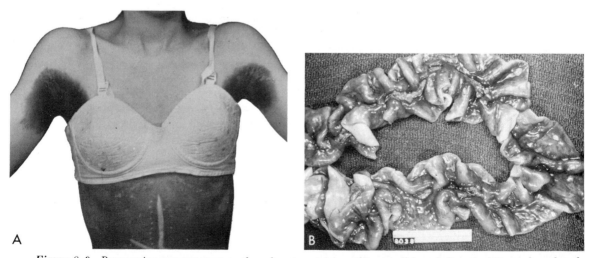

Figure 8–9 Progressive sensory neuropathy, absent gastric motility, small bowel diverticulitis, and profound childhood sensorineural deafness. (A) Acanthosis nigricans in both axillae and over abdomen. *(B)* Thickened ileum together with fibrosed mesentery make full extension of bowel impossible. Note long serpiginous ulcer at mesenteric implantation throughout length of specimen.

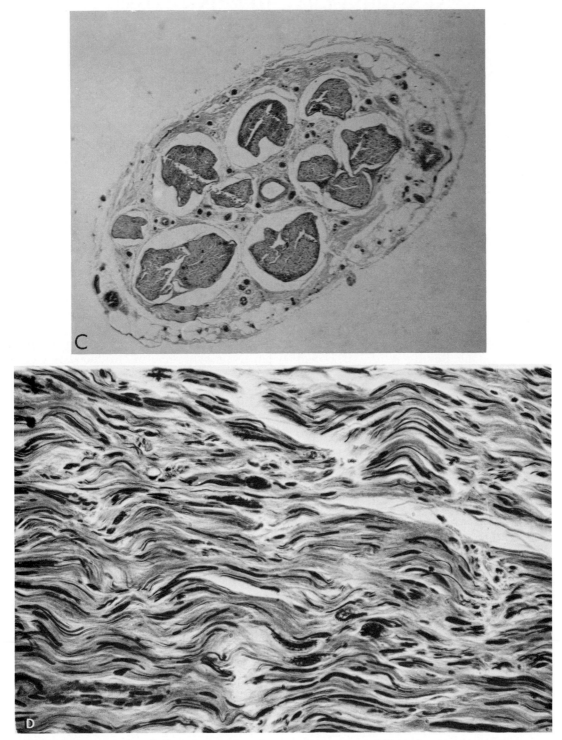

Figure 8–9 Continued. *(C)* Cross section of sural nerve which is thin and fibrosed with nerve bundles separated by connective tissue. *(D)* High-power view showing that only a few axons display remaining, swollen and vacuolated myelin sheaths. *(A–D* from B. I. Hirschowitz *et al., Birth Defects, 8*(2):27, 1972.)

BULBOPONTINE PARALYSIS WITH PROGRESSIVE SENSORINEURAL HEARING LOSS

A syndrome characterized by childhood onset of a very slowly progressive bulbar palsy with facial weakness, dysphagia, dysarthria, and tongue fibrillations, and by progressive sensorineural hearing loss, has been described in three sibships (Vialetto, 1936; van Laere, 1966; Boudin *et al.*, 1971). Several sporadic cases have been described (van Laere, 1967; Arnould *et al.*, 1968; Trillet *et al.*, 1970).

CLINICAL FINDINGS

Nervous System. Generally in the second decade of life, progressive weakness of facial musculature, lips, tongue, larynx, and jaw musculature appears. The facies becomes thin as a result of some muscular atrophy. Patients generally have dysphagia and dysarthria. Vocal-cord paresis was found in two of three sibs described by Vialetto (1936). One of the two affected sisters described by Boudin *et al.* (1971) had tachycardia and radiographic evidence of gastric dilatation, suggesting involvement of the vagus motor nucleus. Thus, the fifth and seventh to twelfth cranial motor nerves are bilaterally affected. Other cranial nerve function was normal.

Later in the course of this disease, other signs developed. One of four sibs described by van Laere (1966) had atrophy of hand musculature and paralysis of the diaphragm; another had discrete steppage gait on the right. A 37-year-old patient had moderate atrophy of the sternocleidomastoid muscles (Vialetto, 1936). The 22-year-old woman described by Boudin *et al.* (1971) had mild atrophy of the shoulder girdle muscles.

Auditory System. A progressive bilateral sensorineural hearing loss was frequently the first symptom of this disease, beginning between 10 and 35 years of age. Two patients had auditory hallucinations (Vialetto, 1936).

Vestibular System. Caloric vestibular tests on four patients showed hypoactive or absent vestibular responses.

HEREDITY

Three affected female sibs in a sibship of 14 were reported by Vialetto (1936). Four involved female sibs in a sibship of 10 were presented by van Laere (1966). Two sisters in a sibship of three were described by Boudin *et al.* (1971). The parents in these sibships were normal. There has been a marked predilection for females. The syndrome has autosomal recessive inheritance.

DIAGNOSIS

This syndrome can be distinguished from juvenile amyotrophic lateral sclerosis because of the striking involvement of bulbar musculature and because of the accompanying hearing loss. Progressive bulbar paralysis syndrome of childhood is characterized by recessive transmission, early onset, malignant course, and normal hearing (Gomez *et al.*, 1962).

TREATMENT

Therapy is symptomatic and is of little help.

PROGNOSIS

Prognosis is poor because of the relentless progression of the disorder.

SUMMARY

The syndrome is characterized by: 1) autosomal recessive inheritance, 2) childhood onset of slowly progressive bulbar paralysis with weakness of facial muscles, lips, tongue, larynx, and muscles of mastication, 3) progressive sensorineural hearing loss, and 4) abnormal vestibular function.

REFERENCES

Arnould, B., Tredon, P., Laxenaire, M., Picard, L., Weber, M., and Brichet, B., Paralysie bulbo-pontine chronique progressive avec surdité. *Rev. Otoneuroophtalmol., 40*:158–161, 1968.
Boudin, G., Pépin, B., Vernant, J. C., Gautier, B., and Gougérou, H., Cas familial de paralysie bulbo-pontine chronique progressive avec surdité. *Rev. Neurol. (Paris), 124*:90–92, 1971.

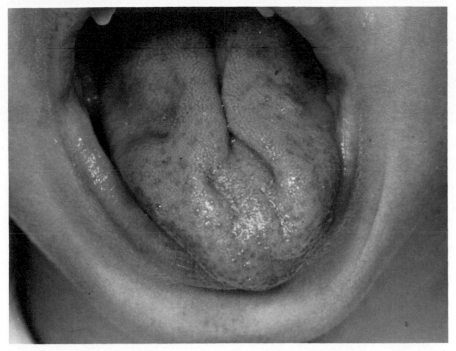

Figure 8-10 *Bulbopontine paralysis with progressive sensorineural hearing loss.* Hypoglossal paralysis of tongue evident in patient seen by one of the authors (R. J. G.).

Gomez, M. R., Clermont, V., and Bernstein, J., Progressive bulbar paralysis in childhood (Fazio-Londe's disorder). *Arch. Neurol.,* 6:317–323, 1962.

Trillet, M., Girard, P. F., Schott, B., Ramel, P., and Woehrle, R., La paralysie bulbo-pontine chronique progressive avec surdité (à propos d'une observation clinique). *Lyon Méd.,* 223:145–153, 1970.

van Laere, J., Paralysie bulbo-pontine chronique progressive familiale avec surdité. *Rev. Neurol.,* 115:289–295, 1966.

van Laere, J., Over een nieuw geval van chronische bulbopontiene paralysis met doofheid. *Verh. K. Vlaam. Acad. Geneeskd. Belg.,* 29:288–308, 1967.

Vialetto, E., Contributo alla forma ereditaria della paralisi bulbare progressiva? *Riv. Sper. Freniatr.,* 40:1–24, 1936.

Chapter 9

GENETIC
HEARING LOSS
WITH METABOLIC
AND OTHER
ABNORMALITIES

Within this section we shall consider a salmagundi of syndromes that did not quite fit into the previous chapters. Pendred syndrome is not uncommon, accounting for perhaps 10 per cent of cases of congenital deafness, but most of the others are rare single-gene disorders or are the result of chromosomal aneuploidy.

GOITER AND PROFOUND CONGENITAL SENSORINEURAL DEAFNESS

(Pendred Syndrome)

Originally described by Pendred (1896), the syndrome of goiter and profound congenital sensorineural deafness received little attention except for occasional sporadic reports (Brain, 1927; Johnsen, 1958; McGirr *et al.,* 1959) until Morgans and Trotter (1958) and Fraser *et al.* (1960) emphasized its importance. The frequency of Pendred syndrome was estimated at 7.5 cases per 100,000 births in the British Isles (Fraser, 1965) and about 1 per 100,000 births in Scandinavia (Nilsson *et al.,* 1964). Possibly the condition accounts for as much as 10 per cent of the cases of congenital deafness (Batsakis and Nishiyama, 1962); this figure is in doubt, however. At least 300 cases have been reported.

Baschieri *et al.* (1963) pointed out that half of the nongoitrous children at a school for the deaf had a positive perchlorate test! Similar results were obtained at Clarke School for the Deaf, Northampton, Massachusetts (Brown, 1967). Obviously then, if the classic clinical criteria for Pendred syndrome are used, a considerab e number of cases will go undetected.

CLINICAL FINDINGS

Endocrine System. The goiter is usually evident before puberty (on the average, at 8 years of age) but in some cases may be observed at birth (Nilsson *et al.,* 1964). At least 50 per cent are noted before 5 years of age. Most are diffuse and soft without a bruit and tend to remain small. Long-standing goiters tend to be nodular, especially in females. After thyroidec-

330

tomy, they often recur, unless thyroid therapy is instituted (Bouchard *et al.*, 1968).

Thyroid enlargement is predicated upon an inborn error in thyroxine synthesis (Morgans and Trotter, 1958), i.e., the organ-binding of the iodine in the thyroid gland. It is this deficiency which probably accounts for the mental retardation that is noted in some cases of Pendred syndrome. Although usually euthyroid, the patient may be somewhat hypothyroid, especially in early life (Safar *et al.*, 1973).

Ocular System. Gomez-Pan *et.* (1974) reported an unusual deposition of pigment in the retina in three sibs. No other authors have mentioned this finding.

Auditory System. Although variations in hearing loss occur, audiometric testing usually shows a congenital bilateral 40 to 100 dB sensorineural hearing loss, more severe in the higher frequencies. It is severe in over 50 per cent of the cases. The average age at which deafness is detected is 2.2 years (Thould and Scowen, 1964). The hearing loss progresses slightly during childhood. Rarely will hearing loss be minimal; occasionally, hearing in one ear may be relatively normal (Fraser, 1965). Speech development is generally poor because of the early severe deafness.

Positive recruitment was found in four of six cases tested by Nilsson *et al.* (1964) and in two cases tested by Fraser (1965). These findings suggest that the auditory defect is in the organ of Corti.

Vestibular System. Caloric vestibular tests generally show depressed vestibular function (Johnsen, 1958; Fraser, 1965), although normal vestibular responses have been found in some cases (Deraemaeker, 1956; von Harnack *et al.*, 1961).

LABORATORY FINDINGS

Tomographic evidence of the Mondini defect of the cochlea has been described in about half of a series of 15 cases (Illum *et al.*, 1972).

The defect in the organic binding of iodine is demonstrable by the perchlorate or thiocyanate test (Morgans and Trotter, 1958), which releases the pooled or unbound iodine, as shown by a sharp decline in the thyroid counting rate when isotopically labeled iodine is employed. An abnormal iodoprotein has been found by Medeiros-Neto *et al.* (1968) but not by Milutinovic *et al.* (1969). Similarly both normal (Bur-

row *et al.*, 1973) and abnormal (Ljunggren *et al.*, 1973) peroxidase activity have been noted in the thyroid gland.

In normal individuals, injected radioactive iodine is incorporated into thyroxine. In patients with Pendred syndrome the iodine is variably discharged (15 to 80 per cent) from the thyroid by perchlorate, resulting in a rapid decrease in radioactivity in the thyroid (Fraser *et al.*, 1960). However, the perchlorate test is not always positive. Bax (1966) described three affected sibs in whom the perchlorate test was positive in two children but normal in the third. The father—otherwise normal—also had a positive perchlorate test. Thus, it appears that the oral perchlorate test is not infallible. The intravenous perchlorate test appears to be much more reliable (Gray *et al.*, 1973).

PATHOLOGY

Grossly, the thyroid is nodular and of variable size. Microscopically, the cells lining the follicles are tall and active; colloid is scanty. At times, nuclear pleomorphism and papillary infoldings are noted, and adenocarcinoma is often erroneously diagnosed (Roberts, 1957; Thieme, 1957; Elman, 1958; Batsakis and Nishiyama, 1962; Wildner and Wittig, 1966).

Temporal bone pathology was described by Hvidberg-Hansen and Balslev-Jørgensen (1968). Changes were bilaterally symmetric and consisted of malformation of the bony inner ear. The osseous semicircular canal system was larger than normal. There were only two cochlear turns in the membranous labyrinth. Occasionally, supporting cells in the organ of Corti were noted, and there was no evidence of hair cells. The tectorial membrane was absent. There were only a few spiral ganglion cells and no fibers in the lamina spiralis. The sensory epithelium was normal with normal innervation and ganglion cells present. The bony changes corresponded to the Mondini defect.

HEREDITY

There have been several families in which several sibs have been involved (Fraser *et al.*, 1964). Consanguinity has been noted by several authors (Deraemaeker, 1956; Fraser *et al.*, 1960; Nilsson *et al.*, 1964; Fraser, 1965). Inheritance is clearly autosomal recessive.

DIAGNOSIS

One must exclude cases of endemic cretinism with deafness, which occur in certain isolated areas, such as the Alps, the Andes, and the Himalayas, where iodine is deficient. This can be done by the absence of cretinoid signs in Pendred syndrome and by a negative perchlorate test in cretinism. The perchlorate test, however, may be positive in Hashimoto's thyroiditis, in sporadic goitrous cretinism, in nontoxic goiter, and in congenital deafness without goiter (Baschieri et al., 1963).

Impairment of hearing is also seen in about half of adult myxedematous patients. This auditory deficiency can be sensorineural, conductive, or mixed (Trotter, 1960; Batsakis and Nishiyama, 1962).

It is difficult to classify the euthyroid female with goiter and deafness reported by Hollander et al. (1964). She was able both to accumulate radioactive iodine normally and to iodinate tyrosine. The authors suggested that she had a partial defect in the condensation of iodotyrosines to form iodothyronines. Although goiter was present in three generations, only the patient had congenital sensorineural deafness. She married a congenitally deaf man. Three of her six children had deafness but no goiter.

A family reported by Thompson et al. (1970) is not sufficiently documented to determine whether members had Pendred syndrome or a separate entity.

The diagnosis of Pendred syndrome is clear when there is a family history that suggests autosomal recessive inheritance, congenital sensorineural deafness, goiter, and a positive perchlorate discharge test.

As mentioned above, there may be a variable degree of hearing loss or goiter in affected persons, and occasionally the perchlorate test is normal. In such cases a positive family history is essential.

TREATMENT

Patients with Pendred syndrome have been subjected to a large number of surgical procedures for removal of the goiter. The goiter invariably returns, following continued stimulation by thyroid-stimulating hormone (TSH). The goiter is best treated by exogenous hormone, which causes a decrease of production of TSH and thyroid stimulation. If therapy is started early, the goiter may regress; hearing does not improve, however (Kitlak and Gebert, 1968).

The hearing loss remains stable with little change over the years. If there is some residual hearing, a hearing aid may be of help.

PROGNOSIS

Patients with Pendred syndrome have a normal life span. With adequate thyroxine therapy, although the hearing does not improve, at least the goiter does not enlarge.

SUMMARY

Characteristics of this syndrome include: 1) autosomal recessive transmission, 2) goiter developing prior to adolescence, 3) positive perchlorate discharge test, and 4) symmetric, generally severe, congenital sensorineural hearing loss.

REFERENCES

Baschieri, L., Benedetti, G., DeLuca, F., and Negri, M., Evaluation and limitations of the perchlorate test in the study of thyroid function. J. Clin. Endocrinol. Metab., 23:786–791, 1963.

Batsakis, J. G., and Nishiyama, R. H., Deafness with sporadic goiter. Pendred's syndrome. Arch. Otolaryngol., 76:401–406, 1962.

Bax, G. M., Typical and atypical cases of Pendred's syndrome in one family. Acta Endocrinol. (Kbh.), 53:264–270, 1966.

Bouchard, R., Guedeney, J., Mazet, P., and Castaing, N., Discussion d'un syndrome de Pendred. Arch. Fr. Pédiatr., 25:453–464, 1968.

Brain, W. R., Heredity in simple goiter. Q. J. Med., 20:203–303, 1927.

Brown, K. W., The genetics of childhood deafness. In Deafness in Childhood. McConnell, F., and Ward, P. H. (eds.), Nashville, Tenn., Vanderbilt University Press, 1967.

Burrow, G. N., Spaulding, S. W., Alexander, N. M., and Bower, B. F., Normal peroxidase activity in Pendred's syndrome. J. Clin. Endocrinol. Metab., 36:522–530, 1973.

Deraemaeker, R., Congenital deafness and goiter. Am. J. Hum. Genet., 8:253–256, 1956.

Elman, D. S., Familial association of nerve deafness with nodular goiter and thyroid carcinoma. N. Engl. J. Med., 259:219–223, 1958.

Fishman, J., Fraser, F. C., Watanabe, M., Sodhi, H. S., and Beck, J. C., Familial nerve deafness and goiter. Can. Med. Assoc. J., 83:889–892, 1960.

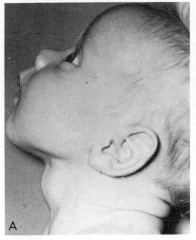

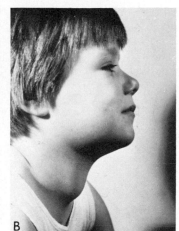

Figure 9–1 *Goiter and profound congenital sensorineural deafness (Pendred syndrome). (A, B)* Two patients with Pendred syndrome showing enlargement of thyroid gland. *(B* courtesy of R. Sacrez, Strasbourg, France.) *(C)* Typical audiogram showing the remaining hearing in the lowest frequencies. Right ear, O– – – – –O; left ear, X– – – – –X; stapedius reflex, right side; ● stapedius reflex, left side. ■. *(D)* Determination of the uptake of radioactive iodine in the thyroid gland with subsequent perchlorate test. **a,** Administration of I 131, 8.1 microcuries; **b,** = I 131, 16 microcuries; **c,** potassium perchlorate, 1 gram. Ordinate indicates counts per minute; abscissa indicates time in hours. Perchlorate test showed a fall in activity of 80 per cent.

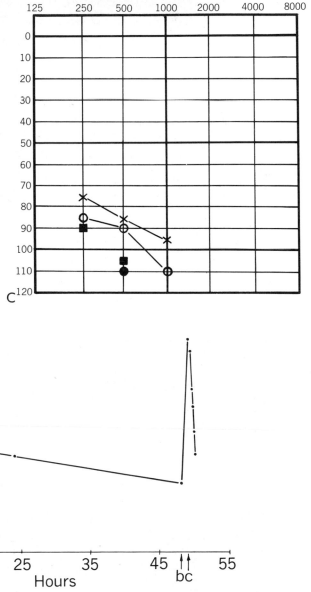

Illustration continued on the following page

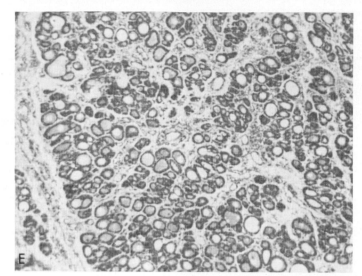

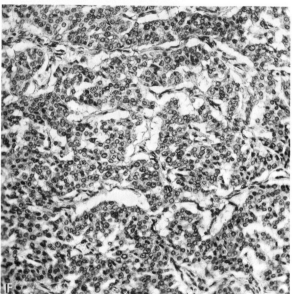

Figure 9–1 Continued. (E) Photomicrograph showing microfollicular adenoma. *(F)* Photomicrograph of trabecular adenoma. (From G. P. Wildner and G. Wittig, *Zentralbl. Allg. Pathol., 109*:52, 1966.) *(G)* Tomograph of right temporal bone, axial-pyramidal projection; midmodiolar cut showing Mondini defect. Only the basal turn can be seen, the apical part of the labyrinth forming a common cavity.

Legend continued on the opposite page

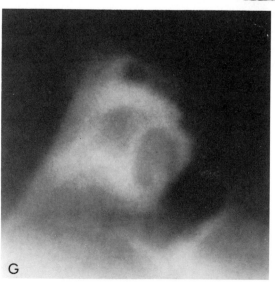

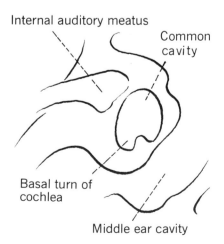

Internal auditory meatus

Common cavity

Basal turn of cochlea

Middle ear cavity

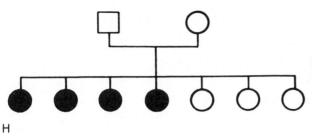

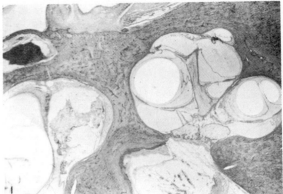

H

Figure 9-1 Continued. (H) Pedigree of affected kindred. (From J. G. Batsakis and R. H. Nishivama, *Arch. Otolaryngol. (Stockh.), 76*:401, 1962.) (I) Section of temporal bone showing defective development of cochlea that has only two turns, a hypoplastic modiolus, and connective tissue formation in the saccule. (*H* from J. Hvidberg-Hansen and M. Balslev Jørgensen, *Acta Otolaryngol. (Stockh.), 66*:129, 1968; *C, D,* and *G* from P. Illum *et al., Arch. Otolaryngol. (Stockh.), 96*: 297, 1972.)

Fraser, G. R., Association of congenital deafness with goiter (Pendred's syndrome). A study of 207 families. *Ann. Hum. Genet., 28*:201–249, 1965.

Fraser, G. R., Morgans, M. E., and Trotter, W. R., The syndrome of sporadic goiter and congenital deafness. *Q. J. Med., 29*:279–295, 1960.

Gomez- Pan, A., Evered, D. C., and Hall, R., Pituitary-thyroid function in Pendred's syndrome. *Br. Med. J., 2*:152–153, 1974.

Gray, H. W., Hooper, L. A., and Greig, W. R., An evaluation of the twenty-minute perchlorate discharge test. *J. Clin. Endocrinol., 37*:351–355, 1973.

Hollander, C. S., Prout, T. E., Rienhoff, M., Ruben, R. J., and Asper, S. P., Jr., Congenital deafness with goiter. *Am. J. Med., 37*:630–637, 1964.

Hvidberg-Hansen, J., and Balslev-Jørgensen, M., The inner ear in Pendred's syndrome. *Acta Otolaryngol. (Stockh.), 66*:129–135, 1968.

Illum, P., Kaier, H. W., Hvidberg-Hansen, J., and Sondergaard, G., Fifteen cases of Pendred's syndrome. *Arch. Otolaryngol., 96*:297–304, 1972.

Johnsen, S., Familial deafness and goiter in persons with a low level of protein-bound iodine. *Acta Otolaryng. (Stockh.) Suppl., 140*:168–177, 1958.

Kitlak, W., and Gebert, P, Klinische und chromosomale Untersuchungen bei angeborener Hypothyreose infolge Thyroxinsynthesestörung und Innenohrschwerhörigkeit (Pendred- oder Kropf-Taubheits-Syndrom). *Arch. Kinderheilkd., 177*:170–183, 1968.

Ljunggren, J. G., Lindström, H., and Hjern, B., The concentration of peroxidase in normal and adenomatous human thyroid tissue with special reference to patients with Pendred's syndrome. *Acta Endocrinol. (Kbh.), 72*:272–278, 1973.

McGirr, E. M., Hutchinson, J. H., and Clement, W. E., Sporadic goitre due to dyshormonogenesis. Impaired utilization of trapped iodine. *Scot. Med. J., 4*:107–114, 1959.

Medeiros-Neto, G. A., Nicolau, W , Kieffer, J., and Ulhoa Cintra, A. G., Thyroidal iodoproteins in Pendred's syndrome. *J. Clin. Endocrinol., 28*:1205–1213, 1968.

Milutinovic, P. S., Stanbury, J. B., Wicken, J V., Thyroid function in a family with the Pendred syndrome. *J. Clin. Endocrinol., 29*:962–969, 1969.

Morgans, M. E., and Trotter, W. R., Association of congenital deafness with goitre; the nature of the thyroid defect. *Lancet, 1*:607–609, 1958.

Nilsson, L. R., Borgfors, N., Gamstorp, I., Holst, H., and Liden, G., Nonendemic goitre and deafness. *Acta Paediatr. Scand., 53*:117–131, 1964.

Pendred, V., Deafmutism and goitre. *Lancet, 2*:532, 1896.

Roberts, K. D., Thyroid carcinoma in childhood in Great Britain. *Arch. Dis. Child., 32*:58–60, 1957.

Safar, A., Chaussain, J. L., Vassal, J. et al., Hypothyroidie précoce majeure, partiellement régressive, dans deux cas de syndrome de Pendred. *Arch. Fr. Pédiatr., 30*:843–848, 1973.

Thieme, E. T., Report of the occurrence of deaf-mutism and goiter in four of six siblings of a North American family. *Ann. Surg., 146*:941–948, 1957.

Thompson, J., Maguire, N. C., and Hurwitz, L. J., A family with deafness, goiter, epilepsy, and low intelligence segregating independently. *Ir. J. Med. Sci., 3*:427–431, 1970.

Thould, A. K., and Scowen, E. F., The syndrome of congenital deafness and simple goiter. *J. Endocrinol., 30*:69–77, 1964.

Trotter, W. R., The association of deafness with thyroid dysfunction. *Br. Med. Bull., 16*:92–98, 1960.

von Harnack, G. A., Horst, W., and Lenz, W., Das erbliche Syndrom: Innenohrschwerhörigkeit und Jodfehlverwertung mit Kropf. *Dtsch. Med. Wochenschr., 88*:2421–2428, 1961.

Wildner, G. P., and Wittig, G., Zur Histomorphologie der Schilddrüse beim Pendredschen Kropf-Taubheits-Syndrom. *Zentralbl. Allg. Pathol., 109*:52–61, 1966.

GOITER, ELEVATED PROTEIN-BOUND IODINE (PBI), STIPPLED EPIPHYSES, AND CONGENITAL SENSORINEURAL DEAFNESS

A syndrome characterized by stippled epiphyses, goiter, elevated circulating thyroid hormone level in the presence of normal thyroxine-binding globulin with apparent euthyroid state, and severe congenital sensorineural hearing loss was described in three of six sibs by Refetoff and colleagues (1967, 1972).

CLINICAL FINDINGS

Physical Findings. The facies of the affected was birdlike or narrow and different from that of other members of the family. Both older sibs had pectus carinatum, winged scapulae, and enlarged thyroid glands (Fig. 9–2A, B). Nystagmus was documented in two of the three sibs. Intelligence was normal.

Endocrine System. The goiters appeared in early to middle childhood and ranged in size from three to four times normal.

Auditory System. Congenital severe bilateral sensorineural deafness was present in all three sibs. The deafness was more marked in the higher frequencies (Fig. 9–2C).

LABORATORY FINDINGS

Roentgenograms. Radiographs showed stippling of the major secondary ossification centers (Fig. 9–2D). Bone age was mildly retarded. With age, the stippling disappeared, but the epiphyseal heads of the humerus and femur were flattened; three were shorter and showed varus deformity of the femoral necks. Laminograms of the petrous bones showed that the internal auditory canal was of decreased length.

Other Findings. Although the patients were clinically euthyroid, some of their laboratory tests suggested hyperthyroidism. PBI levels in two sibs ranged from 12.8 to 20.8 μg. per 100 ml. However, the BMR and the levels of serum lipids and cholesterol were normal. The potassium perchlorate discharge test was normal in both sibs. Because of the presence of high circulating levels of blood thyroxine and normal thyroxine-binding capacity, the authors suggested intracellular resistance to the action of thyroid hormone, which was partially compensated for by excessive hormone production (Refetoff et al., 1972). Unpublished data (1975) suggest peripheral resistance to hormone action.

HEREDITY

There was no family history of goiter, deafness, or other congenital abnormalities in either family. The father was second cousin to his children. Inheritance appeared to be autosomal recessive.

DIAGNOSIS

Elevated PBI levels in the presence of normal thyroid function have been noted in association with thyroxine-binding globulin as an autosomal dominant trait (Torkington et al., 1970). Although resistance to thyroid hormone action in peripheral tissues has been described by Bode et al. (1973) and by Lamberg (1973), in neither case did the patient have deafness or bone abnormalities. Stippled epiphyses may occur in a number of disorders: chondrodysplasia punctata, Zellweger syndrome, multiple epiphyseal dysplasia, and others.

TREATMENT

Treatment of the deafness was ineffective because of the severity of the loss.

PROGNOSIS

There appeared to be no progressive nature to any aspect of the disorder. The stippled epiphyses cleared, and although the femoral heads were flattened, the patients experienced no difficulty in ambulation.

SUMMARY

This syndrome is characterized by: 1) autosomal recessive transmission, 2) stippled epiphyses, 3) goiter with abnormally high PBI, and 4) moderate to severe congenital sensorineural deafness.

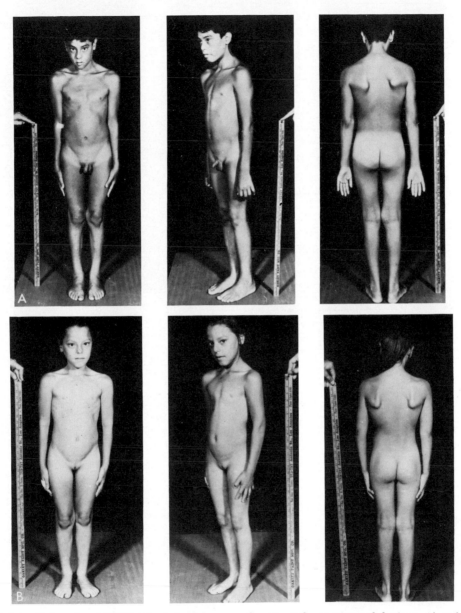

Figure 9–2 *Goiter, elevated PBI, stippled epiphyses, and congenital sensorineural deafness. (A and B)* Twelve and 8-year-old sibs with birdlike facies, pectus carinatum, and winged scapulae.

Illustration continued on the following page

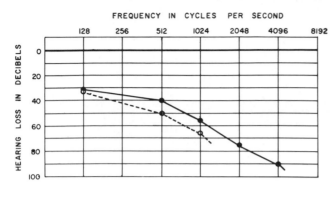

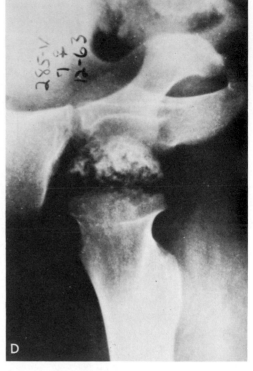

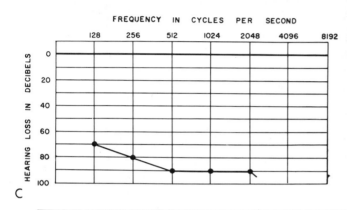

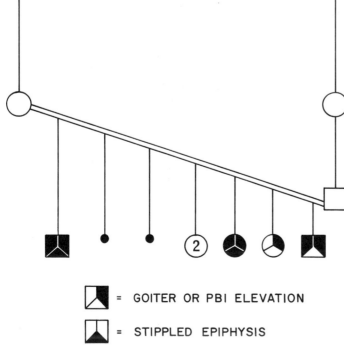

Figure 9–2 Continued. (C) Puretone audiograms of two sibs showing similar hearing loss, more marked in the higher frequencies. (D) Radiograph showing stippled epiphysis of femoral head. Similar changes were present at the knees and in the proximal humerus. (E) Pedigree of affected kindred. (A–D from S. Refetoff *et al.*, *J. Clin. Endocrinol. Metab.*, 27: 279, 1967; E adapted from S. Refetoff *et al.*)

REFERENCES

Bode, H. H., Danon, M., Weintraub, B. D., Maloff, F., and Crawford, J. D., Partial target organ resistance to thyroid hormone. *J. Clin. Invest., 52*:776–782, 1973.

Lamberg, B. A., Congenital euthyroid goitre and partial peripheral resistance to thyroid hormones. *Lancet, 1*:854–857, 1973.

Refetoff, S., DeGroot, L. J., Benand, B., and DeWind, L. T., Studies of a sibship with apparent hereditary resistance to the intracellular action of thyroid hormone. *Metabolism, 21*:723–756, 1972.

Refetoff, A., DeWind, L. T., and DeGroot, L. J., Familial syndrome combining deaf-mutism, stippled epiphyses, goiter and abnormally high PBI: possible target organ refractoriness to thyroid hormone. *J. Clin. Endocrinol., 27*:279–294, 1967.

Torkington, P., Harrison, R. J., Maclagan, N. F., and Burston, D., Familial thyroxine-binding globulin deficiency. *Br. Med. J., 3*:27–29, 1970.

APLASIA OF NASAL ALAE, HYPOTHYROIDISM, GROWTH RETARDATION, MALABSORPTION DUE TO PROTEOLYTIC AND LIPOLYTIC DEFICIENCY, ABSENT PERMANENT TEETH, AND SENSORINEURAL DEAFNESS

Johanson and Blizzard (1971) and Park, Johanson, Jones, and Blizzard (1972) defined a syndrome consisting of aplasia of the nasal alae, growth retardation, malabsorption, hypothyroidism, absent permanent teeth, and sensorineural deafness in three unrelated female children. Morris and Fisher (1967) and Townes (1972) reported less well documented cases in females.

CLINICAL FINDINGS

Physical Findings. Absence of the nasal alae produces a striking appearance. The nasal bridge may be depressed. Midline ectodermal scalp defects have been noted in several patients.

Birth weight is usually low. During infancy there is poor weight gain. Edema ranging from moderate degree over the hands and lower extremities to generalized anasarca has been noted. If the edema is untreated, the patient may develop congestive heart failure. Milestones are usually severely delayed (Johanson and Blizzard, 1971). However, some children appear to have normal intelligence (Townes, 1972).

Urogenital System. There is usually a single urogenital orifice. A double vagina and a double uterus with normal tubes and ovaries have been found. Sexual maturity is retarded (Park *et al.*, 1972). Occasionally, there is an enlarged clitoris with well-formed preputial folds.

Musculoskeletal System. Usually, there is hypotonia and hyperextensibility of joints. Bone age is severely retarded. Most patients are microcephalic. One patient showed somewhat thickened calvaria. Irregularities in ossification of the capital femoral epiphyses, the medial humeral epicondyles, and the epiphyses of the distal femur and proximal tibia were noted (Johanson and Blizzard, 1971). These changes, however, have not been observed in other reported patients.

Gastrointestinal System. Malabsorption, a constant feature, has been shown by Townes (1969) to be associated with absence of trypsin, chymotrypsin, carboxypeptidase, and lipase activity.

With the occasional exception of the mandibular first molars, permanent teeth never develop.

Imperforate anus and rectovaginal fistula have been noted in most reported cases.

Endocrine System. Athyreotic cretinism was present in most, if not all, cases.

Auditory System. The deafness was congenital, profound, and sensorineural in all patients.

Vestibular System. No studies have been reported.

HEREDITY

The disorder to date has been seen only in 46, XX female children. Perhaps the syndrome is lethal in the male. It is likely, however, that one reported male with XXY Klinefelter syndrome had the disorder

(Grand *et al.*, 1966). Along with all of the stigmata of the syndrome he had lung disease. Presumably, he survived by virtue of having the extra X chromosome. A somewhat less certain example of a male with the disorder is the boy reported by Wildervanck (1968). He had small stature, congenital sensorineural deafness, persistent primary teeth, nasal alar hypoplasia, mental retardation, and mild hypospadias. However, he also had microphthalmia and aniridia, and his karyotype was normal.

DIAGNOSIS

Trypsinogen deficiency is associated with severe growth failure, watery diarrhea, hypoproteinemia, and pitting edema of the extremities, but it is not associated with the other anomalies seen in the syndrome under discussion here (Townes, 1972). Park *et al.* (1972) surveyed female pseudohermaphrodites who had a variety of urogenital and anal anomalies but did not have athyreotic cretinism, growth retardation, deafness, pancreatic disorders, or oligodontia, all of which are observed in this syndrome.

TREATMENT

Rhinoplasty may correct the nasal defect. The infant may be maintained on a regimen of protein hydrolysate, pancreatin, and vitamins as supplements to the diet. The athyreotic cretinism may be treated with L-thyroxine or desiccated thyroid. While growth improves, the muscular hypotonia and intelligence do not.

PROGNOSIS

The outlook for these children is poor. The mental retardation is marked, and death may result from heart failure.

SUMMARY

This syndrome is characterized by: (1) limitation largely to females, with possible lethality in males, (2) absence of nasal alae, (3) pancreatic achylia, (4) somatic and mental retardation, (5) athyreotic cretinism, (6) single urogenital orifice, double vagina, and bicornuate uterus, (7) absence of permanent teeth, and (8) congenital profound sensorineural deafness.

REFERENCES

Grand, R. J., Rosen, S. W., Di Sant'Agnese, P. A., and Kirkham, W. R., Unusual case of XXY Klinefelter's syndrome with pancreatic insufficiency, hypothyroidism, deafness, chronic lung disease, dwarfism, and microcephaly. *Am. J. Med., 41*:478–485, 1966.

Johanson, A., and Blizzard, R., A syndrome of congenital aplasia of the alae nasi, deafness, hypothyroidism, dwarfism, absent permanent teeth, and malabsorption. *J. Pediatr., 79*:982–987, 1971.

Morris, M. D., and Fisher, D. A., Trypsinogen deficiency disease. *Am. J. Dis. Child., 114*:203–208, 1967.

Park, I. J., Johanson, A., Jones, H. W., Jr., and Blizzard, R., Special female hermaphroditism associated with multiple disorders. *Obstet. Gynecol., 39*:100–106, 1972 (same as Case 1, Johanson and Blizzard).

Townes, P. L., Trypsinogen deficiency and other proteolytic deficiency diseases. *Birth Defects, 8*(2):95–101, 1972.

Wildervanck, L. S., A first-arch syndrome variant? *Lancet, 2*:350, 1968.

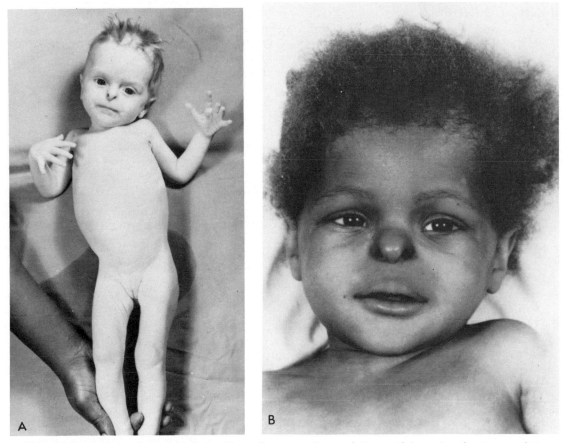

Figure 9–3 *Aplasia of nasal alae, hypothyroidism, growth retardation, malabsorption due to proteolytic and lipolytic deficiency, absence of permanent teeth, and sensorineural deafness. (A and B)* Note striking facies marked by aplasia of the nasal alae. (From A. Johanson and R. Blizzard, *J. Pediatr.,* 79:982, 1971.)

PRENATAL DWARFISM, ELEVATED GROWTH HORMONE LEVELS, MENTAL RETARDATION, AND CONGENITAL DEAFNESS

Van Gemund, Laurent de Angulo, and van Gelderen (1969) reported two male sibs with prenatal dwarfism, elevated serum immunoreactive growth hormone and end-organ unresponsiveness, mental retardation, and congenital deafness.

CLINICAL FINDINGS

Physical Findings. The sibs were prenatally dwarfed (birth weight at term less than 1900 grams), but their extremities and trunk were in proportion. Head circumference was reduced. Pubertal signs, even under therapy, did not appear until 20 years of age.

Nervous System. Both boys had I.Q.s of less than 40.

Auditory System. Both sibs were congenitally deaf, and neither achieved any facility of speech. The deafness was not otherwise described.

Vestibular System. No studies were reported.

LABORATORY FINDINGS

Radiographic study showed severely delayed skeletal maturation. Increased serum immunoreactive growth levels were found. Exogenous human growth hormone (HGH) induced normal responses of serum insulin, glucose, and free fatty acids but failed to increase nitrogen retention and urinary hydroxyproline excretion.

HEREDITY

The normal parents of the two affected male sibs were consanguineous. The disorder probably has autosomal recessive inheritance.

DIAGNOSIS

Laron (1968) described dwarfism with high serum immunoreactive human growth hormone levels. The individuals under study responded normally to exogenous growth hormone. Najjar (1969) reported sibs whose HGH levels were not suppressed by oral intravenous glucose administration. Exogenous HGH failed to increase nitrogen retention and urinary hydroxyproline excretion. In neither family was mental retardation or deafness present.

TREATMENT

Anabolic steroid therapy may be initiated to promote growth.

PROGNOSIS

Although the disorder is not life-threatening, prognosis is poor since treatment is ineffective.

SUMMARY

Characteristics of this syndrome include: 1) autosomal recessive inheritance, 2) prenatal dwarfism, 3) elevated serum immunoreactive growth hormone and end-organ unresponsiveness, 4) mental retardation, and 5) severe congenital deafness, probably sensorineural.

REFERENCES

Laron, Z., Pertzelan, A., and Karp, M., Pituitary dwarfism with high serum level of growth hormone. *Isr. J. Med. Sci., 4*:883–894, 1968.

Najjar, S. S., Pituitary dwarfism with elevated serum HGH levels. *Acta Endocrinol. Suppl., 138*:144, 1969.

Van Gemund, J. J., Laurent de Angulo, M. S., and van Gelderen, H. H., Familial prenatal dwarfism with elevated serum-reactive growth hormone levels and end-organ unresponsiveness. *Maandschr. Kindergeneeskd., 37*:372–382, 1969.

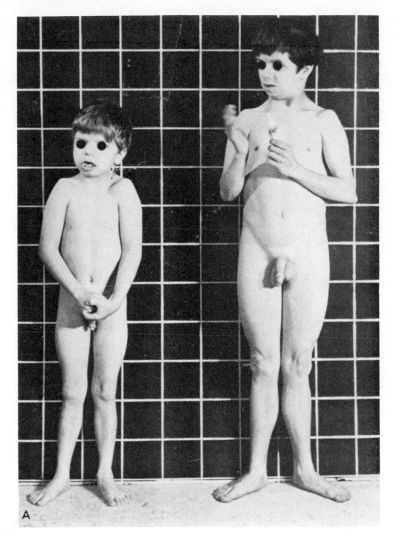

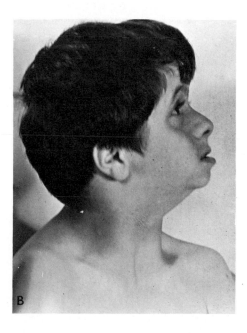

Figure 9–4 *Prenatal dwarfism, elevated growth hormone levels, mental retardation, and congenital deafness. (A) Sibs at 12 years of age (height, 97 cm.) and 22 years of age (height, 117 cm.). (B) Note hypoplasia of midface. (From J. J. Van Gemund et al., Maandschr. Kindergeneeskd., 37:372, 1969.)*

HYPOTHALAMOHYPOPHYSEAL DWARFISM AND SENSORINEURAL DEAFNESS

Winkelmann *et al.* (1972) reported two sisters with hypothalamohypophyseal dwarfism and sensorineural deafness.

CLINICAL FINDINGS

Physical Findings. The dwarfism was proportionate. Birth weight and size were normal. The growth retardation was first noted at the time of school registration. Adult height was 139 cm. in one sister and 146 cm. in the other.

Endocrine System. Neither girl achieved sexual maturity, i.e., neither developed pubic hair or breasts, both had primary amenorrhea. The external and internal genitalia were infantile.

Auditory System. At the age of approximately 6 to 8 years, loss of hearing, which rapidly progressed, was noted. By 12 years of age both sisters were totally deaf.

Vestibular System. No studies were reported.

LABORATORY FINDINGS

Radiographic examination of the sisters as adults showed generalized retarded bone age (open cranial sutures and absence of epiphyseal fusion).

Radioimmunologic assays of plasma levels of growth hormone (HGH) were 3.0 ng./ml. (normal levels are 30.0 ± 10.0 ng./ml.), rising no higher than 5.0 ng./ml. on insulin stimulation. Follicle-stimulating hormone (FSH) and luteinizing hormone (LH) assays were at prepubertal levels.

Radioactive iodine uptake, cortisol, and corticosterone excretion were normal. Urinary 17-hydroxy- and 11-hydroxycortico-steroid levels were normal, even after ACTH stimulation.

Serum cholesterol and triglycerides were elevated in one girl but were normal in the other.

HEREDITY

The parents and one sister of the patients were normal. There was no known parental consanguinity. Inheritance appears to be autosomal recessive.

DIAGNOSIS

There are several types of pituitary dwarfism, but none has been associated with sensorineural deafness (McKusick, 1975).

TREATMENT

It should be possible to treat such patients with growth hormone or with anabolic steroids.

PROGNOSIS

For treatment of the deafness the prognosis is poor. Hormonal therapy for the dwarfism should be effective.

SUMMARY

Characteristics of the syndrome include: 1) autosomal recessive inheritance, 2) somatic and sexual infantilism due to deficiency of growth hormone and gonadotropins, 3) normal intelligence, and 4) sensorineural hearing loss, appearing at about 6 to 8 years of age and progressing rapidly to complete deafness.

REFERENCES

McKusick, V. A., *Mendelian Inheritance in Man*, 4th ed. Baltimore, Md., Johns Hopkins Press, 1975.

Winkelmann, W., Solbach, H. G., Wiegelmann, W., Bethge, H., and Pfeiffer, R. A., Hypothalamo-hypophysärer Minderwuchs mit Innenohrschwerhörigkeit bei zwei Schwestern. *Internist,* *13*:52–56, 1972.

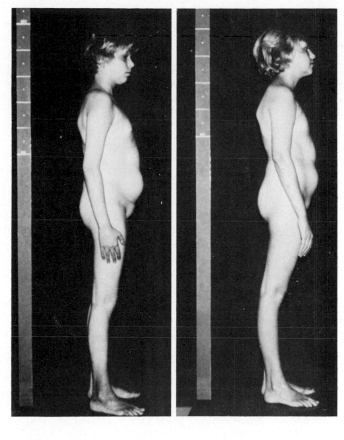

Figure 9–5 *Hypothalamohypophyseal dwarfism and sensorineural deafness.* Sisters at 22 and 19 years of age, respectively, exhibiting reduced height and lack of sexual maturity. (From W. Winkelmann *et al., Internist, 13*:52, 1972.)

MUCOPOLYSACCHARIDOSES

The mucopolysaccharidoses are inherited disorders of mucopolysaccharide metabolism. Defective activity of various genetically controlled pathways of lysosomal degradation lead to intracellular storage of undegraded acid mucopolysaccharides and to relatively similar clinical and skeletal changes. The phenotype is most pronounced in the Hurler and Maroteaux-Lamy syndromes and less severe in other mucopolysaccharidoses (McKusick, 1972; Spranger, 1972).

Within the brief scope of this text, we can only briefly outline clinical and laboratory findings in those mucopolysaccharidoses that are associated with deafness.

CLINICAL FINDINGS

Hurler syndrome (MPS I-H) is the classic prototype of the mucopolysaccharidoses.

It has the following cardinal features: growth failure after infancy, marked mental retardation, progressive coarsening of facial features beginning toward the end of the first year of life, corneal clouding, chronic nasal discharge and repeated upper respiratory infections, hernias, progressive lack of mobility of joints resulting, for example, in clawhand deformity, hepatosplenomegaly, marked somatic and mental retardation, and biochemical evidence of intracellular storage and excessive urinary excretion of acid mucopolysaccharides. Death usually occurs before 10 years of age from pneumonia and/or cardiac failure (Fig. 9–6*A*).

In *Scheie syndrome* (MPS I-S), an allelic form of Hurler syndrome, the facies is somewhat coarsened and shows mandibular prognathism and downturned oral commissures. The nose is broad. Progressive corneal clouding begins in early life and by the fourth decade usually curtails vision. Stature is mildly retarded. Intelligence is normal. The hands and feet are broad, and the fingers and toes are fixed in a clawlike position. Mobility in all joints is limited. The carpal-tunnel syndrome is common. Most affected individuals have aortic regurgitation.

Hunter syndrome (MPS II) occurs in mild (type A) and severe (type B) forms. Type A patients usually survive to adulthood. Type B patients suffer rapid psychomotor deterioration and usually die before puberty. In type A, intelligence is mildly impaired. Stature is less severely retarded than in MPS I-H. In contrast to patients with Hurler syndrome, patients with Hunter syndrome usually do not show gross evidence of corneal clouding (Fig. 9–6*B*).

Sanfilippo syndrome (MPS III) occurs in two nonallelic forms. The facies is far less marked than in MPS I-H, and the corneas are clear. Height is almost normal. The children become aggressive and restless prior to school years. Death usually occurs in the second decade.

Morquio syndrome (MPS IV) is characterized by marked growth failure after the first year of life, short neck, pigeon breast, progressive spinal deformity, and other skeletal anomalies, such as knock-knees and flat feet. The facies is normal. The extremities appear disproportionately long. Usually there is excessive joint mobility. Intelligence is nearly always normal.

Maroteaux-Lamy syndrome (MPS VI) patients exhibit a severe Hurler-like appearance but have normal intelligence. There are two forms—mild and severe. In the mild form the first changes appear about 6 years of age when small stature and spinal alterations are noted; these patients survive to adulthood. The severe form is identified in early childhood by severe facial and skeletal changes, severely impaired vision, hearing loss, and cardiac defects that lead to death in adolescence (Fig. 9–6*C*).

Auditory System. Perhaps this has been the most difficult section to write in the entire text since virtually no hard data are available on deafness in the many different types of mucopolysaccharidoses. Although there have been earlier surveys of

about 75 examples, the approximately 25 per cent who showed hearing loss or deafness represented a pooled group of persons with mucopolysaccharidoses. This percentage does not, in any sense, reflect the frequency in each form (Ricci and Ancetti, 1955; Kittel, 1963). Therefore, we have read over 200 case reports of the various types of hearing loss. This is obviously an unsatisfactory approach, since mental retardation, lack of cooperation, and early death have sharply biased the data. Many case reports have not mentioned deafness—either because it was not considered to be marked or because it was not noticed since it was minimal. Therefore, with few exceptions most of our comments are merely impressions. It is our fervent hope that this confession of ignorance shall serve heuristic purpose.

Probably most Hurler syndrome patients have some degree of progressive conductive deafness. The deformed nasopharynx and the increased susceptibility to upper respiratory illness lead to middle ear infection. Although other investigators described conductive deafness, only Kelemen (1966) reported temporal bone findings. His patient suffered a 60 dB loss, mostly in the middle range. The air cells of the tegmen and epitympanum were filled with reticular mesenchymal tissue. The mucous membrane of the middle ear was high and papillomatous, blocking the niches of the oval and round windows, which were sites of bony overgrowth. These changes were considered to be the prenatal result of the disease (Fig. 9–6*D, E*).

A systematic audiometric study has not been carried out in Scheie syndrome. From our tabulation, possibly not more than 10 to 20 per cent exhibit hearing loss, usually not severe, in middle age. Although not adequately documented, the loss is probably mixed (Koskenoja and Suvanto, 1959; Murray, 1959; Scheie *et al.*, 1962).

Hunter syndrome has been accompanied by deafness in about half of the cases, although the loss is usually not severe (Leroy and Crocker, 1966). Although other researchers have stated that the deafness is sensorineural in type, on the basis of our limited experience we suggest that the hearing loss is more often mixed. Kittel (1963) illustrated mixed hearing loss in his patient. Wolff (1942) found no joint cavity between the malleus and incus. Although she did not describe typical otosclerotic foci, she noted in the round window area irregular bony nodules that protruded into the lowermost portion of the scala tympani as well as alterations reminiscent of those reported by Kelemen (1965) in Hurler syndrome. There were changes in the organ of Corti, but these appeared to be postmortem artifacts.

Zechner and Altmann (1968) found the middle ear mucosa to be edematous and to contain large foamy PAS-positive cytoplasm. The malleus and incus were normal in shape but contained large hyperemic marrow spaces. The stapes and pneumatic cellular system appeared normal. PAS-positive cells were inside the mastoid air cells, and thick PAS-positive mantles surrounded smaller blood vessels. In the semicircular canal region, numerous blue mantles were seen. Otosclerotic foci were noted near the oval and round windows. The organ of Corti was normal. Beneath the stria vascularis, a broad PAS-positive zone was noted. The cytoplasm of the spiral and vestibular ganglia was engorged with foamy PAS-positive material.

In Sanfilippo syndrome, deafness has rarely been reported. It was evident in only 1 of 10 patients documented by Spranger *et al.* (1967) and in two or possibly 3 of 8 patients studied by Rampini (1969). However, the aggressive nature and lack of cooperation among these patients has made audiometric testing difficult to impossible. Sparse evidence suggests that, when present, the hearing loss appears at about 6 to 7 years of age and becomes progressive.

Most patients with Morquio syndrome exhibit mixed deafness. It usually has its onset during the second decade, and in most cases it is not severe (Robins *et al.*, 1963; Von Noorden *et al.*, 1968).

About 25 per cent of the patients with Maroteaux-Lamy syndrome exhibit deafness, probably conductive, which appears at about 6 to 8 years of age and results from frequent bouts of otitis media (Liebenam, 1938; Stoeckel, 1941; Maroteaux *et al.*, 1963; Sarrouy *et al.*, 1965; Fallis *et al.*, 1968; Spranger *et al.*, 1970).

Vestibular System. The only study in which vestibular function was described — that of a patient with Hunter syndrome — indicated that it was reduced bilaterally.

LABORATORY FINDINGS

Roentgenograms. Radiographically, all but the Morquio syndrome show dysostosis multiplex to varying degrees. The most severe form is seen in the Hurler (MPS I-H) and Maroteaux-Lamy (MPS IV) syndromes. The skull becomes large and deformed, and the sella assumes a J-shape. The ribs are wide, and the vertebral bodies are dysplastic with biconvex end plates and hook-shaped configurations of the lower thoracic and upper lumbar bodies after 12 to 18 months of age. The long tubular bones exhibit marked diaphyseal widening, distortion, and deformities of the epiphyses. The shafts of the short tubular bones are underconstricted and have bullet-shaped phalanges and proximal pointing of the second to fifth metacarpals (Fig. 9–6*F, G*).

Radiologic alterations in Scheie syndrome are minimal. There is clawlike deformity of the fingers and small, often cystic, carpal bones.

In Hunter syndrome (MPS II) the dysostosis multiplex is less severe than in Hurler syndrome (MPS I-H).

In Sanfilippo syndrome (MPS III) the calvaria is thickened posteriorly, the mastoids are sclerotic, and the vertebral bodies are ovoid. The hands are normal.

The radiologic changes in Morquio syndrome (MPS IV) are marked by platyspondyly, hypoplasia of the odontoid, coxa valga, flared ilia, and femoral head dysplasia. The bases of the second to fifth metacarpals are pointed, and the carpals are small and irregular.

Other Findings. The enzyme defects currently identified are deficiency of α-L-iduronidase in the Hurler and Scheie syndromes. Both types of Hunter syndrome patients have sulfoiduronate sulfatase deficiency. In Sanfilippo syndrome (MPS III-A) there is deficient activity of heparan-N-sulfatase; in MPS-III-B, N-acetyl-β-D-glucosaminidase. In MPS VI there is a deficiency in aryl sulfatase B.

The various conditions are characterized by excessive urinary excretion of the following mucopolysaccharides: MPS I — dermatan sulfate and heparan sulfate, mostly the former; MPS II — dermatan sulfate and heparan sulfate, in about equal amounts; MPS III — heparan sulfate; MPS IV — keratan sulfate; and MPS VI — dermatan sulfate.

HEREDITY

With the exception of Hunter syndrome, which is X-linked, all of the other conditions considered in this section have autosomal recessive inheritance.

DIAGNOSIS

The mucopolysaccharidoses most often are confused with the mucolipidoses. In the latter group of conditions, excessive storage and/or excretion of acid mucopolysaccharides does not occur. Among the classic mucopolysaccharidoses, differential diagnosis is not usually difficult. Patients with the Hurler and Hunter syndromes are usually mentally retarded but appear normal for the first year of life. Maroteaux-Lamy syndrome patients have normal mental development but cloudy corneas. In Hunter syndrome the corneas are grossly clear.

TREATMENT

No satisfactory long-term therapy has been devised for the mucopolysaccharidoses.

PROGNOSIS

See above for discussion.

SUMMARY

In general, the characteristics of these syndromes include: 1) autosomal recessive inheritance, except for X-linked Hunter syndrome, 2) coarsening of facial features and dysostosis multiplex, except in Morquio syndrome, 3) storage and urinary excretion of one or more specific mucopolysaccharides, and 4) deafness, varying in type and degree with the mucopolysaccharidosis.

REFERENCES

de Lange, C., Gerlings, P. G., de Kleyn, A., and Lettinga, T. W., Some remarks on gargoylism. II. Otological and laryngological findings. *Acta Paediatr., 31*:398–416, 1944.
Fallis, N., Barnes, F. L., and DiFerrante, N., A case of polydystrophic dwarfism with urinary excretion of dermatan sulfate and heparan sulfate. *J. Clin. Endocrinol., 28*:26–33, 1968.
Kelemen, G., Hurler's syndrome and the hearing organ. *J. Laryngol., 80*:791–803, 1966.
Kittel, G., Pfaundler-Hurlersche Krankheit oder Gargoylismus unter HNO-ärztlicher Sicht. *Z. Laryng. Rhinol. Otol., 42*:206–217, 1963.
Koskenoja, M., and Suvanto, E., Gargoylism. Report of adult form with glaucoma in two sisters. *Acta Ophthalmol. (Kbh.), 37*:234–240, 1959.
Leroy, J. G., and Crocker, A. C., Clinical definition of Hunter-Hurler phenotypes. A review of 50 patients. *Am. J. Dis. Child., 112*:518–530, 1966.
Liebenam, L., Beitrag zur Dysostosis multiplex. *Z. Kinderheilkd., 59*:91–123, 1938.
McKusick, V. A., *Heritable Disorders of Connective Tissue,* 4th Ed. St. Louis, C. V. Mosby Company, 1972, pp. 521–686.
Maroteaux, P., Lévêque, B., Marie, J., and Lamy, M., Une nouvelle dysostose avec élimination urinaire de chondroitine-sulfate B. *Presse Méd., 71*:1849–1852, 1963.
Meyer, S. J., and Okner, H. B., Dysostosis multiplex with special reference to ocular findings. *Am. J. Ophthalmol., 22*:713–722, 1939.
Murray, J. F., Pulmonary disability in the Hurler syndrome. *N. Engl. J. Med., 261*:378–382, 1959.
Rampini, S., Das Sanfilippo-Syndrom. *Helv. Paediatr. Acta, 24*:55–91, 1969.
Ricci, V., and Ancetti, A., Considerazioni sulle anomalie del l'osso temporale in un caso di gargoilismo. *Arch. Ital. Otol., 66*:734–744, 1955.
Robins, M. M., Stevens, H. F., and Linker, A., Morquio's disease: an abnormality of mucopolysaccharide metabolism. *J. Pediatr., 62*:881–889, 1963.
Sarrouy, C., Farouz, S., Roche, M., Sabatini, R., Villaud, J., and Révol, A., A propos d'une nouvelle observation de maladie de Hurler. *Presse Méd., 73*:3219–3222, 1965.
Scheie, H. G., Hambrick, G. W., Jr., and Barness, L. A., A newly recognized forme fruste of Hurler's disease (gargoylism). *Am. J. Ophthalmol., 53*:753–769, 1962.
Spranger, J. W.. The systemic mucopolysaccharidoses. *Ergeb. Inn. Med. Kinderheilkd., 32*:166–265, 1972.
Spranger, J. W., Koch, F., McKusick, V. A., Natztchka, J., Wiedemann, H. R., and Zellweger, H., Mucopolysaccharidosis VI. (Maroteaux-Lamy's disease). *Helv. Paediatr. Acta, 25*:337–362, 1970.
Spranger, J. W., Teller, W., Kosenow, W., Murken, J., and Eckert-Husemann, E., Die HS—

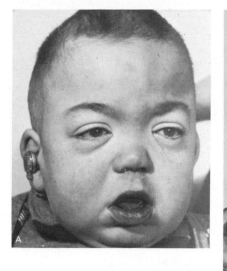

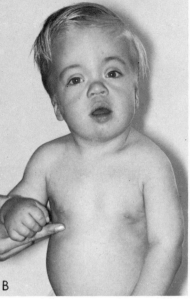

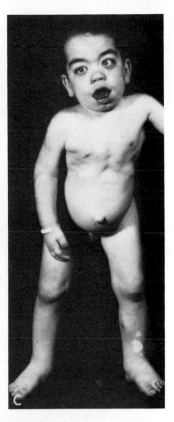

Figure 9-6   *Mucopolysaccharidoses.* (A) Patient with Hurler syndrome. (B) Patient with Hunter syndrome. (C) Patient with Maroteaux-Lamy syndrome. (C from D. A. Stumpf *et al., Am. J. Dis. Child.,* 126:747, 1973.) (D) Pneumatic cells of tegmen filled by reticular tissue.

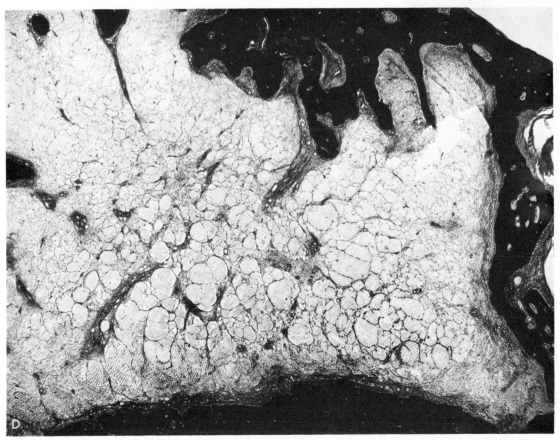

Illustration continued on the following page

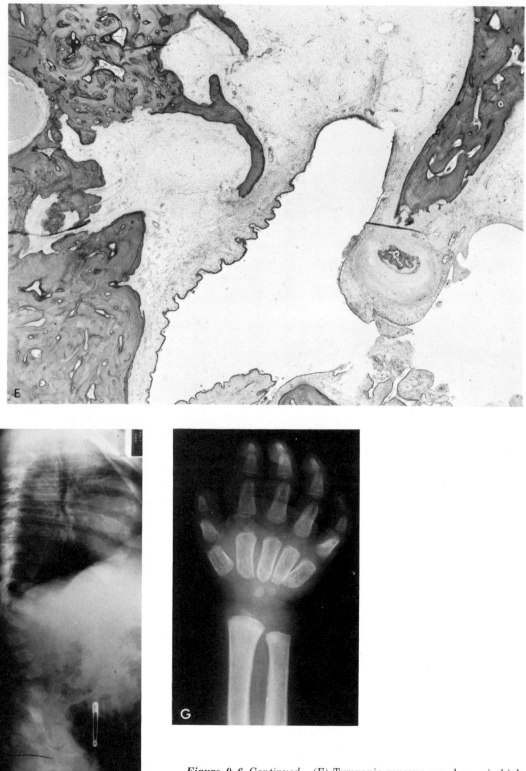

Figure 9–6 Continued. *(E)* Tympanic mucous membrane is high and papillomatous. The long process of the incus is disintegrated. *(F* and *G)* Radiographs showing dysostosis multiplex. *F,* Hook-shaped vertebral bodies; *G,* bullet-shaped metacarpals, pointed phalanges, and delayed bone age.

Mukopolysaccharidose von Sanfilippo (Polydystrophie Oligophrenie). Bericht über 10 Patienten. *Z Kinderheilkd., 101*:71–84, 1967.

Stoeckel, K. H., Über zwei Fälle von Chondro-osteodystrophie von Typus Hurler. *Mschr. Kinderheilkd., 86*:348–368, 1941.

Von Noorden, G. K., Zellweger, H., and Ponseti, I. V., Ocular findings in Morquio-Ullrich's disease. *Arch. Ophthalmol., 64*:585–591, 1960.

Wolff, D., Microscopic study of temporal bones in dysostosis multiplex (gargoylism). *Laryngoscope, 52*:218–22, 1942.

Zechner, G., and Altmann, F., The temporal bone in Hunter's syndrome (gargoylism). *Arch. Klin. Exp. Ohren-, Nasen-, Kehlkopfheilkd., 192*:137–144, 1968.

MANNOSIDOSIS

Mannosidosis was first characterized in 1967 by Öckerman. Autio *et al.* (1973) described several other cases, and in personal communication (March 1974), Autio indicated that he had studied adult patients with the disorder. Booth *et al.* (1975) and Farriaux *et al.* (1975) reported three affected sibs; Spranger *et al.* (1976) studied 12 children. Other cases were noted by Beaudet and Nichols (1975), Tsay *et al.* (1974), and Perelman *et al.* (1975). Loeb *et al.* (1969) described a probable case of mannosidosis, and we have seen a single example.

The children are essentially normal for the first year of life but exhibit a propensity toward recurrent respiratory infections.

CLINICAL FINDINGS

Facies. The coarsening of the facies noted after the first few years of life progresses but neither to the degree noted in MPS I nor as early as found in ML II. The nasal bridge tends to be low, whereas the forehead and mandible are prominent. The neck is somewhat short.

Musculoskeletal System. There is general mild hypotonia. Kyphoscoliosis is common. The abdomen is protuberant. The liver may be enlarged. Umbilical or inguinal hernia is common.

Nervous System. There is delayed early motor development, which becomes manifest as clumsy motor function. Speech is delayed. All known patients have mental retardation that apparently is progressive (Autio *et al.*, 1973).

Ocular System. Wheel-like lens opacities have been noted in a few patients (Öckerman, 1967; Autio *et al.*, 1973; Spranger *et al.*, 1976).

Oral Findings. Macroglossia and widely spaced teeth have been noted (Öckerman, 1967.)

Other Findings. Bilateral testicular hydrocele has been described in two of three children (Autio *et al.*, 1973).

Auditory System. Severe high-frequency sensorineural deafness is a frequent feature (Öckerman, 1967; Loeb *et al.*, 1969; Booth *et al.*, 1975; Spranger *et al.* 1976).

Vestibular Findings. No vestibular studies have been reported.

LABORATORY FINDINGS

Roentgenograms. The calvaria is thick. The long bones are osteoporotic, and the ulna and radius are broad, with curved diaphyses and a thin cortex. There is mild expansion of the tubular bones of the hand. The vertebral bodies are somewhat ovoid, flattened, or hook-shaped in form. The inferior portions of the ilia are hypoplastic. The skeletal pattern is that of mild to moderate dyostosis multiplex (Spranger *et al.*, 1976).

Other Findings. A great number of the peripheral lymphocytes may be vacuolated (Spranger *et al.*, 1976). Coarse, dark granules are present in the neutrophils.

HEREDITY

Inheritance is autosomal recessive.

DIAGNOSIS

The phenotype becomes evident after the first few years of life. To be excluded are the mucopolysaccharidoses, the mucolipidoses, aspartylglycosaminuria, and other storage diseases. The condition is diagnosed by finding mannose-rich components in the urine and by reduced α-mannosidase activity at pH 4 in liver, plasma, and white blood cells (Autio *et al.*, 1973).

TREATMENT

Treatment is symptomatic.

PROGNOSIS

Many children succumb to respiratory infections. The deafness and mental retardation are progressive.

SUMMARY

The disorder is characterized by: 1) autosomal recessive inheritance, 2) coarse facies and short neck, 3) recurrent respiratory infections, 4) kyphoscoliosis, mild hypotonia, protuberant abdomen, inguinal and/or umbilical hernia, 5) progressive mental retardation, 6) mild dysostosis multiplex, 7) reduced mannosidase activity in liver, plasma, and leukocytes, 8) vacuolated lymphocytes, and 9) severe high-frequency sensorineural deafness.

REFERENCES

Autio, S., Norden, N. E., Öckerman, P. A., Riekkinen, P., Rapola, J., and Louhimo, T., Mannosidosis: Clinical, fine-structural, and biochemical findings in three cases *Acta Paediatr. Scand., 62*:555–565, 1973.

Beaudet, A., and Nichols, B. L., Diagnosis of alpha-mannosidase deficiency. *Pediatr. Res., 9*:311, 1975.

Booth, C. W., Chen, K., and Nadler, H. L., Radiologic and biochemical abnormalities in mannosidosis. *Pediatr. Res., 9*:312, 1975.

Farriaux, J. P., Legouis, I., Humbel, R., Dhondt, J. L., Richard, P., Strecker, G., Fourmaintroux, A., Ringel, J., and Fontaine, G., La mannosidosis; à propos de 5 observations. *Nouv. Presse Méd., 4*:1867–1870, 1975.

Loeb, H., Tondeur, M., Toppet, M., and Cremer, N., Clinical, biochemical, and ultrastructural studies of an atypical form of mucopolysaccharidosis. *Acta Paediatr. Scand., 58*:220–228, 1969.

Öckerman, P. A., A generalized storage disorder resembling Hurler's syndrome. *Lancet, 2*:239–241, 1967.

Perelman, R., Nathanson, M., Lepastier, G., Lesavre, P., Plainfosse, B., Chirazi, S., and Seringe, P., Mannosidose associée à l'absence d'alpha-1-antitrypsine. *Ann. Pédiatr., 22*:385–396, 1975.

Spranger, J., Gehler, J., and Cantz, M., The radiographic features of mannosidosis. *Radiology, 119*:401–407, 1976.

Tsay, G. C., Dawson, G., and Matalon, R., Excretion of mannose-rich complex carbohydrates by a patient with alpha-mannosidase deficiency (mannosidosis). *J. Pediatr., 84*:865–868, 1974.

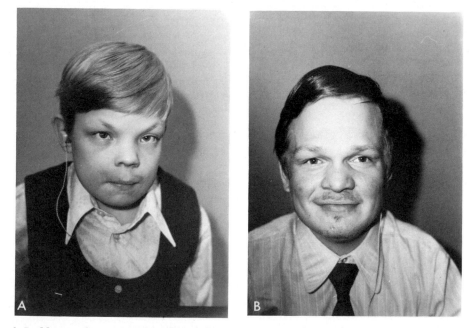

Figure 9–7 *Mannosidosis. (A* and *B)* Coarse features in child and in adult with mannosidosis. (Courtesy of S. Autio, Helsinki, Finland.)

SKELETAL DYSPLASIA, MENTAL RETARDATION, SKIN GRANULOMATA, AND PROFOUND CONGENITAL SENSORINEURAL DEAFNESS

Fountain (1974) reported four mentally retarded sibs with severe congenital deafness. Two developed cutaneous granulomata.

CLINICAL FINDINGS

Physical Findings. Birth weight and length were apparently normal, but adult height was less than 153 cm.

Skeletal System. Although there was thickening of the calvaria and poor modeling of the long bones, these were not clinically manifested (see Laboratory Findings). One sib who had died had exhibited spina bifida.

Integumentary System. One sib had a cyst of the cheek, buccal mucosal tags, and gingival enlargement when she was examined at 15 years of age. At 22 years of age, her lower lip became progressively swollen and granulomatous. Her brother had inguinal hernia repair, followed by a foreign body granulomatous reaction. At about the age of 22 years, he manifested enlargement of the upper lip. A third sib, presently 21 years old, exhibited no granulomata.

Nervous System. All affected sibs were mentally retarded. An I.Q. of 75 was reported for one sib.

Auditory System. All three sibs as well as one who died were described as congenitally deaf. The deafness was not otherwise characterized.

Vestibular System. No mention was made of any vestibular studies.

LABORATORY FINDINGS

Roentgenograms. Radiographic studies showed thickened calvaria and lack of modeling of the distal femur and distal radius. The acetabula were shallow.

Other Findings. A host of laboratory studies yielded normal values. In personal communication with the authors (September 1975), Fountain indicated that mannosidosis and aspartylglycosaminuria had been excluded.

PATHOLOGY

Gingival biopsy showed a granulomatous infiltrate marked by large, foamy cells that did not contain fat. PAS stain was mildly positive and diastase-resistant.

HEREDITY

Four sibs exhibited mental retardation, severe congenital sensorineural deafness, and skeletal abnormalities. Two of the four had granulomatous enlargement of the lips and gingiva. The parents were normal. The disorder appears to have autosomal recessive inheritance.

DIAGNOSIS

The syndrome most closely resembles asparty glycosaminuria, an autosomal recessive disease characterized by mental retardation, coarse facial features, sagging cheeks, frequent infections, diarrhea, and vacuolated lymphocytes (Pollitt *et al.,* 1968; Autio, 1972; Autio *et al.,* 1973). Deafness does not appear to be part of that disorder.

TREATMENT

Therapy is unknown. The deafness is profound.

PROGNOSIS

Although the disorder is not life-threatening, the general outlook is poor.

SUMMARY

The syndrome is characterized by: 1) autosomal recessive inheritance, 2) mental retardation, 3) somewhat reduced height, 4) skin granulomata, 5) thickened calvaria and poor modeling of bones, and 6) severe congenital deafness, probably sensorineural.

REFERENCES

Autio, S., Aspartylglycosaminuria. Analysis of thirty-four patients. *J. Ment. Def. Res. (Monograph Ser.), 1*:1–93, 1972.

Autio, S., Visakorpi, J. K., and Järvinen, H., Aspartylglycosaminuria (AGU). Further aspects on its clinical picture, mode of inheritance, and epidemiology based on a series of 57 patients. *Ann. Clin. Res., 5*:149–155, 1973.

Fountain, R. B., Familial bone abnormalities, deaf mutism, mental retardation, and skin granulomas. *Proc. R. Soc. Med., 67*:878–879, 1974.

Pollitt, R. J., Jenner, F. A., and Merskey, H., Aspartylglycosaminuria. An inborn error of metabolism associated with mental defect. *Lancet, 2*:253–255, 1968.

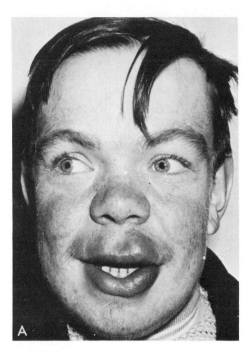
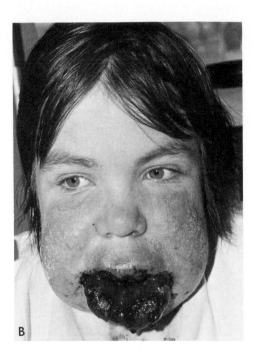

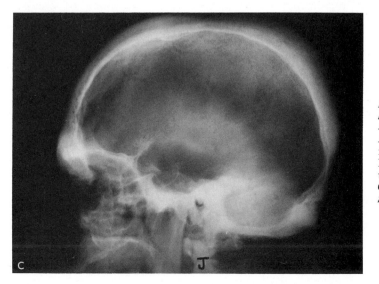

Figure 9-8   *Skeletal dysplasia, mental retardation, skin granulomata, and profound sensorineural deafness. (A* and *B)* Affected sibs exhibiting coarse facies and skin granulomata. *(C)* Radiograph showing marked thickening of calvaria. *(A, B,* and *C* from R. B. Fountain, *Proc. R. Soc. Med., 67*:878, 1974.)

MISCELLANEOUS STORAGE DISEASES AND DEAFNESS

We have suggested that there is a paucity of hard data on hearing loss in the various mucopolysaccharidoses. At the risk of sounding captious, we must say that there is even less information available on deafness in the several mucolipidoses and sphingolipidoses. In large part, this lack is due to the severe accompanying psychomotor retardation and early death.

Tay-Sachs disease, according to Kelemen (1965), who reviewed the literature and studied two cases, is frequently accompanied by hyperacusis and otitis media. This was borne out by Boies (1963).

G_{M1} gangliosidosis, type 1 patients exhibit sensorineural deafness (R. Desnick, personal communication, 1975).

Goldberg et al. (1971) found bilateral sensorineural deafness in a storage disease characterized by growth retardation, coarse features, mental retardation, seizures, corneal clouding, macular cherry-red spot, dysostosis multiplex, β-galactosidase deficiency, and autosomal recessive inheritance.

Couchot et al. (1974) in review of the literature and study of three cases of metachromatic leukodystrophy noted a hearing deficit in 10 of 13 cases.

Mucolipidosis III patients, in our experience, have often manifested a mild conductive deafness.

About 50 per cent of patients with Fabry disease have a mild sensorineural hearing loss (R. Desnick, personal communication, 1975).

REFERENCES

Boies, L. R., Tay-Sachs disease in its relation to otolaryngology. *Arch Otolaryngol.,* 77:166–173, 1963.

Couchot, J., Pluot, M., Schmauch, M. A., Pennaforte, F., and Fandre, M., La mucosulfatidose. *Arch. Fr. Pédiatr.,* 31:775–795, 1974.

Goldberg, M. F., Cotlier, E., Fischenscher, L. G., Kenyon, K., Enat, R., and Borowsky, S. A., Macular cherry-red spot, corneal clouding, and β-galactosidase deficiency. *Arch. Intern. Med.,* 128:387–398, 1971.

Kelemen, G., Tay–Sachs–Krankheit und Gehörorgan. *Z. Laryngol. Rhinol. Otol.,* 44:728–738, 1965.

CHRONIC LACTIC ACIDEMIA, METABOLIC MYOPATHY, GROWTH RETARDATION, AND SENSORINEURAL DEAFNESS

Hackett, Bray, Ziter, Nyhan, and Creer (1973) described two sisters with this apparently unique syndrome.

CLINICAL FINDINGS

Musculoskeletal System. The children were asymptomatic until 6 to 8 years of age at which time there was insidious onset of muscle weakness—first in the neck, later in the trunk and the extremities.

Growth retardation was marked, being below 3 S D. in both sisters.

Nervous System. Intelligence was normal. One sister manifested photoconvulsive epilepsy.

Endocrine System. The sister who is living manifested retarded sexual maturation. The other girl died prior to puberty.

Auditory System. Both sisters exhibited moderate sensorineural deafness, otherwise uncharacterized.

Vestibular System. No vestibular function tests were carried out.

LABORATORY FINDINGS

Large amounts of alanine were found in the urine and blood. Loading tests with oral alanine demonstrated reduced clearance. Blood pyruvate and lactic acid concentrations were markedly elevated. The urine was low in creatine, but the serum showed normal levels of creatinine phosphokinase.

Electromyographic studies demonstrated a myopathy.

PATHOLOGY

Areas of "granular necrosis" were seen in skeletal and cardiac muscle under light microscopy. On ultrastructural study, these regions were found to be numerous large mitochondria with degenerating myofibrils (D'Agostino *et al.*, 1968).

HEREDITY

Inheritance is probably autosomal recessive.

DIAGNOSIS

There are some similarities to the syndrome of *progressive external ophthalmoplegia, retinal pigmentary degeneration, cardiac conduction defects, and mixed hearing loss,* and to several of the disorders discussed under *Diagnosis* of that condition (Chapter 4).

TREATMENT

Therapy consists of treatment of lactic acidosis as indicated.

PROGNOSIS

Prognosis apparently is not good. The lactic acidosis resulted in death in one sister.

SUMMARY

The syndrome is characterized by: 1) autosomal recessive inheritance, 2) muscle weakness with insidious onset at 6 to 8 years of age, 3) growth retardation, 4) possible retarded sexual maturation, 5) chronic lactic acidemia, and 6) moderate sensorineural deafness.

REFERENCES

Hackett, T. N., Jr., Bray, P. F., Ziter, F. A., Nyhan, W. L., and Creer, K. M., A metabolic myopathy associated with chronic lactic acidemia, growth failure, and nerve deafness. *J. Pediatr., 83*: 426–431, 1973.
D'Agostino, A. M., Ziter, F. A., Rallison, M. L., and Bray, P. F., Familial myopathy with abnormal muscle mitochondria. *Arch. Neurol., 118*:388–401, 1968.

HYPERPROLINEMIA AND HYPERPROLINURIA (IMINOGLYCINURIA) AND SENSORINEURAL DEAFNESS

Hyperprolinemia is characterized by elevation of the plasma proline concentration. Two types have been described (Selkoe, 1969). In type I there is decreased activity of the enzyme, proline oxidase (Efron, 1965). In type II there is deficiency of pyrroline-5-carboxylate dehydrogenase (Selkoe, 1969). Hearing loss has been described only in some individuals affected with type I hyperprolinemia.

Compounding the difficulty in unraveling this skein is the shared pathway in renal tubular active transport of glycine, proline, and hydroxyproline. Iminoaciduria appears to be the homozygous recessive state of a gene that is concerned with renal tubular resorption of glycine and iminoacids. Heterozygotes may exhibit hyperglycinuria without iminoaciduria. However,

several genes may be involved in intestinal and renal transport of iminoacids and glycine (Scriver, 1968; Rosenberg *et al.*, 1968).

We have doubts about the relationship between deafness and proline metabolism. For example, Schafer, Scriver, and Efron (1962) described a 5-year-old-boy with mental retardation, a large left kidney and a hypoplastic right kidney, marked hearing loss, and seizures. The child, who had persistent hematuria and repeated urinary tract infections, finally died of uremia at 5 years of age. One of the patient's five sibs had only hyperprolinemia; another had hyperprolinemia and hematuria; a third had hyperprolinemia, hematuria, and renal hypoplasia. Two sibs were completely normal. The mother had hematuria, deafness, and renal hypoplasia, but her blood proline levels were normal. Several of his maternal aunts and uncles were deaf. The maternal grandmother had hematuria. We suspect that the family had *Alport syndrome* with dominant transmission and that the children had entirely independent autosomal recessive hyperprolinemia.

Efron (1965) and Perry *et al.* (1968) presented other families in which affected persons had hyperprolinemia and renal disease but no hearing loss.

Prolinuria (iminoglycinuria) has been described in the syndrome of *renal disease, hyperprolinuria, ichthyosis, and sensorineural deafness.*

Rosenberg *et al.* (1968) reported a 6-year-old male with severe congenital sensorineural deafness. His sibs and parents were not affected. Although studies were normal, the boy exhibited persistent iminoaciduria. Renal clearance studies showed a tubular defect in reabsorption of glycine,

proline, and hydroxyproline. Plasma levels of these amino acids were normal.

Fraser *et al.* (1968) described a male, the probable offspring of a brother-sister mating, who suffered from congenital sensorineural deafness, iminoglycinuria, and tapetoretinal degeneration, each of which may have been separately inherited as autosomal recessive traits.

Blehová *et al.* (1973) reported a mentally retarded infant with elevated urinary but normal blood levels of proline, hydroxyproline, and glycine. Both parents and the paternal aunt's mentally retarded child exhibited excessive glycinuria. The father, his sister, and the paternal grandfather and great-grandfather were congenitally partially deaf.

Rokkones and Løken (1968) described a mentally retarded patient with elevated urinary levels of proline and hydroxyproline and renal dysplasia but no deafness.

REFERENCES

Blehová, B., Pažoutová, N., Hyanek, J., and Jirásek, J., Iminoglycinuria in a child in Czechoslovakia. *Humangenetik, 19*:207–210, 1973.

Efron, M. L., Familial hyperprolinemia. *N. Engl. J. Med., 272*:1243–1254, 1965.

Fraser, G. R., Friedmann, A. I., Patton, V. M., Wade, D. N., and Wolff, L. I., Iminoglycinuria — a "harmless" inborn error of metabolism? *Humangenetik, 6*:362–367, 1968.

Perry, T. L., Hardwick, D. F., Lowry, R. B., and Hansen, S., Hyperprolinemia in two successive generations of a North American Indian family. *Ann. Hum. Genet., 31*:401–408, 1968.

Rokkones, T., and Løken, A. C., Congenital renal dysplasia, retinal dysplasia, and mental retardation associated with hyperprolinuria and hyper-OH-prolinuria. *Acta Paediatr. Scand., 57*:225–229, 1968.

Rosenberg, L. E., Durant, J. L., and Elasas, L. J., Familial iminoglycinuria. An inborn error of renal tubular transport. *N. Engl. J. Med., 278*:1407–1413, 1968.

Schafer, I. A., Scriver, C. R., and Efron, M. L., Familial hyperprolinemia, cerebral dysfunction, and renal anomalies occurring in a family with hereditary nephropathy and deafness. *N. Engl. J. Med., 267*:51–60, 1962.

Scriver, C. R., Renal tubular transport of proline, hydroxyproline, and glycine. *J. Clin. Invest., 47*:823–835, 1968.

Selkoe, D. J., Familial hyperprolinemia and mental retardation. *Neurology (Minneap.), 19*:494–502, 1969.

ELECTROCARDIOGRAPHIC ABNORMALITIES, FAINTING SPELLS, AND SUDDEN DEATH WITH CONGENITAL SENSORINEURAL DEAFNESS

(Jervell and Lange-Nielsen Syndrome, Cardioauditory Syndrome, Surdocardiac Syndrome)

Jervell and Lange-Nielsen (1957) described a syndrome of profound congenital deafness, electrocardiographic abnormalities characterized by a prolonged QT interval, fainting attacks, and, occasionally, sudden unexplained death in childhood. The syndrome was subsequently noted by numerous authors (Levine and Woodworth, 1958; Fraser, Froggatt, and James, 1964; Jervell, Thingstad, and Endsjö, 1966; Lisker and Finkelstein, 1966; Kallfelz, 1968; Sanchez Cascos *et al.*, 1969; van Bruggen *et al.*, 1969; Fauchier *et al.*, 1969; Athanasiou and Weiner, 1972). Fraser, Froggatt, and Murphy (1964) estimated its frequency at 3 to 4 cases per 1 million births. They further stated that the syndrome may account for 1 per cent of hereditary deafness; Sanchez Cascos *et al.* (1969), however, found only 1 case among 511 deaf-mute children. Fay *et al.* (1971) found one example among 1100 deaf children. An additional four patients had syncope without a prolonged QT interval, whereas five had a prolonged QT interval without syncope.

CLINICAL FINDINGS

Cardiovascular System. All affected children had "fainting spells" and sudden lapses of consciousness, beginning between infancy and adolescence, but usually appearing between 3 and 5 years of age. Death occurred between 3 and 14 years of age in over half of the cases as a result of cardiac arrhythmia, which leads to ventricular and/or asystolic fibrillation (Olley and Fowler, 1970). Usually, the fainting spells are precipitated by nervousness or physical exertion (Jervell *et al.*, 1966). The attacks vary in severity from a mild fainting spell to loss of consciousness for 5 to 10 minutes with temporary residual disorientation. They also vary in frequency; in some patients, several occur in a day.

Auditory System. All patients had congenital bilateral severe sensorineural hearing loss.

Vestibular System. In no case have vestibular findings been described.

LABORATORY FINDINGS

The electrocardiographic changes are characterized by a prolonged QT interval with large T waves, which can be upright, notched, biphasic, or inverted. The degree of QT prolongation varies both within and between families, but it almost always exceeds 0.5 seconds (maximum normal: 0.4 seconds). Since the QT interval varies with heart rate, a simple formula for calculation of the interval is QT = (RR × 0.2) + 0.18 ± 0.04 (Ljung, 1949) (Fig. 9–9A).

A mild hypochronic anemia has been found in several cases (Jervell and Lange-Nielsen, 1957; Fraser, Froggatt, and James, 1964; Jervell *et al.*, 1966; Lamy *et al.*, 1967; Kallfelz, 1968).

PATHOLOGY

Autopsies have been done in numerous cases. Gross and histologic examinations of the heart have exhibited no abnormalities in most cases. Special examination of the conducting system of the heart showed marked narrowing of a major branch of the sinus node artery with resultant infarction of the node (Friedmann *et al.*, 1966, 1968). Fraser, Froggatt, and James (1964) found the normal glycogen-containing perinuclear zone to be absent in the Purkinje nerve fibers in the hearts of these children.

Temporal bone changes were described by Friedmann *et al.* (1966, 1968). The most unique change was the accumulation of PAS-positive hyaline aggregates in an atrophic stria vascularis. There was almost complete degeneration of the organ of Corti and loss of sensory cells. The tectorial membrane was shrunken or retracted, and the Reissner's membrane was adherent to the basilar membrane, practically obliterating the cochlear duct. The sensory epithelium of the utricle and saccule was atrophic, and the cristae were disorganized. There was moderate loss of spiral ganglion cells.

HEREDITY

The syndrome is clearly inherited as an autosomal recessive trait. Consanguinity is common (Fraser, Froggatt, and Murphy, 1964; Lamy *et al.*, 1967; Sanchez Cascos *et al.*, 1969). The heterozygote may exhibit moderate prolongation of the QT interval (Fraser, Froggatt, and Murphy, 1964). A possible linkage with the Rh factor has been suggested (Friedmann, Fraser, and Froggatt, 1968).

DIAGNOSIS

The same electrocardiographic changes (that is, a prolonged QT interval) have been described without deafness (Johansson and Jorming, 1972; van der Straaten and Bruins, 1973; Singer *et al.*, 1974). There was sudden death and/or attacks of unconsciousness. However, in these families, the abnormality was inherited as a dominant trait. Jervell (1973) described another dominantly inherited syndrome of multiple extrasystoles with attacks of ventricular fibrillation but with normal QT interval. There were certain similarities to changes seen in *Refsum syndrome.* In both syndromes there are sensorineural deafness, anomalies of cardiac conduction with prolongation of the QT interval and abnormal T waves, and occasionally sudden death. The deafness in Refsum syndrome, however, has its onset in adulthood; in addition, serum phytanic acid levels are elevated.

The fainting spells in the Lange-Nielsen syndrome may be erroneously diagnosed as epileptic seizures. However, the electroencephalogram is normal, whereas the electrocardiogram is grossly bizarre. Furthermore, the children do not have profound stupor following the fainting episodes. There are several atypical cases. Mathews *et al.* (1972) reported an autosomal dominant form with mild, high frequency deafness. The deafness and cardiac abnormalities may have been inherited as independent dominant traits. Furlanello *et al.* (1972) and Athanasiou and Muller-Seydlitz (1972) also described a dominant form in adults with mild deafness. It is also conceivable that these kindreds had the *leopard syndrome.*

The reader should bear in mind that prolonged QT interval may be caused by hypokalemia, hypocalcemia, hypomagnesemia and quinidine and phenothiazine administration.

TREATMENT

A hearing aid may be of some help for minimizing the hearing loss. Jervell *et al.* (1966) suggested that digitalization is helpful in decreasing the electrocardiographic abnormalities that accompany exercise and in reducing the number of syncopal attacks. Olley and Fowler (1970) and Vincent *et al.* (1974) have had considerable success with the β-adrenergic blocker propanolol. Singer *et al.* (1974) described the efficacious use of bretylium tasylate, which is selectively taken up by the peripheral sympathetic nerve fibers where it inhibits efferent adrenergic transmission peripheral to the ganglion without parasympathetic blockage.

PROGNOSIS

There is little progression of the hearing loss over the years. Affected persons have a variable number of syncopal attacks. In about half of the cases the patient has died by the age of 15 years; few patients older than 21 years of age have been identified.

SUMMARY

The major features of this syndrome include: 1) autosomal recessive transmission, 2) prolonged electrocardiographic QT intervals, 3) recurrent Stokes-Adams attacks beginning in early childhood and occasionally resulting in sudden death, and 4) congenital severe sensorineural deafness.

REFERENCES

Athanasiou, D. J., and Müller-Seydlitz, P. M., Weitere Beobachtungen zum Jervell und Lange-Nielsen-Syndrom. *Münch. Med. Wochenschr., 114*:1961–1965, 1972.

Athanasiou, D. J., and Weiner, C., Das Jervell-und Lange-Nielsen-Syndrom. *Münch. Med. Wochenschr., 114*:698–706, 1972.

Fauchier, C., Regy, J. M., and Combe, P., Syndrome de Jervell et Lange-Nielsen. *Pédiatrie, 24*:843–852, 1969.

Fay, J. E., Olley, P. M., Partington, M. W., and Kavetz, V. B., Surdo-cardiac syndrome; incidence among children in schools for the deaf. *Can. Med. Assoc. J., 105*:718–720, 1971.

Fraser, G. R., Froggatt, P., and James, T. N., Congenital deafness associated with electrocardiographic abnormalities, fainting attacks, and sudden death. *Q. J. Med., 33*:361–385, 1964.

Fraser, G. R., Froggatt, P., and Murphy, T., Genetical aspects of the cardioauditory syndrome of Jervell and Lange-Nielsen (congenital deafness and electrocardiographic abnormalities). *Ann. Hum. Genet., 28*:133–157, 1964.

Friedmann, I., Fraser, G. R., and Froggatt, P., Pathology of the ear in the cardioauditory syndrome of Jervell and Lange-Nielsen (Recessive deafness with electrocardiographic abnormalities). *J. Laryngol. Otol., 80*:451–470, 1966.

Friedmann, I., Fraser, G. R., and Froggatt, P., Pathology of the ear in the cardioauditory syndrome of Jervell and Lange-Nielsen. Report of a third case with an appendix on possible linkage with the Rh blood group locus. *J. Laryngol. Otol., 82*:883–896, 1968.

Furlanello, F., Maccà, F., and Dal Palù, C., Observation on a case of Jervell and Lange-Nielsen syndrome in an adult. *Br. Heart J., 34*:648–652, 1972.

Jervell, A., Surdocardiac and related syndromes in children. *Adv. Intern. Med., 17*:425–438, 1973.

Jervell, A., and Lange-Nielsen, F., Congenital deaf-mutism, functional heart disease with prolongation of the QT interval, and sudden death. *Am. Heart J., 54*:59–68, 1957.

Jervell, A., Thingstad, R., and Endsjö, T., The surdo-cardiac syndrome. *Am. Heart J., 72*:582–593, 1966.

Johansson, B. W., and Jorming, B., Hereditary prolongation of QT interval. *Br. Heart J., 34*:744–751, 1972.

Kallfelz, H. C., Über ein neues EKF-Syndrome bei Kindern mit synkopalen Anfällen und plötzlichen Tod. *Dtsch. Med. Wochenschr., 93*:1046–1052, 1968.

Lamy, M., Frezal, J., Fessard, C., and Roy, C., Le syndrome de Jervell et Lange-Nielsen. *Arch. Fr. Pédiatr., 24*:415–425, 1967.

Levine, S., and Woodworth, C. R., Congenital deaf-mutism, prolonged QT interval, syncopal attacks, and sudden death. *N. Engl. J. Med., 259*:412–417, 1958.

Lisker, S. A., and Finkelstein, D., The cardioauditory syndrome of Jervell and Lange-Nielsen: report of an additional case with radioelectrocardiographic monitoring during exercise. *Am. J. Med. Sci., 252*:458–464, 1966.

Ljung, O., A simple formula for clinical interpretation of the QT interval. *Acta Med. Scand., 134*:79–86, 1949.

Mathews, E. C., Jr., Blount, A. W., Jr., and Townsend, J. I., QT prolongation and ventricular arrhythmias, with and without deafness, in the same family. *Am. J. Cardiol., 29*:702–711, 1972.

Olley, P. M., and Fowler, R. S., Surdocardiac syndrome and therapeutic observations. *Br. Heart J., 32*:467–471, 1970.

Sanchez Cascos, A., Sanchez-Harguindey, L., and DeRabago, P., Cardioauditory syndromes. Cardiac and genetic study of 511 deaf-mute children. *Br. Heart J., 31*:26–33, 1969.

Singer, B. A., Crampton, R. S., and Bass, N. H., Familial QT prolongation syndrome. *Arch. Neurol., 31*:64–66, 1974.

van Bruggen, H. W., Sebus, J., and van Heyst, A. N. P., Convulsive syncope resulting from arrhythmia in a case of congenital deafness with ECG abnormalities. *Am. Heart J., 78*:81–86, 1969.

van der Straaten, P. J. C., and Bruins, C. L. D., A family with heritable electrocardiographic QT prolongation. *J. Med. Genet., 10*:158–160, 1973.

Vincent, G. M., Abildskov, J. A., and Burgess, M. J., Q-T interval syndromes. *Progr. Cardiovasc. Dis., 16*:523–530, 1974.

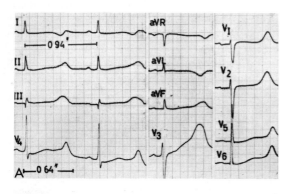

Figure 9–9 *Electrocardiographic abnormalities, fainting spells, and sudden death with congenital sensorineural deafness.* *(A)* Electrocardiogram of a patient showing QT interval of 0.64 sec. (0.41 sec. is upper limit of normal). (From A. Jervell *et al., Am. Heart J., 72*:582, 1966.) *(B)* Photomicrograph of cochlea showing adherent Reissner's membrane, degenerated organ of Corti, atrophic stria vascularis, and deposit of PAS-positive material. (From I. Friedmann *et al., J. Laryngol. Otol., 80*:451, 1966.)

OTODENTAL DYSPLASIA

Levin and Jorgenson (1972, 1974) and Jorgenson *et al.* (1975) described a syndrome of dental abnormalities and sensorineural hearing loss in two large kindreds.

CLINICAL FINDINGS

Dental Findings. Dental abnormalities were found in 30 of 34 affected members. Delayed eruption of deciduous teeth and absence of premolars were noted in half the patients. The crowns of the posterior teeth were bulbous and malformed, the relation between cusps and major grooves being eliminated (Fig. 9–10*A, B*). Similar changes were seen in the deciduous molars, but in contrast to the normal permanent canine the deciduous canine was also affected. The same dental abnormalities (globodontia) were found in another kindred in variable association with high frequency sensorineural deafness (Witkop *et al.*, 1976).

Auditory System. Bilateral high-tone sensorineural hearing loss to about 65 dB was noted in 28 of 30 affected individuals. The age of onset ranged from early childhood to middle age. The pinnae were described as outstanding in some affected individuals (Jorgenson *et al.*, 1975).

LABORATORY FINDINGS

Radiologic examination of the teeth has demonstrated taurodontism of molar teeth with large calcifications in the pulp chambers and root canals. In some individuals the deciduous molars appeared to have two separate pulp chambers, the extra one in the distolingual aspect.

Vestibular System. Caloric tests were normal.

PATHOLOGY

No pathologic studies were described.

HEREDITY

The syndrome is inherited as an autosomal dominant trait with variable expressivity.

DIAGNOSIS

Premolars are absent in about 5 per cent of the general population. Taurodontism may occur as an isolated finding or may be part of a syndrome (Gorlin *et al.*, 1976).

TREATMENT

A hearing aid may be employed.

SUMMARY

This syndrome is characterized by: 1) autosomal dominant inheritance, 2) dental changes, which include globoid posterior teeth and taurodontism, and 3) bilateral high-tone sensorineural hearing loss.

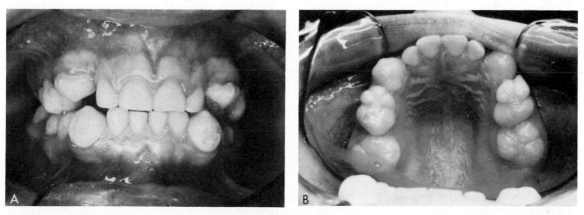

Figure 9–10 *Otodental dysplasia. (A* and *B)* Anterior and occlusal views of teeth exhibiting "globodontia." Note enlarged and bulbous canine and molar teeth. Grooves are shallow. (Courtesy of C. J. Witkop, Minneapolis, Minnesota.)

REFERENCES

Gorlin, R. J., Pindborg, J. J., and Cohen, M. M., Jr., *Syndromes of the Head and Neck.* 2nd Ed. New York, McGraw-Hill Book Company, 1976.

Jorgenson, R., March, S. J., and Farrington, F. H., Otodental dysplasia. *Birth Defects* 11(5):115–120, 1975.

Levin, L. S., and Jorgenson, R. J., Familial otodental dysplasia: a "new" syndrome. *Am. J. Hum. Genet., Suppl. 61a,* 1972.

Levin, L. S., and Jorgenson, R. J., Otodental dysplasia: a previously undescribed syndrome. *Birth Defects, 10*(4):310–312, 1974.

Levin, L. S., Jorgenson, R. J., and Cook, R., Otodental syndrome. A new ectodermal dysplasia. Clin. Genet., *8*:136–144, 1975.

Witkop, C. J., Jr., Gundlach, K., Streed, W. J., and Sauk, J. J., Jr., Globodontia in the otodental syndrome. *Oral Surg., 41*:472–483, 1976.

PROGRESSIVE LIPODYSTROPHY OF THE FACE AND ARMS, MULTIPLE BONE CYSTS, AND CONDUCTION DEAFNESS

VanLeeuwen (1933) described conductive deafness with lipodystrophy of the face and arms, bone cysts, and mild mental retardation in three adult sisters.

CLINICAL FINDINGS

Physical Findings. The facies, with its gaunt, deathlike look, was striking.

Integumentary System. Lipodystrophy of the face and arms began at about 5 to 6 years of age and progressed for about the next 5 years. One girl was stated to have little axillary hair, but the normal pattern of distribution of pubic hair. However, the patient showed generalized lanugo-like hirsutism.

Skeletal System. The three sibs had small adult stature (57 to 59 inches). Small defects or bone cysts filled with red marrow were scattered throughout the tibia, ilium, humerus, and fibula of the three girls.

Endocrine System. Breast development was poor, and menses were delayed and irregular in all three sibs. One girl was found to have a hypoplastic uterus.

Auditory System. All three sisters manifested conduction deafness at about 5 to 6 years of age—approximately the same time that the lipodystrophy became evident. Although the degree of deafness was not stated, it was implied that it was severe.

Vestibular System. No studies were reported.

LABORATORY FINDINGS

Radiographic studies showed numerous bone defects. Although the sibs were stated to be mildly mentally retarded, no testing evidence was presented. It is conceivable that the profound deafness and the shyness resulting from the unusual facies produced a false impression of retardation.

HEREDITY

The parents and five other sibs were normal. There was parental consanguinity. Although an uncle and a cousin were stated to be similarly affected they had not been examined, and there was no documentation of their condition. Inheritance appears to be autosomal recessive.

DIAGNOSIS

Generalized lipodystrophy (Seip syndrome) is an autosomal recessively inherited disorder characterized by loss of subcutaneous, mesenteric, and retroperitoneal fat, and by hyperlipemia, acanthosis nigricans, and insulin-resistant diabetes mellitus. The subcutaneous fat is lost over the entire body. Deafness and bone defects are not components of the disorder. However, a family having "cystic angiomatosis" of bone and generalized lipodystrophy has been documented (Brunzell *et al.*, 1968). To be excluded is partial lipodystrophy, which involves the upper half of the body with marked adiposity below the waist. It occurs far more frequently in females (4 females: 1 male) and is probably heritable. Associated nephropathy is common (Senior and Gellis, 1964; Piscatelli *et al.*, 1970). Senior and Gellis (1964) noted unilateral sensorineural deafness in 2 of their 14 patients.

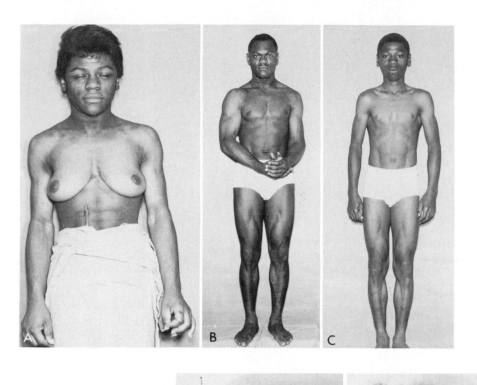

Figure 9-11 *Progressive lipodys-trophy of the face and arms, multiple bone cysts, and conductive deafness. (A-C)* Patients at ages 22, 20, and 14, respec-tively. *(D-E)* Six-month-old affected sib. These individuals had many of the signs reported by van Leeuwen, but no deafness was mentioned.

Illustration continued on the following page

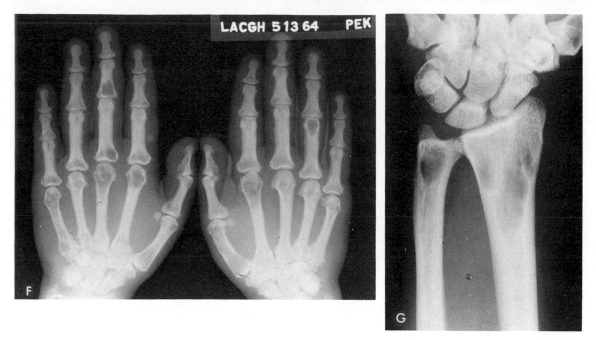

Figure 9-11 *Continued.* *(F)* Cystic angiomatosis of phalanges and metacarpals. *(G)* Similar lesions of distal radius and ulna. (From J. D. Brunzell *et al., Ann. Intern. Med., 69*:501, 1968.)

TREATMENT

Stapedectomy could be performed to correct the deafness.

PROGNOSIS

One sister died of osteosarcoma, which had metastasized to the lung.

SUMMARY

The syndrome is characterized by: 1) autosomal recessive inheritance, 2) progressive lipodystrophy of face and arms, beginning in the first decade, 3) multiple bone cysts, and 4) severe conduction deafness.

REFERENCES

Brunzell, J. D., Shankle, S. W., and Bethune, J. E., Congenital generalized lipodystrophy accompanied by systemic cystic angiomatosis. *Ann. Intern. Med., 69*:501–576, 1968.

Piscatelli, R. L., Vieweg, W. V., and Havel, R. J., Partial lipodystrophy: metabolic studies in three patients. *Ann. Intern. Med., 73*:963–970, 1970.

Senior, B., and Gellis, S. S., The syndromes of total lipodystrophy and of partial lipodystrophy. *Pediatrics, 33*:593–612, 1964.

van Leeuwen, H. C., Über familiäres Vorkommen von Lipodystrophia progressiva zusammen mit Otosklerose, Knochencysten und geistiger Debilität. *Z. Klin. Med., 123*:534–547, 1933.

FAMILIAL STREPTOMYCIN OTOTOXICITY

There have been several reports of familial ototoxicity to streptomycin, suggesting that in these cases there is a heritable increased sensitivity to this drug (Pražić *et al.*, 1964; Podvinec and Stefanovic, 1966; Tsuiki and Murai, 1971; Johnsonbaugh *et al.*, 1974).

Pražić *et al.* (1964) reported a family in which four female sibs experienced permanent hearing loss following streptomycin injections. One grain per day for five days produced signs of deafness in all sibs.

Tsuiki and Murai (1971) observed 16 families in which two or more members had their hearing affected by administration of dihydrostreptomycin. Sensorineural hearing loss was of a moderate to marked degree. Dosage in various families ranged from 3 to 40 grams, total dosage.

Johnsonbaugh et al. (1974) described moderate to severe high-tone sensorineural loss in a mother and son. While the mother received a considerable dose of streptomycin for a prolonged period, her son received only 19 mg. per kg. of the drug intramuscularly for seven doses at 12 hour intervals.

Vestibular disturbances were found in about 25 per cent of children receiving large doses of streptomycin (Pražić and Salaj, 1975).

Inheritance is probably autosomal dominant with incomplete penetrance. However, there has been no male-to-male transmission and one cannot exclude multifactorial inheritance.

REFERENCES

Johnsonbaugh, R. E., Drexler, H. G., Light, I. J., and Sutherland, J. M., Familial occurrence of drug-induced hearing loss. *Am. J. Dis. Child., 127*:245–247, 1974.

Podvinec, S., and Stefanovic, P., Surdité par la streptomycine et prédisposition familiale. *J. Fr. Otorhinolaryngol., 15*:61–67, 1966.

Pražić, M., and Salaj, B., Ototoxicity with children caused by streptomycin. *Audiology, 14*:173–176, 1975.

Pražić, M., Salaj, B., and Subotić, R., Familial sensitivity to streptomycin. *J. Laryngol. Otol., 78*:1037–1043, 1964.

Tsuiki, T., and Murai, S., Familial incidence of streptomycin hearing loss and hereditary weakness of the cochlea. *Audiology, 10*:315–322, 1971.

TURNER SYNDROME AND DEAFNESS

Turner syndrome is characterized by short stature, sexual infantilism, streak gonads, elevated urinary gonadotropin levels, and various physical stigmata, such as pterygium colli, cubitus valgus, short fourth metacarpal, osteoporosis, and increased cutaneous nevi. Negative nuclear sex chromatin and XO karyotype or other abnormalities of sex chromatin pattern are found.

Otitis media occurs frequently in Turner syndrome (Stratton, 1965). Ferguson-Smith et al., (1964) noted decreased auditory function in about one third of 30 patients with gonadal dysgenesis. These included 4 of 10 with XO karyotype and 3 of 10 with XO/XX mosaicism. Engel and Forbes (1965) found hearing loss in 8 of 11 patients and otitis media in 6 of 12 XO patients. Hearing loss was noted in 3 of 3 XO/XX₁ patients. Several other variants manifested deafness. In all, 18 of 48 Turner syndrome patients had either sensorineural or conductive hearing loss or both. Valkov et al. (1975) found sensorineural hearing loss in patients with Turner syndrome mosaicism but not in those with 45,XO karyotypes.

Goldberg et al. (1968), studying a large series of patients with Turner syndrome, noted that 14 of 24 (58 per cent) with an XO karyotype had a history of frequent otitis and that about 35 per cent manifested a hearing deficit. Four of six patients with XX₁ or XX/XX₁ karyotype had hearing loss. Similar findings were reported by Matteri et al. (1971).

Anderson et al. (1969) found that of 76 patients about 68 per cent experienced middle ear infection (usually in childhood) and that about 20 per cent showed a conductive or mixed hearing deficit. Since the external auditory meatus was caudally displaced, abnormal orientation of the Eustachian tubes was probable and also predisposed the patient to middle ear infection.

Sensorineural loss with recruitment was found in about 65 per cent of cases, generally as a bilaterally symmetric dip in the audiogram and centered about 2000 Hz. Anderson et al. suggested that this was due to a defect in the outer hair cells in the organ of Corti in the upper part of the basal and in the lower part of the middle coils of the cochlea. There was no striking progress of hearing loss with older age. However, since severe deafness in children with Turner syndrome was noted only in about 10 per cent, these changes were considered to be degenerative rather than congenital. Similar findings were reported in about 20 per cent of patients with XXY Klinefelter syndrome (Anderson *et al.*, 1971).

Vestibular function was found to be normal.

REFERENCES

Anderson, H., Filipson, R., Fluur, E., Koch, B., Lindsten, J., and Wedenberg, E., Hearing impairment in Turner's syndrome. *Acta Otolaryngol. Suppl., 247*:1–26, 1969.

Anderson, H., Lindsten, J., and Wedenberg, E., Hearing defects in males with sex chromosome anomalies. *Acta Otolaryngol. (Stockh.), 72*:55–58, 1971.

Engel, E., and Forbes, A. P., Cytogenetic and clinical findings in 48 patients with congenitally defective or absent ovaries. *Medicine, 44*:135–164, 1965.

Ferguson-Smith, M. A., Alexander, D. S., Bowen, P., Goodman, R. M., Kaufmann, B. N., Jones, H. W., Jr., and Heller, R. H., Clinical and cytogenetical studies in female gonadal dysgenesis and their bearing on the cause of Turner's syndrome. *Cytogenetics, 3*:355–383, 1964.

Goldberg, M. B., Scully, A. L., Solomon, J. L., and Steinbach, H. L., Gonadal dysgenesis in phenotypic female subjects. A review of eighty-seven cases, with cytogenetic studies in fifty-three. *Am. J. Med., 45*:529–543, 1968.

Lindsten, J., *The Nature and Origin of X Chromosome Aberrations in Turner's Syndrome. A Cytogenetical and Clinical Study of 57 Patients.* Stockholm, Almqvist and Wiksell Förlag AB, 1963, pp. 1–167.

Matteri, M. S., Wolff, H., Salzano, F. M., and Mallmann, M. L., Cytogenetic, clinical, and genealogical analyses in a series of gonadal dysgenesis patients and their families. *Humangenetik, 13*:126–143, 1971.

Stratton, H. J. M., Gonadal dysgenesis and the ears. *J. Laryngol. Otol., 79*:343–346, 1965.

Valkov, I. M., Dukomov, S. I., Genkova, P. I., and Dimov, D. S., Olfactory, auditory, and gustatory function in patients with gonadal dysgenesis. *Obstet. Gynecol., 46*:417–418, 1975.

XX GONADAL DYSGENESIS AND CONGENITAL SENSORINEURAL DEAFNESS

"XX gonadal dysgenesis" refers to individuals of female phenotype whose height is greater than 152 cm. and who exhibit sexual infantilism, primary amenorrhea, and eunuchoid habitus. They are often tall and slender with increased arm span and absence of Turner syndrome–like features.

Streak gonads, i.e., absence of primordial follicles, are present in most cases, but in some individuals even these have been absent. Mesonephric rests but no Leydig cells have been found in nearly all cases. Fallopian tubes and a uterus are present but are hypoplastic. Usually, urinary gonadotropins are elevated and estrogen excretion is decreased.

A high proportion of cases of XX gonadal dysgenesis may be due to a single autosomal recessive gene, since it has been reported in sibs. Parental consanguinity has also been noted (Christakos *et al.*, 1969; Perez-Ballester *et al.*, 1970; Simpson *et al.*, 1971).

In a few cases, deafness has been noted. Josso *et al.* (1963) described sisters with XX gonadal dysgenesis and severe congenital deafness. Christakos *et al.* (1969) reported three sisters with XX gonadal dysgenesis. Two of these sisters and their male sib manifested sensorineural hearing loss. All three girls were mildly mentally retarded. Perez-Ballester *et al.* (1970) described three sisters with XX gonadal dysgenesis and severe congenital sensorineural deafness.

REFERENCES

Christakos, A. C., Simpson, J. L., Younger, J. B., and Christian, C. D., Gonadal dysgenesis as an autosomal recessive condition. *Am. J. Obstet. Gynecol., 104*:1027–1030, 1969.

Josso, N., de Grouchy, J., Frézal, J., and Lamy, M., Le syndrome de Turner familial. Étude de deux familles avec caryotypes XO et XX. *Ann. Pédiatr., 10*:163–167, 1963.

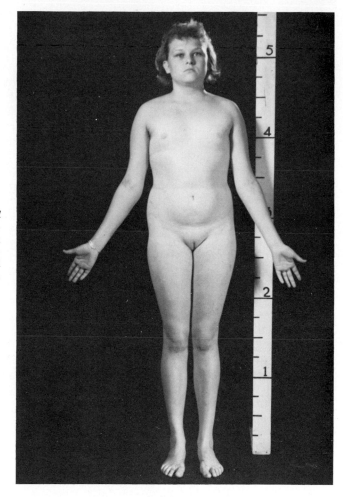

Figure 9–12 *XX gonadal dysgenesis and congenital sensorineural deafness.* Seventeen-year-old patient was one of three sisters with XX gonadal dysgenesis and congenital sensorineural deafness. Note normal height and lack of sexual development. (Courtesy of R. B. Greenblatt, Augusta, Georgia.)

Perez-Ballester, B., Greenblatt, R. B., and Byrd, J. R., Familial gonadal dysgenesis. *Am. J. Obstet. Gynecol., 107*:1262–1263, 1970.

Simpson, J. L., Christakos, A. C., Horwith, M., and Silverman, F. S., Gonadal dysgenesis in individuals with apparently normal chromosomal complements: tabulation of cases and compilation of genetic data. *Birth Defects, 7*(6):215–228, 1971.

TRISOMY 21 AND MIXED DEAFNESS

The signs of trisomy 21 (Down syndrome) are too numerous and too familiar to the reader to merit review.

There is little documentation available on the frequency of deafness in this condition. Glovsky (1966), in a study of 38 children with trisomy 21, found 50 per cent with sensorineural hearing loss, 20 per cent with mixed loss, and 3 per cent with conductive deafness. In contrast, Fulton and Lloyd (1968) found conductive deafness in 20 per cent, mixed loss in 10 per cent, and sensorineural hearing loss in 10 per cent.

REFERENCES

Fulton, R. T., and Lloyd, L. L., Hearing impairment in a population of children with Down's syndrome. *Am. J. Ment. Defic., 73*:298–302, 1968.

Glovsky, L., Audiological assessment of a mongoloid population. *Train. Sch. Bull. (Vinel.), 63*:27–36, 1966.

TRISOMY 13 AND DEAFNESS

Clinical stigmata include mental retardation, apneic spells, sloping forehead, microphthalmos and/or colobomata, cleft lip and/or palate, abnormal pinnae, postaxial polydactyly, and congenital heart disease.

Although it has been stated that about 85 per cent of infants with trisomy 13 have "apparent deafness" and further, in spite of the abbreviated life span of these infants (nearly always less than 3 months), there have been very few audiologic and/or pathologic studies performed (Kos *et al.*, 1966; Maniglia *et al.*, 1970; Black *et al.*, 1972; Lindsay, 1973; Saito *et al.*, 1974; Sando *et al.*, 1975).

The external auditory canals have been normal. Changes have been limited to the middle ear and the inferior part of the inner ear. The middle ear exhibits thickened mucosa due to unresolved embryonic mesenchymal tissue. Generally, the ossicles have been normal.

Careful analysis of the temporal bones in 7 cases (14 ears) of trisomy 13 showed the following vestibular anomalies in decreasing order of frequency: abnormalities of the horizontal semicircular canal; a flat, horizontal canal crista; anomaly of posterior semicircular canal; absence or shortening of utriculoendolymphatic valve; and utricular macular and saccular anomalies (3 ears). Cochlear findings (also in decreasing order of frequency) consisted of shortening of mean length, widened cochlear aqueduct, cystic stria vascularis in part of basal turn, anomaly of modiolus, absence of bony interscalar septum in upper cochlear turns, vessels running through perilymphatic spaces, and lack of communication of cochlear aqueduct with scala tympani. The organ of Corti, tectorial membrane, Reissner's membrane, and cochlear nerve in cochlear and internal auditory canals were normal (Sando *et al.*, 1975).

By contrast, neither Mottet and Jensen (1965) nor Kelemen *et al.* (1968) found anomalies of the inner ear.

REFERENCES

Black, F. O., Sando, I., Wagner, J. A., and Hemenway, W. G., Middle and inner ear abnormalities 13–15 D₁ trisomy. *Arch. Otolaryngol.,93*:615–619, 1971.

Kelemen, G., Hooft, C., and Kluyskens, P., The inner ear in autosomal trisomy. *Pract. Otorhinolaryngol., 30*:251–258, 1968.

Kos, A. O., Schuknecht, H. F., and Singer, A. J., Temporal bone studies in 13–15 and 18 trisomy syndrome. *Arch. Otolaryngol., 83*:439–445, 1966.

Lindsay, J. R., Profound childhood deafness. Inner ear pathology. *Ann. Otol. Rhin. Laryngol., 82, Suppl. 5*:1–115, 1973.

Maniglia, J. M., Wolff, D., and Herques, A. J., Congenital deafness in 13–15 syndromes. *Arch. Otolaryngol., 92*:181–188, 1970.

Mottet, N. K., and Jensen, H., The anomalous embryonic development associated with trisomy 13–15. *Am. J. Clin. Pathol., 43*:334–341, 1965.

Saito, H., Okano, Y., Furuta, M., Asamoto, H., Fujita, H., and Takeuchi, T., Temporal bone findings in trisomy D. *Arch. Otolaryngol.,100*:386–389, 1974.

Sando, I., Leiberman, A., Bergstrom, L., Izumi, S., and Wood, R. P., Temporal bone histopathologic findings in trisomy 13 syndrome. *Ann. Otol. Rhinol. Laryngol., 84, Suppl. 21*:1–20, 1975.

TRISOMY 18 AND DEAFNESS

Infants with trisomy 18 frequently die within the first few weeks of life. Clinical characteristics include hypertonia, severe mental retardation, malformed pinnae, micrognathia, talipes, overlapping flexed fingers, short sternum, and cardiac abnormalities.

Histopathologic study of the ears has been documented in only a few cases (Kelemen, 1966; Kos *et al.*, 1966; Sando *et al.*, 1970; Gacek, 1971; Miglets *et al.*, 1975). Middle ear anomalies have varied: abnormal form of ossicles, and abnormal course of facial nerve and chorda tympani. Inner ear anomalies have included absence of semicircular canals and cristae, poorly developed modiolus, defective cochlear partitions, and decreased or absent spiral ganglion cells.

Miglets *et al.* (1975) noted complete bony atresia of the external canal, aberrant tensor tympani muscle, wide short utricular and saccular ducts and widely patent cochlear aqueduct. Wolf *et al.* (1965), on the other hand, found no significant changes in the inner ear in four examples of trisomy 18.

REFERENCES

Gacek, R., The pathology of hereditary sensorineural hearing loss. *Ann. Otol. Rhin. Laryngol., 80*:289–298, 1971.

Kelemen, G., Rubella and deafness. *Arch. Otolaryngol., 83*:520–532, 1966 (Case 5).

Kos, A. O., Schuknecht, H. F., and Singer, J. O., Temporal bone studies in 13–15 and 18 trisomy syndrome. *Arch. Otolaryngol., 83*:439–445, 1966.

Lindsay, J. R., Profound childhood deafness. Inner ear pathology. *Ann. Otol. Rhin. Laryngol., 822, Suppl. 5*:1–115, 1973.

Miglets, A. W., Schuller, D., Ruppert, E., and Lim, D. J., Trisomy 18. A temporal bone report. *Arch. Otolaryngol., 101*:433–437, 1975.

Sando, I., Bergstrom, L., Wood, R. P., and Hemenway, W. G., Temporal bone findings in trisomy 18 syndrome. *Arch. Otolaryngol., 91*:552–559, 1970.

Wolf, V., Reinwein, H., and Schroeter, R., Bericht über vier Trisomen 18 une eine Trisomie 18-Mosaik. *Humangenetik, 1*:232–245, 1965.

CHROMOSOME 18 LONG ARM DELETION (18q-) SYNDROME AND DEAFNESS

Deletion of the long arm of chromosome 18 is associated with short stature, psychomotor retardation, muscular hypotonia, microcephaly, midfacial hypoplasia, hypertelorism, epicanthal folds, spindle-shaped fingers, congenital heart disease, and an increased number of fingertip whorls.

The pinnae are often dysplastic with prominent anthelix and antitragus. The external auditory canals are stenosed with hearing loss. Kunze *et al.* (1972) in their survey of 38 cases of ring 18 chromosome (18r) and 52 cases of deletion of the long arm of chromosome 18 (18q-) noted that in over 50 per cent of the cases atresia or stenosis of the auditory canals was found, and deafness was reported in about 65 per cent. Bergstrom *et al.* (1974) reported conductive hearing loss due to atresia or hypoplasia of the external auditory canals in three of four 18q- or 18r syndrome patients. Petrous pyramid polytomography showed atresia plates in the region of the tympanic membrane. They reviewed auditory findings in other reported cases: rudimentary tympanic membrane, absent annular sulcus, and fused and/or malformed ossicles.

REFERENCES

Bergstrom, L., Stewart, J., and Kenyon, B., External auditory atresia and the deletion chromosome. *Laryngoscope, 84*:1905–1917, 1974.

Kunze, J., Stephan, E., and Tolksdorf, M., Ring-Chromosom 18. Ein 18p-/18q- Deletionssyndrom. *Humangenetik, 15*:289–318, 1972.

SICKLE CELL DISEASE AND SENSORINEURAL HEARING LOSS

Sickle cell disease is a relatively common hemoglobinopathy of blacks. It has been estimated that about 7 to 9 per cent of American blacks are heterozygotes (hemoglobin S trait). Thus, about 1 in 400 would be homozygous.

Homozygotes may initially exhibit only anemia and little or no splenomegaly.

However, there is extramedullary hemopoiesis and hyperplastic marrow. Patients may develop recurrent attacks of weakness, fatigue, abdominal pain, anorexia, jaundice, and pallor. With age, there may be enlargement of the heart, leg ulcers, aseptic necrosis of the hip, and hematuria.

Morgenstein and Manace (1969) reported moderate bilateral hearing loss, somewhat more marked in the higher frequencies. Temporal bone studies showed degenerative changes in the organ of Corti and the stria vascularis consistent with ischemia. Within the ossicles the marrow was hyperplastic and erosive. Todd *et al.* (1973) found at least a 25 dB sensorineural hearing loss in 22 per cent of Jamaicans with sickle cell disease compared to 4 per cent of controls. Males were affected as often as females. Onset was insidious and primarily affected the high tones. They postulated that the hearing deficit resulted from a thromboembolic process. Serjeant *et al.* (1975) ruled out narrowing of the internal auditory canal as an etiologic factor.

REFERENCES

Morgenstein, K. M., and Manace, E. D., Temporal bone histopathology in sickle cell disease. *Laryngoscope,* 79:2172–2180, 1969.

Serjeant, G. R., Norman, W., and Todd, G. B., The internal auditory canal and sensorineural hearing loss in homozygous sickle cell disease. *J. Laryngol. Otol.,* 89:453–456, 1975.

Todd, G. B., Serjeant, F. R., and Larson, M. R., Sensorineural hearing loss in Jamaicans with SS disease. *Acta Otolaryngol. (Stockh.),* 76:268–272, 1973.

AUTHOR INDEX

Note: Coauthors are listed even when not specifically named on a given page.

SUBJECT INDEX

Note: Syndromes described in detail in the text are in italics. Illustrations, audiograms, pedigrees, and micrographs are also in italics.

385